Natural Cycle and Minimal Stimulation IVF

Michael von Wolff
Editor

Natural Cycle and Minimal Stimulation IVF

From Physiology to Clinical Practice

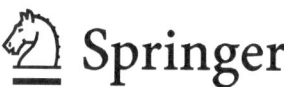 Springer

Editor
Michael von Wolff
Inselspital
University Women's Hospital
Bern, Bern, Switzerland

ISBN 978-3-030-97570-8   ISBN 978-3-030-97571-5   (eBook)
https://doi.org/10.1007/978-3-030-97571-5

This Springer imprint is published by the registered company Springer Nature Switzerland AG
The registered company address is: Gewerbestrasse 11, 6330 Cham, Switzerland

This book is dedicated to all those who are willing to leave the trodden path of conventional IVF to offer their patients a broad spectrum of up-to-date, individualized and patient-orientated IVF treatments.

Foreword

The first child born following IVF in 1978, Louise Brown, was from an unstimulated cycle. Professor Bob Edwards previous attempts using IVF along with ovarian stimulation using clomiphene citrate failed, which he contributed to the induced luteal phase abnormalities. Subsequent mainstream development of IVF—chiefly in Australia and the USA—led to the belief that ovarian stimulation should be considered an integral part of IVF. In an attempt to overcome shortcomings in the in vitro fertilization laboratory procedures, the general principle became—and by some still is—the more oocytes to start with wasteful laboratory procedures the better.

Hence, extremely complex, costly and hazardous ovarian stimulation regimens have been developed over the last three decades involving multiple drugs and creating the need for frequent hospital visits and intense monitoring of ovarian response. In quite a few programmes, the total cost associated with ovarian stimulation exceeds the expenses of the IVF procedure itself.

Indeed, numerous studies confirmed that IVF cycles starting with a greater number of available oocytes is associated with higher pregnancy rates. This is often erroneously used to justify high dose intense ovarian stimulation protocols. The wisdom that high oocyte numbers following stimulation primarily represent good prognosis patients, no matter what you do, is often ignored.

Current IVF with much improved laboratory performance can certainly be performed in cycles with no ovarian stimulation. This approach renders IVF much faster, cheaper and with less burden of treatment and reduced chances for complications. Overall, pregnancy rates per IVF cycle are certainly reduced which should be viewed in the context of the many advantages. Moreover, cumulative pregnancy rates over a given period of time (involving multiple IVF cycles) may run favourable, especially in good prognosis patients.

Over the years many mild (or minimal) ovarian stimulation protocols have been developed using different compounds and dosing regimens. In addition, multiple studies have now shown comparable pregnancy rates, reduced dropouts, and the association with reduced cost and complications. A more holistic approach on infertility care cannot only focus on "success" of treatment, completely ignoring induced side effects, chances for complications, and cost rendering IVF treatment out of reach for many throughout the world.

The current book is a well-timed, comprehensive attempt to cover this rapidly developing and now more accepted field of natural cycle and mild (or minimal) stimulation IVF.

Bart C. J. M. Fauser
University of Utrecht & Utrecht Medical Center
Utrecht, Netherlands

Preface

The first pregnancies and births after in vitro fertilisation (IVF) occurred in 1978 and 1979 after natural cycle IVF (NC-IVF) [1]. The IVF treatments were led by Robert Geoffrey Edwards, a geneticist who received the Nobel Prize in Physiology and Medicine in 2010 for his contributions to IVF, and Patrick Steptoe, a gynaecologist.

Interestingly, Edwards and Steptoe had already developed IVF therapy with gonadotropin stimulation. As these treatments did not result in pregnancy, they continued their IVF programme with NC-IVF therapies in 1977. As a result, four clinical pregnancies and two births developed, including that of Louise Brown, who was born on 25 July 1978 (see Chap. 4).

These first NC-IVF treatments cannot be compared to the NC-IVF therapies used today. For example, Edwards and Steptoe retrieved an oocyte laparoscopically, and the effectiveness of IVF was much lower at that time. The effectiveness of IVF increased by leaps and bounds after it was recognised that a gonadotropin-induced polyfollicular response led to luteal phase insufficiency. Luteal phase support was introduced, and the chances of IVF success increased significantly due to the large number of oocytes availability.

In recent years, however, it has become apparent that conventional IVF with high-dose gonadotropin stimulation is not the best approach for all couples for the following reasons:

- The proportion of women with a low ovarian reserve increases, in whom only a few oocytes can be obtained despite high-dose gonadotropin stimulation.
- High-dose gonadotropin stimulation can be disadvantageous in patients with a high ovarian reserve as the cumulative live birth rate decreases with a very high number of collected oocytes.
- An increasing proportion of women are critical of hormone therapy because of concerns about side effects.
- The cost per treatment cycle is significantly lower with NC-IVF or minimal stimulation IVF, so some patients might prefer to start with cheaper treatment cycles.

It is also significant that IVF laboratories have made such considerable progress that the chances of success per oocyte have increased to the point where a high success rate is possible even with only one or with a few oocytes. Accordingly, studies now show that the success rate with low-dose gonadotropin stimulation, also called minimal stimulation IVF, or even NC-IVF can be just as effective as conventional IVF therapy with high-dose gonadotropin stimulation. Since NC-IVF or minimal stimulation IVF therapy cycles can be performed monthly, the success rate per therapy time may even be higher in some patients.

Accordingly, NC-IVF or minimal stimulation IVF therapies are becoming increasingly widespread. The spread is currently still hampered by the reimbursement of IVF therapies, which is no longer up to date in most countries. In most cases, only a few IVF cycles are paid for, irrespective of the stimulation dose. Because of this, many couples choose high-dose stimulation in the hope of a higher cumulative success rate. However, a rethink is also taking place here. In Germany, for example, some health insurers already pay for unstimulated IVF cycles, and in Switzerland there are signs that NC-IVF therapies will become an elementary part of IVF reimbursement by health insurers.

However, NC-IVF and minimal stimulation IVF treatments will never be able to replace high-dose gonadotropin-stimulated IVF treatments, as these are still more beneficial in several cases. All these IVF therapies are therefore to be understood as complementary techniques with different indications, which together enable an individualised and thus optimal IVF therapy with low risks and high success rates [2].

The International Society for Mild Approaches in Assisted Reproduction, ISMAAR, has been advocating a lower stimulation dose since 2007. ISMAAR has published several position papers summarising and evaluating the above-mentioned positive effects of lower stimulation doses [3].

Every reproductive physician and embryologist should be aware that these therapies are independent forms of therapy. Transferring the logistics of conventional IVF therapy without reflection to NC-IVF or minimal stimulation IVF therapy leads to frustration for all involved and makes it impossible to realise the full potential of these therapies.

Because of this, the idea was born to provide reproductive health professionals and embryologists with practical guidance from centres specialising in NC-IVF and/or minimal stimulation IVF therapies.

Since a basic understanding of reproductive endocrinology is essential for NC-IVF or minimal stimulation IVF, this book first teaches the endocrinological and technical principles relevant to IVF, and only then, based on this knowledge, explains the practically relevant therapeutic procedures. The topic is rounded off by chapters such as costs, risks, history of NC-IVF and minimal stimulation IVF and their future prospects.

The aim of the book is to provide the widest possible expertise. As a result, specialists from different centres, from different continents such as Europe, Asia and North America and thus from regions with different cultural, financial and health policies have agreed to present their clinical-practical strategies in order to adapt NC-IVF and minimal stimulation IVF therapy to local conditions and so that it can be performed worldwide.

The representatives of these centres are sure that every reproductive specialist who gets involved with these techniques and offers them to many couples, instead of only using them as a stopgap in desperate cases, will be amazed and enthusiastic about the potential these techniques have.

I hope you enjoy reading the book and implementing the contents in your fertility centre.

References

1. Steptoe PC, Edwards RG. Birth after the reimplantation of a human embryo. Lancet. 1978;2(8085):366.
2. von Wolff M. The role of Natural Cycle IVF in assisted reproduction. Best Pract Res Clin Endocrinol Metab. 2019;33:35–45.
3. Nargund G, Datta AK, Campbell D, Patrizio P, Chian RC, Obelet W, von Wolff M, Lindenberg S, Frydman R, Fauser B. ISMAAR recommendations on ovarian stimulation for IVF. Submitted.

Bern, Switzerland   Michael von Wolff

Contents

Editor and Contributors

About the Editor

Michael von Wolff is a reproductive physician and the head of the university-based IVF centre in Berne, Switzerland. He has set up a large programme of natural cycle IVF and minimal stimulation IVF in Germany, Switzerland and Austria. His main goal was to optimize and introduce these techniques in many centres due to their manifold advantages. To achieve this goal, he published this practical guide, based on around 30 studies from his centre and based on the expertise of other specialists from Japan and the United States, such as K. Kato and J. Zhang. This guide allows any reproductive physician and embryologist to better understand, introduce and optimize these techniques.

Contributors

Keiichi Kato, MD, PhD Kato Ladies Clinic, Tokyo, Japan

Isotta Magaton, MD Division of Gynecological Endocrinology and Reproductive Medicine, University Women's Hospital, University of Bern, Bern, Switzerland

Markus Montag, PhD ilabcomm GmbH, Sankt Augustin, Germany

Annemarie Schweizer-Arau, MD Insula-Institut, Hannover, Germany

Satoshi Ueno, PhD Kato Ladies Clinic, Tokyo, Japan

Michael von Wolff, MD Division of Gynecological Endocrinology and Reproductive Medicine, University Women's Hospital, University of Bern, Bern, Switzerland

John Zhang, MD New Hope Fertility Center, New York, USA

Abbreviations

AFC	Antral follicle count
AMH	Anti-mullerian hormone
ART	Assisted reproductive technologies
BMI	Body mass index
CI	Confidence interval
cIVF	conventional IVF (IVF with high-dose gonadotropin stimulation)
COC	Cumulus oophorus complex
d	day
D	Day
E2	Oestradiol
ESHRE	European Society of Human Reproduction and Embryology
FSH	Follicle-stimulating hormone
GnRH	Gonadotropin-releasing hormone
GnRHa	Gonadotropin-releasing hormone agonist
GnRHant	Gonadotropin-releasing hormone antagonist
h	hour
HCG	Human chorionic gonadotropin
HMG	Human menopausal gonadotropin
ISMAAR	International Society for Mild Approaches in Assisted Reproduction
ICSI	Intracytoplasmic sperm injection
IL	Interleukin
IU	International unit
IUI	Intrauterine insemination
IVF	In vitro fertilisation (includes fertilisation by insemination and by intracytoplasmic sperm injection)
LGA	Large-for-gestational-age
LH	Luteinising hormone
NC-IVF	Natural cycle IVF
NSAID	Non-steroidal anti-inflammatory drug
OHSS	Ovarian hyperstimulation syndrome
OR	Odds ratio

P4	Progesterone
PCOS	Polycystic ovary syndrome
PG	Prostaglandin
PGT	Preimplantation genetic testing
PGT-A	Preimplantation genetic testing for aneuploidy
POI	Premature ovarian insufficiency
RNA	Ribonucleic acid
RR	Relative risk
SD	Standard deviation
SGA	Small-for-gestational-age

Part I
Basics

Chapter 1
How to Use This Book

Michael von Wolff

1.1 Background

The book "Natural Cycle IVF and Minimal Stimulation IVF—from physiology to clinical practice" was written to enable other reproductive health professionals to perform natural Cycle IVF and minimal stimulation IVF treatments effectively. For conventional, i.e. gonadotropin-stimulated IVF, there are fixed stimulation protocols that are easy to apply. However, natural cycle IVF and minimal stimulation IVF require individualisation of the treatment protocols, therefore the use of fixed treatment protocols is only of limited use. Good knowledge of physiology and reproductive endocrinology, as well as a different set of aspiration needles, medications and logistics are also required.

Because of this, it makes sense that you approach the subject matter systematically to have the best sense of achievement and chances of success. In the following we will show you how the book can support this process.

1.2 The Thorough Systematic Approach

The thorough systematic approach follows the principle of "to put the cart behind the horse". This means that you first familiarise yourself with the basics and background and then plan the first therapy. The book has been structured accordingly. It would therefore be best if you first read the book in chronological order from beginning to end, which might take a weekend, and only then start.

M. von Wolff (✉)
Division of Gynecological Endocrinology and Reproductive Medicine,
University Women's Hospital, University of Bern, Bern, Switzerland
e-mail: Michael.vonwolff@insel.ch

3

Of course, you have just looked up how many pages the book has and asked yourself how and when you are supposed to finish it. We understand this perfectly, as it is not different for us. Nevertheless, we maintain that a thorough systematic approach would be the best way.

However, if you are too busy to read the whole book, we have put together a fast-track programme below that will get you started in 10 steps, which might just take a few hours.

1.3   The (Supposedly) Quick Approach in 10 Steps

The quick approach follows the principle: "to put the cart before the horse". This means that you follow the ten steps below and as the 8th step you read the chapter "Treatment protocols". You will select a protocol and start the treatment. The treatment protocols are then adjusted during the course of the treatment. However, it remains to be seen whether this is really the faster way. Natural cycle IVF and minimal stimulation IVF therapy that satisfies the patient and the doctor, and is even enjoyable, always requires an understanding of the basics.

The 10 Most Important Chapters for a Quick Approach
1. Chapter "How to use this book?"
   Well done. You have already completed this most important step by opening this central chapter. Stay tuned and follow the further chapter suggestions.
2. Chapter "Definitions"
   This chapter gives you an overview of how natural cycle IVF and minimal stimulation IVF are defined in the book. You should know what we are actually talking about in the chapters.
3. Chapter "Indications"
   This chapter gives you an orientation for whom natural cycle IVF and/or minimal stimulation IVF is indicated and for whom it is not. The viewpoint of the editor is presented. This is relevant because frustration is inevitable if natural cycle IVF is only offered to women with a very poor prognosis and therefore as a last straw. Natural cycle IVF is also unlikely to help a 42-year-old woman with a high ovarian reserve who wants to undergo natural cycle IVF after several frustrating conventional IVF treatment cycles.
4. Chapter "Laboratory aspects"
   Monofollicular (natural cycle IVF) or oligofollicular (minimal stimulation IVF) requires laboratory processes that are adapted to the low oocyte count. For example, in monofollicular IVF, no oocyte may be retrieved, which negates all the preparations made by the laboratory. Follicular flushing is also useful in many cases, which must be prepared by the laboratory. You should therefore involve your embryologist and the laboratory in your considerations and planning. A disgruntled and therefore rebellious laboratory is no fun.

5. Chapter "Costs"

   Natural cycle IVF and minimal stimulation IVF are cheaper per treatment cycle. However, you should calculate the costs over approx. 3 treatment cycles to enable a comparison with conventional IVF. IVF therapies also have special billing requirements. If only one oocyte is retrieved and it is successfully fertilised, but degenerates shortly before transfer, then you need to decide whether the entire laboratory process should be charged to the couple. From a laboratory point of view it is correct, but from a patient motivation point of view it is very awkward. A mixed calculation is conceivable, for example, in which the laboratory costs are only incurred if a transfer is also achieved. These things have to be clarified in advance, especially if you have an economist or a CEO breathing down your neck.

6. Chapter "Success rates"

   A central point in counselling the couple is the success rate. This must be calculated individually based on the medical history. However, it makes sense not to calculate it per cycle, but per three-month therapy interval. This is because in three months you carry out three natural cycle IVF or minimal stimulation IVF treatments, whereas you would only manage around one conventional IVF treatment in this period. This procedure also allows a cross-comparison with conventional IVF therapy.

7. Part VIII "Case discussions"

   The procedure for natural cycle IVF or minimal stimulation IVF therapy is not standardised, but depends on the medical history and the cause of infertility. It is therefore useful to look at the procedures suggested by other centres/networks and then decide how to proceed with your couple. We have chosen leading centres/networks to give room not only for different treatment philosophies, but also for different cultures.

8. Chapter "Treatment protocols"

   If you have decided to perform natural cycle IVF or minimal stimulation IVF, turn to this chapter and choose one of the treatment protocols. The descriptions are detailed and geared towards clinical practice, so the protocols should be a good guide.

9. Chapter "Follicular aspiration"

   The chapters on "Physiology" (Part II) and on "Technical aspects" (Part III) can be put on hold if necessary. You must, however, read the chapter on "Follicular aspiration". Follicular aspiration in mono- or oligofollicular IVF is quite different from that in conventional IVF. Or rather, it should be different. To perform analgesia or anaesthesia for 1–2 follicles is as nonsensical as a follicle aspiration for 1–2 follicles with a thick puncture needle commonly used in conventional IVF.

10. The other chapters

    With this minimal programme, you can certainly carry out a first natural cycle IVF or minimal stimulation IVF treatment cycle. However, after this first treatment cycles at the latest, you should also turn to the other chapters.

    The biggest mistake is to assume that natural cycle IVF or minimal stimulation is "small IVF" in the sense of "simple IVF". For the woman it is certainly simple, but for the reproductive physician it can be intellectually and logistically challenging.

Chapter 2
Definitions for Natural Cycle and Minimal Stimulation IVF

Michael von Wolff

2.1 Background

The first IVF treatment in the world was natural cycle IVF. Shortly after, different stimulation treatments were introduced, and new names were coined for the various IVF therapies. Most physicians understand IVF therapies as treatments with gonadotropin stimulation at a dosage of usually 150–300 IU per day. Such stimulation generates a sufficient number of oocytes to allow a high chance of success with low risks. The stimulation protocols have been widely evaluated and standardised. Since these IVF stimulations have been used for years, they can be referred to conventional IVF treatments.

However, no uniform definitions are used for IVF treatments without or with a lower level of stimulation. This makes these IVF treatments confusing and difficult to compare. Because of this, various definitions of IVF treatments without or with a low level of stimulation are presented in this chapter and the definitions used specifically in this book are described.

2.2 Definitions According to ISMAAR, 2007

The International Society for Mild Approaches in Assisted Reproduction (ISMAAR) (http://www.ismaar.org/) was founded in 2007. It promotes a more physiological, less drug-oriented, lower risk, less expensive and more patient friendly approach to

M. von Wolff (✉)
Division of Gynecological Endocrinology and Reproductive Medicine,
University Women's Hospital, University of Bern, Bern, Switzerland
e-mail: Michael.vonwolff@insel.ch

© The Author(s), under exclusive license to Springer Nature Switzerland AG 2022
M. von Wolff (ed.), *Natural Cycle and Minimal Stimulation IVF*,
https://doi.org/10.1007/978-3-030-97571-5_2

Table 2.1 Definitions, aims and methodology of IVF treatments according to the International Society for Mild Approaches in Assisted Reproduction, ISMAAR [1]

Treatment	Aim	Methodology
Natural cycle IVF	1 oocyte	No medication.
Modified natural cycle IVF	1 oocyte	HCG, FSH/HMG only as add back if GnRH antagonists are used.
Mild IVF	2–7 oocytes	GnRH antagonists, low dose FSH/HMG, oral compounds.
Conventional IVF	≥8 oocytes	GnRH agonist or antagonists, conventional FSH/HMG dose.

assisted reproduction embracing not only natural cycle treatment, but also mild stimulation protocols and in vitro maturation of oocytes [1].

ISMAAR had proposed a terminology for ovarian stimulation for IVF in 2007. The terminology, aim and methodology are shown in Table 2.1. The terminology of ISMAAR is basically very good, but shows some weaknesses in clinical practice.

According to ISMAAR, natural cycle IVF is defined as treatment without any medication, i.e. without an ovulation trigger and without individual doses of GnRH antagonists or non-steroidal anti-inflammatory drugs (NSAID). In practice, however, this makes little sense, as natural cycle IVF therapy cannot be carried out effectively without such medication.

According to ISMAAR, modified natural cycle IVF includes gonadotropin stimulation if GnRH antagonists are also given. This raises the question of whether the term "natural cycle" is still justified with the administration of gonadotropins.

Mild IVF is defined by ISMAAR as IVF therapy with gonadotropin stimulation of up to 150 IU per day administered as part of an antagonist cycle. According to the publications from the last few years, an IVF with approx. 150 IU gonadotropin is referred to as mild IVF in almost all studies. The studies compared a mild IVF with mostly 150 IU gonadotropin with a conventional IVF with >150 IU [2].

What is missing from the terminology is a term for very mild stimulations that do not require a fixed antagonist protocol and that can be performed logistically like natural cycle IVF, i.e. without analgesia or anaesthesia during the follicle aspiration.

2.3   Definitions According to the International Glossary on Infertility and Fertility Care, 2017

A group of 25 professionals from all parts of the world set up a consensus-based and evidence-driven set of 283 terminologies used in infertility and fertility in 2017 [3]. The terminology developed by the expert group is presented in Table 2.2.

The definitions in the International Glossary on Infertility and Fertility Care are relatively well suited for clinical practice, but also have a few weaknesses.

Table 2.2 Definitions according to the International Glossary on Infertility and Fertility Care, 2017 [3]

Treatment	Definition
Natural cycle IVF	An ART procedure in which one or more oocytes are collected from the ovaries during a menstrual cycle without the use of any pharmacological compounds.
Modified natural cycle IVF	An ART procedure in which one or more oocytes are collected from the ovaries during a spontaneous menstrual cycle. Pharmacological compounds are administered with the sole purpose of blocking the spontaneous LH surge and/or inducing final oocyte maturation.
Mild ovarian stimulation IVF	A protocol in which the ovaries are stimulated with gonadotropins, and/or other pharmacological compounds, with the intention of limiting the number of oocytes following stimulation for IVF.

Even with this terminology, a natural cycle IVF (ART) therapy is understood as a treatment without any medication. However, such an IVF, i.e. an IVF without an ovulation trigger, cannot be effectively implemented.

This terminology also lacks a term for very light stimulations that do not require a fixed antagonist protocol and that can be performed logistically like a natural cycle IVF, i.e. without analgesia or anaesthesia during the follicle aspiration.

2.4 Terminology Used in This Book

In this book, an attempt is made to use basically modified definitions of the already established terminology from ISMAAR and the International Glossary on Infertility and Fertility Care. The definitions used here are derived from the developments in the field of these IVF techniques (see Chap. 4, Fig. 4.2). However, they had to be adapted to the requirements of everyday clinical practice (Table 2.3).

The main difference is that "Natural cycle IVF" is defined as any IVF with natural folliculogenesis and a mostly natural luteal phase, but with the inclusion of medication to prevent premature ovulation. Since folliculogenesis is not relevantly influenced by medication to prevent premature ovulation, no luteal phase support is required (see Chap. 8). The definition of "Natural cycle IVF" thus corresponds to the "Modified Natural cycle IVF" of the "International Glossary on Fertility and Fertility Care" presented in Table 2.2.

The term "Minimal stimulation IVF" was also introduced. This term refers to treatments with light stimulation, be it with clomiphene citrate, aromatase inhibitors or gonadotropins with a dose of ≤ 100 IU per day. The aim of this light stimulation is to grow fewer oocytes without analgesia/anaesthesia and to perform monthly cycles. Cryopreservation is usually not necessary.

Conventional IVF is defined as all gonadotropin stimulations with a stimulation dose of ≥ 150 IE per day. Conventional IVF treatments usually require anaesthesia during aspiration and all aim to retrieve a relatively large number of oocytes, carry

10 M. von Wolff

Table 2.3 Principles, aims and methodology of IVF treatments used in this book

Treatment	Principle	Aim	Methodology
Natural cycle IVF (Modified natural cycle IVF according to the International Glossary terminology, Table 2.2).	Monofollicular IVF	1 oocyte; aspiration without analgesia/ anaesthesia	Medication to trigger ovulation or to avoid premature ovulation (low dose clomiphene citrate, NSAIDs, single injections of GnRH antagonists); usually no luteal phase support.
Minimal stimulation IVF	Oligofollicular IVF	1–3 oocytes; aspiration usually without analgesia/ anaesthesia.	Stimulation with clomiphene citrate, aromatase inhibitors, gonadotropins ≤100 IU per day; GnRH antagonists only if required; luteal phase support.
Conventional IVF (Includes mild IVF according to ISMAAR, Table 2.1, and the International Glossary terminologies, Table 2.2).	Polyfollicular IVF	>3 oocytes; aspiration mostly with analgesia/ anaesthesia.	Gonadotropin stimulation ≥150 IE gonadotropin per day; GnRH agonists or GnRH antagonist protocols or progestin-primed ovarian stimulation (PPOS); luteal phase support.

out embryo selection, preserve surplus embryos and allow preimplantation genetic testing for aneuploidy (PGT-A) if necessary.

In summary,

The definitions proposed worldwide are basically good, but they are of limited applicability for clinical practice when performing natural cycle IVF treatments and IVF treatments with minimal stimulation. Therefore, slightly adapted definitions are used in this book. It should be noted that the definitions from the centres "Kato Ladies Clinic, Tokyo, Japan" and "New Hope Fertility Center, New York, United States" may differ somewhat (for centre-specific definitions see chapters in "Part VII, Worldwide programs").

References

1. Nargund G, Fauser BC, Macklon NS, Ombelet W, Nygren K, Frydman R. Rotterdam ISMAAR Consensus Group on Terminology for Ovarian Stimulation for IVF. The ISMAAR proposal on terminology for ovarian stimulation for IVF. Hum Reprod. 2007;22:2801–4.
2. Datta AK, Maheshwari A, Felix N, Campbell S, Nargund G. Mild versus conventional ovarian stimulation for IVF in poor, normal and hyper-responders: a systematic review and meta-analysis. Hum Reprod Update. 2021;27:229–53.
3. Zegers-Hochschild F, Adamson GD, Dyer S, Racowsky C, de Mouzon J, Sokol R, Rienzi L, Sunde A, Schmidt L, Cooke ID, Simpson JL, van der Poel S. The international glossary on infertility and fertility care, 2017. Hum Reprod. 2017;32:1786–801.

Chapter 3
Indications for Natural Cycle and Minimal Stimulation IVF

Michael von Wolff

3.1   Background

In a review article about natural cycle IVF published in 2019 [1], von Wolff concluded that "Natural Cycle-IVF and conventional gonadotropin stimulated IVF are basically different forms of treatment .... The treatments should not compete with each other but should be seen as complementary".

This statement applies not only to natural cycle IVF, but also to minimal stimulation IVF treatments and, of course, conventional IVF treatments. In practical terms, this means that the indications for the treatments are partly the same, some of indications overlap and some indications apply exclusively to only one of the therapies.

This becomes particularly clear with the following two examples:

In a woman with an incipient premature ovarian insufficiency with increased FSH concentrations but still regular cycles, conventional IVF does not make sense. On the other hand, in a 42-year-old woman with a still high ovarian reserve, NC-IVF does not make sense.

An indication for IVF therapy is made based on the individual medical requirements. However, the indication is also influenced by the couple's wishes, the logistical possibilities of the centre and the regional or personal cultural circumstances. Thus, the indication for or against a specific IVF therapy is made up of several factors. In this chapter, the factors that speak for, but also against one of the therapies are presented.

M. von Wolff (✉)
Division of Gynecological Endocrinology and Reproductive Medicine,
University Women's Hospital, University of Bern, Bern, Switzerland
e-mail: Michael.vonwolff@insel.ch

Natural Cycle IVF is Especially Suitable If:
- Good prognostic factors (female age ca. <38 years, short duration of infertility, andrological infertility)
- Regular cycles
- Follicle aspiration without analgesia/anaesthesia possible
- Ovaries for aspiration easily accessible
- Longer time to pregnancy acceptable
- High risk with gonadotropin stimulation (thrombosis, lupus erythematosus, etc.)
- Poor responder with very low ovarian reserve

Natural Cycle IVF is Rather Not Suitable If:
- Bad prognostic factors (female age ca. ≥40 years, idiopathic infertility, several previous IVF treatments and embryo transfers without pregnancies) in combination with still high ovarian reserve
- Irregular cycles
- Follicular aspiration very painful, requiring analgesia/anaesthesia
- Ovaries for aspiration hardly accessible

Minimal Stimulation IVF is Especially Suitable If:
- Good prognostic factors (female age ca. <38 years, short duration of infertility, andrological infertility)
- Follicle aspiration without analgesia/anaesthesia possible
- Ovaries for aspiration easily accessible
- High risk with gonadotropin stimulation (thrombosis, lupus erythematosus, etc.)
- Poor responder with very low ovarian reserve

Minimal Stimulation IVF is Rather Not Suitable If:
- Bad prognostic factors (female age ca. ≥40 years, idiopathic infertility, several previous IVF treatments and embryo transfers without pregnancies) in combination with still high ovarian reserve
- Follicular aspiration very painful, requiring analgesia/anaesthesia
- Ovaries for aspiration hardly accessible
- Wish not to use hormone injections

Conventional IVF is Especially Suitable If:
- Bad prognostic factors (female age ca. ≥40 years, idiopathic infertility, several previous IVF treatments and embryo transfers without pregnancies) in combination with still high ovarian reserve
- Preimplantation genetic testing (PGT) required

Conventional IVF is Rather Not Suitable If:
- Low ovarian reserve
- Poor responder
- High risk with gonadotropin stimulation (thrombosis, lupus erythematosus etc.)
- Wish not to use hormone injections

Practical Conclusions

- The indication for IVF therapy is influenced by the individual medical conditions, the wishes of the couple, the logistical possibilities of the centre and the regional or personal cultural circumstances.
- The indications for the different treatments are partly the same but can also overlap. There are also indications that apply exclusively to one of the therapies.
- The indication for one of the IVF therapies must be made individually and may change during the course of the IVF therapy.

Reference

1. von Wolff M. The role of natural cycle IVF in assisted reproduction. Best Pract Res Clin Endocrinol Metab. 2019;33:35–45.

Chapter 4
History of Natural Cycle and Minimal Stimulation IVF

Michael von Wolff

4.1 Background

The first pregnancies and births after in vitro fertilisation (IVF) occurred in 1978 and 1979 after natural cycle IVF (NC-IVF). The IVF treatments were carried out by, among others, Robert Geoffrey Edwards, a geneticist who received the Nobel Prize in Physiology and Medicine in 2010 for his services in the field of IVF, and Patrick Steptoe, a gynaecologist.

The successful path to the first birth was the result of several years of joint research by Edwards and Steptoe, which began in 1968. Together they solved a multitude of elementary challenges. Edwards brought in his interest and knowledge in genetics and embryology and Steptoe his interest and knowledge in infertility and laparoscopy.

Edwards and Steptoe first developed IVF therapy with gonadotropin or clomiphene citrate stimulation. As these treatments did not result in pregnancies, they continued their IVF programme with natural cycle IVF therapies in 1977. As a result, 4 clinical pregnancies and 2 live births developed, including that of Louise Brown, who was born on 25 July 1978.

Thus, from the very beginning of the first IVF pregnancies, the realisation that a natural and unstimulated cycle can be beneficial was crucial.

After following many years of successful development of IVF therapy with high-dose gonadotropin stimulation, the realisation is now spreading again that a return to natural cycle IVF or to IVF with only mild or minimal stimulation can be beneficial.

M. von Wolff (✉)
Division of Gynecological Endocrinology and Reproductive Medicine,
University Women's Hospital, University of Bern, Bern, Switzerland
e-mail: Michael.vonwolff@insel.ch

© The Author(s), under exclusive license to Springer Nature Switzerland AG 2022
M. von Wolff (ed.), *Natural Cycle and Minimal Stimulation IVF*,
https://doi.org/10.1007/978-3-030-97571-5_4

This chapter describes the development of IVF up to the birth of the first IVF child as well as the subsequent developmental steps in the field of natural cycle IVF and minimal stimulation IVF.

4.2   The Years before the Birth of the First IVF Child

The history of mammalian IVF began in the 1930s in den USA. Pincus and Enzmann [1] claimed 1934 to have successfully produced rabbit offspring after fertilisation of rabbit eggs in vitro. Rock and Menkin [2] claimed 1944 the fertilisation and cleavage of three human oocytes. In 1951, Chang [3] and Austin [4] independently discovered sperm capacitation and therefore questioned the claims by Pincus and Enzmann [1] and Rock and Menkin [2]. This discovery led to the first definite successful IVF in rabbits and viable rabbit offspring in 1959 [5].

For the introduction of human IVF there were major challenges to be solved in establishing IVF in the human system:

• Ovulation induction
• Timing of laparoscopy for follicle aspiration after ovulation induction
• Technique of follicle aspiration
• Sperm preparation and capacitation
• Insemination procedure
• Oocyte and embryo culture
• Technique of embryo transfer
• Luteal phase support

A first major challenge was that of oocyte maturation. Since this occurs in mammals after 12 h, it took 6 years until Edwards was able to publish in 1965 that the time span in humans is approx. 36 h [6].

Another challenge was sperm capacitation. Edwards had already been working on this for four years when Steptoe offered to isolate sperm from the fallopian tubes, as he assumed that they were activated there by various substances from the genital tract. This was ultimately not necessary as Bavister described in 1969 [7] that full fertilisation capacity could be achieved in vitro by exposing sperm to raised pH.

Steptoe solved the challenge of oocyte collection by introducing laparoscopy to diagnose sterility [8]. He also developed a "suction device" with Edwards for the collection of follicular fluid [9] which is similar to the aspiration systems still used. No follicular flushing was performed.

After the introduction of laparoscopic oocyte aspiration, it was important to optimise the timing of the laparoscopy. The laparoscopy was initially performed on cycle day 10–12, 28.75–29.5 h after HCG administration. As oocyte yield was initially only 33% and as most oocytes were immature, the timing was first extended to 29.5–30.0 and then to 32.0–33.5 h in the late 1970 [10].

Edwards and Steptoe believed that, as in the animal model, the chance of successful IVF could be increased by human menopuasal gonadotropins (HMG) stimulation. Accordingly, most IVF therapies were initially carried out with HMG. The shortening of the luteal phase by HMG stimulation prompted Edwards in 1973 to use clomiphene citrate 50 mg twice a day instead of HMG and to trigger ovulation with HCG. Due to the low oocyte recovery rate, the use of clomiphene citrate was rejected and HMG was used again from 1975 to 1977 [10]. Although it was recognised that the luteal phase was deficient under HMG stimulation and various therapies such as luteal administration of HCG and progesterone were introduced, pregnancy did not occur.

Because of this, the decision was made in 1977 to initially work only in the natural cycle and only trigger oocyte maturation with HCG.

As a result, 4 clinical pregnancies and 2 live births developed. The mother of the first IVF baby, Leslie Brown, underwent IVF therapy due to bilateral tubal occlusion. Laparoscopic egg retrieval was performed on 10th November 1977 and embryo transfer of an 8-cell embryo took place 2 days later. Louise Brown was born by caesarean section to her 31-year-old mother on July 25th, 1978 at Oldham General Hospital, Oldham, U.K [11]. This event led to much media interest at the press conference (Fig. 4.1) but also to much criticism.

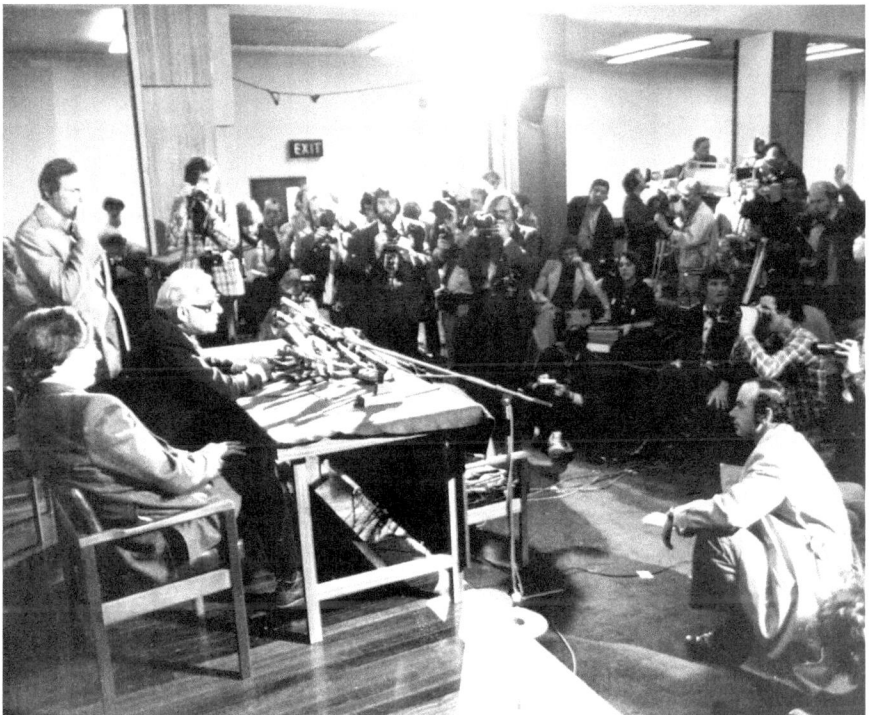

Fig. 4.1 Robert G. Edwards (right) and Patrick C. Steptoe (left, speaking) announcing the birth of the first IVF baby at a press conference (Reprinted with permission from Alamy Limited, U.K.)

4.3   The First Years After the Birth of the First IVF Baby

After these initial IVF successes, IVF therapies in the U.K. were halted until 1982, when Bourn Hall was built in Cambridgeshire. The reason was that Steptoe retired, which is why Edwards, Steptoe and Purdy needed to be relocated from Oldham. However, the relocation was not supported by Cambridge University. This gap was filled by two groups in Melbourne, Australia, who had been working on the IVF technique since the early 1970s and were able to report a first clinical pregnancy (generated by natural cycle IVF) in 1980 [12]. This pregnancy resulted in the birth of the 3rd IVF baby and the first IVF baby in Australia.

In the following years further ground-breaking successes were achieved (Fig. 4.2), which paved the way for the widespread use of IVF.

The following should be mentioned in particular:

- the introduction of transvaginal follicle aspiration (Lenz and Lauritsen, 1982) [13],
- the first pregnancy after embryo donation (Trounson et al., 1983) [14],
- the first birth after intracytoplasmic sperm injection (Van Steirteghem et al., 1993) [15],
- the first birth after preimplantation genetic testing (Handyside et al., 1990) [16],
- the first pregnancy after cryopreservation of an embryo (Trounson and Mohr, 1983) [17],
- the successful cryopreservation of oocytes (Cobo et al., 2010) [18].

The developments in IVF led to great scientific interest from various working groups. Accordingly, the world's first IVF meeting was held in Bourn Hall on 3–5 September 1981 (Fig. 4.3).

The European Society of Human Reproduction and Embryology, ESHRE, was founded on 2 September 1985 by Robert Edwards and Jean Cohen (Paris, France). The American Society for Reproductive Medicine (ASRM) was founded in 1944 as the American Fertility Society (AFS).

4.4   The Development of Natural Cycle and Minimal Stimulation IVF

As the world's first three births after IVF therapy in Oldham, U.K. and in Melbourne, Australia were the result of natural cycle IVF, the proof of principle of natural cycle IVF had been impressively demonstrated.

To mention success rates of the first IVF attempts at this point actually makes little sense, as IVF was just being established. Nevertheless, it is interesting to note that 457 laparoscopic egg collections were performed in Oldham from 1969 to 1978 in at least 281 women. Oocytes were obtained in 388 of 436 documented egg collections. 331 of the oocytes underwent fertilisation, the development of 167

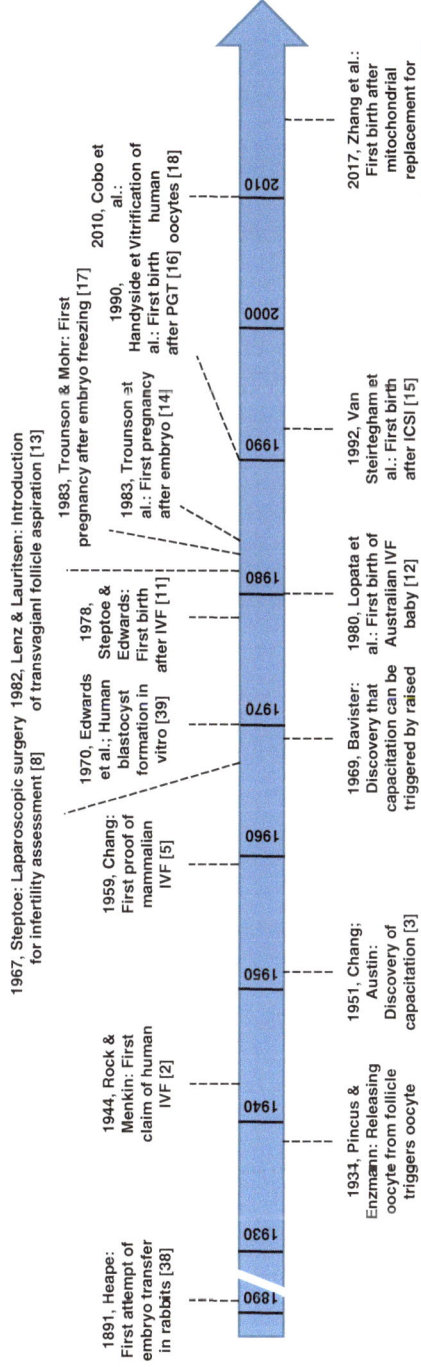

Fig. 4.2 Key events in the development of IVF with the year of publication

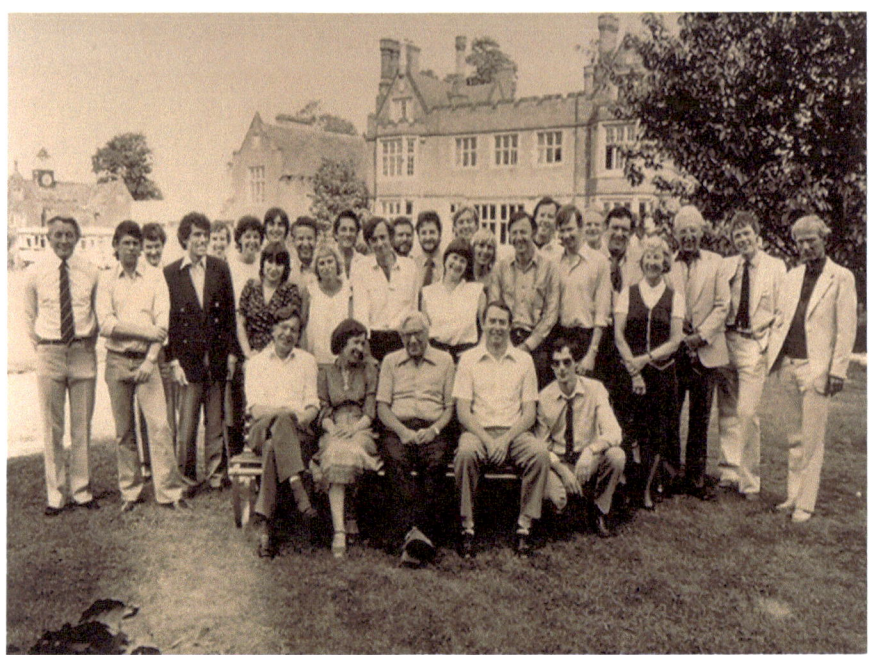

Fig. 4.3 The first IVF meeting in the world, held at Bourn hall, the first IVF clinic worldwide, September 3rd–5th 1981. In the middle the geneticist Robert G. Edwards (1925–2013), flanked by the laboratory assistant Jean M. Purdy (1945–1985) and the gynaecologist Patrick C. Steptoe (1913–1988). (With permission of Bourn hall clinic)

embryos was documented and 112 embryo transfers were performed. A maximum of 11 biochemical/preclinical and five clinical pregnancies were documented, two of which resulted in live births in 1978 and 1979 [9]. Accordingly, the overall clinical pregnancy rate per initiated cycle was in the very initial stage of IVF just 1.1%.

However, after solving the problem of luteal phase insufficiency due to gonadotropin stimulation, the majority favoured gonadotropin-stimulated IVF treatment over the following decades.

Only Lenton initially still ran a programme with an all-natural IVF, i.e. even without the use of HCG to trigger ovulation. However, the great effort to detect the onset of LH surge and the low success rate led to this programme being stopped. According to Lenton et al., 2007 [19], 534 cycles were started in 1991–1992. 495 cycles were scheduled for egg collection. In 403 cycles (81%), an oocyte was collected. In 43 cycles (8.7%) an oocyte could not be collected due to premature ovulation. In 48 cycles (9.7%) no oocyte was aspirated. An embryo transfer was achieved in 257 cycles (64%). 38 clinical pregnancies were counted, which corresponds with a pregnancy rate of 14.8% per embryo transfer, 9.4% per aspirated oocyte and 7.7% per cycle scheduled for oocyte collection. The clinical pregnancy rate per initiated cycle was 7.1% (see also Chap. 12).

Mild approaches, including natural cycle IVF and minimal stimulation IVF, were only systematically introduced again at the turn of the millennium in some centres as shown by the following studies:

In 1996, Nargund and Wei [20] published the use of indomethacin to inhibit ovulation in a natural cycle IVF. Teramoto and Kato published a study in 2007 [21] in which they evaluated 44,345 minimal stimulation IVF cycles. The evaluation period was from January 2001 to December 2005.

This development over time is also reflected in the number of publications when entering the search term "Natural Cycle In vitro fertilization" in the PubMed database (www.ncbi.nlm.nih.gov). In 1995 there were around 15 publications per year, in 2000 around 20 publications and since 2018 around 100 publications annually.

The first book on minimal stimulation IVF was published in 2011. A second book was published in 2014 and this book is the third book and the first practical guide (Table 4.1).

Table 4.1 Books published about natural cycle IVF and/or minimal stimulation IVF

Title	Language	Publisher	Editors	Year of publication	Number of pages	Characteristics
Textbook of minimal stimulation IVF. Milder, mildest or back to Nature.	English	Jaypee Brothers Medical Publishers	Alejandro Chavez Badiola, Gautam N. Allahbadia	2011	190	Textbook on minimal stimulation IVF. Written by many authors.
Minimal stimulation and natural cycle in vitro fertilisation	English	Springer	Gautam N. Allahbadia, Markus Nitzschke	2015	101	Collection of monographies presenting many aspects of natural cycle IVF. Written by many authors.
Natural cycle and minimal stimulation IVF – from physiology to clinical practice	English	Springer	Michael von Wolff	2022	see this book	Practically oriented book providing basic endocrinological, physiological and technical knowledge and practical guidance on natural cycle IVF and minimal stimulation IVF. Written by few authors to publish a book as one piece and to link the contents of the chapters.

4.5   The International Society for Mild Approaches in Assisted Reproduction (ISMAAR)

The International Society for Mild Approaches in Assisted Reproduction, ISMAAR (www.ismaar.org) was founded in 2007. In 2006 a 1st World congress on natural cycle and minimal stimulation IVF was organised in London by ISNAR, the preliminary society with Geeta Nargund as President and René Frydmann as Chairman (Fig. 4.4). This very first conference on more natural approaches in IVF received very much attention with attendants from all over the world.

The conference was opened by Robert Edwards with an introduction entitled "IVF Strategy—Time for a Re-Think" which led to his publication "IVF, IVM, natural cycle IVF, minimal stimulation IVF—time for a rethink", published in 2007 [22]. This opening was a powerful message to make IVF safer, affordable and physiological. This conference motivated several physicians, including the editor of this book, to embark on natural cycle IVF with all its modifications.

Fig. 4.4 The cover of the program of the legendary 1st World congress on natural cycle and minimal stimulation IVF in London in 2006 organised by ISNAR, the International Society of Natural Cycle Assisted Reproduction with Geeta Nargund as president and René Frydmann as chairman. In 2007 the society was renamed ISMAAR. (With permission of G. Nargund)

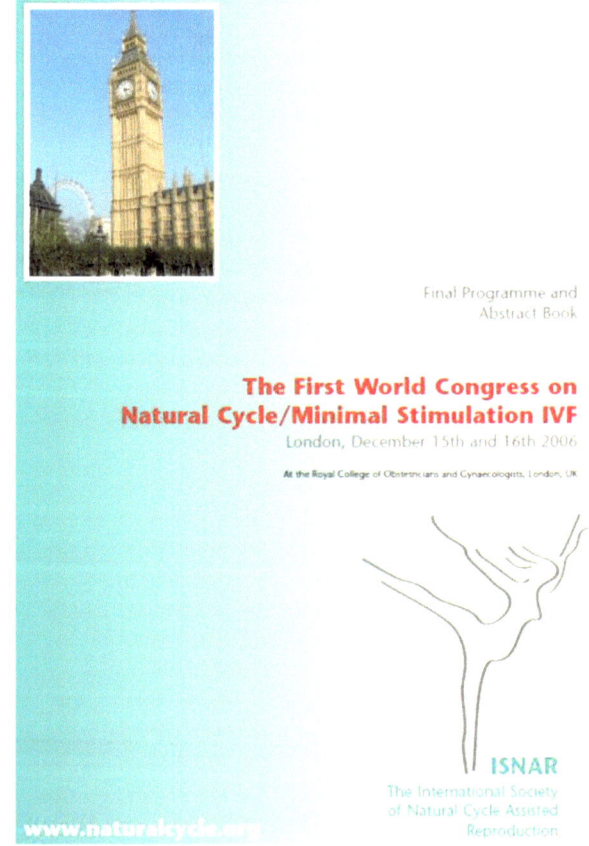

Final Programme and
Abstract Book

**The First World Congress on
Natural Cycle/Minimal Stimulation IVF**
London, December 15th and 16th 2006

At the Royal College of Obstetricians and Gynaecologists, London, UK

ISNAR
The International Society
of Natural Cycle Assisted
Reproduction

www.naturalcycle.org

In 2007 the society was renamed ISMAAR. ISMAAR is a non-profit making organisation and a UK Charity, organised by 8 board members with Geeta Nargund as the president. It was set up to promote a more physiological, less drug-oriented, lower risk, less expensive and more patient friendly approach to assisted reproduction embracing not only natural cycle treatment but also mild stimulation protocols and in vitro maturation of oocytes.

Since 2007 ISMAAR has organised several World congresses and symposia around the world to spread its philosophy. ISMAAR also proposed a terminology for ovarian stimulation for IVF which was set up by the Rotterdam ISMAAR Consensus Group in 2007 [23].

The 9th World congress was again held in London in 2018, the 40th birthday of Louise Brown who also attended the conference dinner.

4.6   New Approaches in the Field of Natural Cycle IVF and Minimal Stimulation IVF

Following the remarkable first 3 deliveries after natural cycle IVF, proving that this technique is a feasible option, several improvements were necessary to increase the efficacy of natural cycle IVF and minimal stimulation therapies. Interestingly, some of these improvements and endocrinological and technical aspects were already discussed before the first IVF baby was born (Table 4.2).

The key for the success was certainly the numerous small improvements in the IVF lab which have significantly increased the success rate per aspirated oocyte. However, apart from these many improvements which have been beneficial for all kinds of IVF treatments, many natural cycle IVF and minimal stimulation IVF specific modifications needed to be evaluated and improved. The main steps which were essential for the success of these techniques are described in the following chapters.

Table 4.2 Endocrinological and technical aspects already recognized before the first IVF baby was born and current status of knowledge

Aspects	As discussed before the first IVF baby was born[a]	As discussed and known nowadays
Effects of clomiphene citrate	Clomiphene citrate was introduced in 1973 (50 mg twice a day) to reduce the apparently unfavourable supraphysiological oestrogen concentrations induced by hMG stimulation, but still to get a polyfolliclar response. However, clomiphene resulted in very low egg recovery rates and was therefore abandoned.	Clomiphene citrate has several effects such as: • increase in the number of follicles and oocytes, • thinning of the endometrium, • possibly reducing implantation rate at doses higher than 25mg/d • inhibiting ovulation and thereby decreasing premature ovulation. (see also Chap. 11)

(continued)

Table 4.2 (continued)

Aspects	As discussed before the first IVF baby was born[a]	As discussed and known nowadays
Flushing of the follicles	Flushing was not performed until the first IVF baby was born, but was later introduced in Bourn Hall.	The effect of follicle flushing seems to depend on the number of follicles such as: • flushing is not favourable in oligofollicular and polyfollicular ovaries • flushing does seem to be favourable in monofollicular ovaries. (see also Chap. 13)
Timing of follicle aspiration	Laparoscopic follicle aspiration was first performed 28.75–29.5 h after HCG and was then extended to 32.0–33.5 h in 1973.	HCG is commonly administered in natural cycle and in minimal stimulation IVF 34–36 h before aspiration. (see also Chap. 12).
Effect of supraphysiological E2 levels on endometrial function	It was realised that high oestrogen concentrations in the follicular phase were unfavourable for the luteal phase endometrium.	Supraphysiological oestrogen concentrations lead to endometrial and placental dysfunction, thereby: • reducing the implantation rate • increasing the risk of gestational hypertension disorders and preeclampsia • reducing the birth weight of the babies (see also Chap. 9)
Effect of supraphysiological E2 levels on the luteal phase	It was realised that high oestrogen concentrations in the follicular phase shortened the luteal phase.	We now know that: • luteal phase support is not required in natural cycle IVF • luteal phase support is not required in low dose clomiphene-stimulated IVF • luteal phase support is required in gonadotropin-stimulated IVF. (see also Chap. 14).

[a] Johnson. Int. J.Dev. Biol 2019, 63: 83–92

4.6.1 Definition of Indications for Natural Cycle IVF and Minimal Stimulation IVF

Since conventional IVF therapies with high-dose gonadotropin stimulation as well as natural cycle IVF and minimal stimulation IVF therapies should be considered complementary therapies, it is important to know for which indications the therapies have particularly high success rates.

Von Wolff et al. (2019) [24] systematically investigated potential factors for the success of natural cycle IVF therapy, which are already known before the start of IVF therapy. They were able to show that only a low age of the woman and a short duration of infertility are statistically measurable success factors (see also Chap. 19).

4.6.2 Medication to Avoid Premature Ovulation

Clomiphene citrate was already described as a stimulant in IVF therapy in 1978 [25]. MacDougall et al., 1994 [26] showed for the first time in a prospective randomised controlled study with IVF treatment cycles that the use of clomiphene citrate, at a dosage of 100 mg of clomiphene per day, inhibits the LH surge and thereby decrease the risk of premature ovulations. In a retrospective controlled study in 2014 with natural cycle IVF treatment cycles, von Wolff et al. showed that even a low clomiphene citrate dose of 25 mg per day reduces the rate of premature ovulation [27].

The use of non-steroidal anti-inflammatory drug, NSAID, to inhibit ovulation was first described as a case report by Nargund and Wei 1996 [20] using indomethacin. The group of von Wolff et al. confirmed the effect of NSAIDs in a prospective controlled study using ibuprofen. (See also Chap. 11).

4.6.3 Ovulation Triggering with GnRH Agonist Nasal Spray

In conventional IVF therapy, in egg donation and in medical and social freezing, ovulation induction with GnRH agonists in freeze-all cycles is now a routine therapy [28].

The use of GnRH agonists in minimal stimulation IVF therapies without freeze-all was first described by Teramoto et al. in 2007 [21].

Whether ovulation can also be triggered in natural cycle IVF cycles without the need for luteal phase support, which would make IVF therapy less stressful than with HCG injections, will be shown by the outcome of a randomised controlled study initiated in 2022 (ClinicalTrials.gov: NCT04850261).

4.6.4 Flushing of Follicles

Large meta-analyses have shown that follicular flushing in conventional IVF thera-pies and thus in predominantly polyfollicular ovaries does not lead to a higher IVF success rate [29]. The same was demonstrated in a small meta-analysis in poor responders and thus in oligofollicular ovaries [30].

Méndez Lozano et al. (2009) [31] were the first to show in a prospective con-trolled study of minimal stimulation therapies that follicular flushing increases the chance of IVF success. In the case of natural cycle IVF therapies, such evidence was achieved in 2013 with a retrospective study [32] and in 2022 with a prospective randomised controlled study [33] (see also Chap. 13).

4.6.5 Luteal Phase Support

Large meta-analyses have shown that luteal phase support in conventional IVF ther-apies increases IVF success rates [34].

However, it was unclear whether luteal phase support is also necessary in natural cycle IVF or minimal stimulation IVF, as follicle aspiration and flushing could theo-retically lead to corpus luteum insufficiency due to the loss of granulosa cells.

In a prospective controlled study in 2017, von Wolff et al. [35] demonstrated that luteal phase support is not required in natural cycle IVF, even after follicular flush-ing. Length of the luteal phase and luteal phase oestradiol and progesterone concen-trations were not affected (see also Chap. 14).

4.6.6 Treatment Stress

Conventional IVF therapy is accompanied by a high level of treatment stress, which can lead to discontinuation of IVF therapy [36]. The causes are manifold and cannot be clearly attributed to individual therapy elements.

In 2018, Haemmerli Keller et al. [37] showed in a prospective controlled study that psychological stress is lower in natural cycle IVF therapy than in conventional IVF with high-dose gonadotropin stimulation, despite the larger number of cycles (see also Chap. 23).

References

1. Pincus G, Enzmann EV. Can mammalian eggs undergo normal development in vitro? Proc Natl Acad Sci U S A. 1934;20:121–2.
2. Rock J, Menkin MF. In vitro fertilization and cleavage of human ovarian eggs. Science. 1944;100:105–7.

3. Chang MC. Fertilizing capacity of spermatozoa deposited into the fallopian tubes. Nature. 1951;168:697–8.

4. Austin CR. Observations on the penetration of the sperm in the mammalian egg. Aust J Sci Res B. 1951;4:581–96.

5. Chang MC. Fertilization of rabbit ova in vitro. Nature. 1959;184(Suppl 7):466–7.

6. Edwards RG. Maturation in vitro of human ovarian oocytes. Lancet. 1965;2:926–9.

7. Bavister BD. Environmental factors important for in vitro fertilization in the hamster. J Reprod Fertil. 1969;18:544–5.

8. Steptoe PC. Laparoscopy in gynaecology. Edinburg, U.K.: E and S Livingstone; 1967.

9. Edwards RG, Steptoe PC. Induction of follicular growth, ovulation and luteinization in the human ovary. J Reprod Fertil Suppl. 1975;22:121–63.

10. Elder K, Johnson MH. The Oldham notebooks: an analysis of the development of IVF 1969-1978. II. The treatment cycles and their outcomes. Reprod Biomed Soc Online. 2015;1:9–18.

11. Steptoe PC, Edwards RG. Birth after the reimplantation of a human embryo. Lancet. 1978;2:366.

12. Lopata A, Johnston IW, Hoult IJ, Speirs AI. Pregnancy following intrauterine implantation of an embryo obtained by in vitro fertilization of a preovulatory egg. Fertil Steril. 1980;33:117–20.

13. Lenz S, Lauritsen JG. Ultrasonically guided percutaneous aspiration of human follicles under local anesthesia: a new method of collecting oocytes for in vitro fertilization. Fertil Steril. 1982;38:673–7.

14. Trounson A, Leeton J, Besanko M, Wood C, Conti A. Pregnancy established in an infertile patient after transfer of a donated embryo fertilised in vitro. Br Med J (Clin Res Ed). 1983;286:835–8.

15. Van Steirteghem AC, Nagy Z, Joris H, Liu J, Staessen C, Smitz J, Wisanto A, Devroey P. High fertilization and implantation rates after intracytoplasmic sperm injection. Hum Reprod. 1993;8:1061–6.

16. Handyside AH, Kontogianni EH, Hardy K, Winston RM. Pregnancies from biopsied human preimplantation embryos sexed by Y-specific DNA amplification. Nature. 1990;344:768–70.

17. Trounson A, Mohr L. Human pregnancy following cryopreservation, thawing and transfer of an eight-cell embryo. Nature. 1983;305:707–9.

18. Cobo A, Meseguer M, Remohí J, Pellicer A. Use of cryo-banked oocytes in an ovum donation programme: a prospective, randomized, controlled, clinical trial. Hum Reprod. 2010;25:2239–46.

19. Lenton EA. Natural cycle IVF with and without terminal HCG: learning from failed cycles. Reprod Biomed Online. 2007;15:149–55.

20. Nargund G, Wei CC. Successful planned delay of ovulation for one week with indomethacin. J Assist Reprod Genet. 1996;13:683–4.

21. Teramoto S, Kato O. Minimal ovarian stimulation with clomiphene citrate: a large-scale retrospective study. Reprod Biomed Online. 2007;15:134–48.

22. Edwards RG. IVF, IVM, natural cycle IVF, minimal stimulation IVF—time for a rethink. Reprod Biomed Online. 2007;15:106–19.

23. Nargund G, Fauser BC, Macklon NS, Ombelet W, Nygren K. Frydman R; Rotterdam ISMAAR Consensus Group on Terminology for Ovarian Stimulation for IVF. The ISMAAR proposal on terminology for ovarian stimulation for IVF. Hum Reprod. 2007;22:2801–4.

24. von Wolff M, Schwartz AK, Bitterlich N, Stute P, Fäh M. Only women's age and the duration of infertility are the prognostic factors for the success rate of natural cycle IVF. Arch Gynecol Obstet. 2019;299:883–9.

25. Lopata A, Brown JB, Leeton JF, Talbot JM, Wood C. In vitro fertilization of preovulatory oocytes and embryo transfer in infertile patients treated with clomiphene and human chorionic gonadotropin. Fertil Steril. 1978;30:27–35.

26. MacDougall MJ, Tan SL, Hall V, Balen A, Mason BA, Jacobs HS. Comparison of natural with clomiphene citrate-stimulated cycles in in vitro fertilization: a prospective, randomized trial. Fertil Steril. 1994;61:1052–7.

27. von Wolff M, Nitzschke M, Stute P, Bitterlich N, Rohner S. Low-dosage clomiphene reduces premature ovulation rates and increases transfer rates in natural-cycle IVF. Reprod Biomed Online. 2014;29:209–15.
28. Mizrachi Y, Horowitz E, Farhi J, Raziel A, Weissman A. Ovarian stimulation for freeze-all IVF cycles: a systematic review. Hum Reprod Update. 2020;26:118–35.
29. Georgiou EX, Melo P, Brown J, Granne IE. Follicular flushing during oocyte retrieval in assisted reproductive techniques. Cochrane Database Syst Rev. 2018;4:CD004634.
30. Neumann K, Griesinger G. Follicular flushing in patients with poor ovarian response: a systematic review and meta-analysis. Reprod Biomed Online. 2018;36:408–15.
31. Méndez Lozano DH, Fanchin R, Chevalier N, Feyereisen E, Hesters L, Frydman N, Frydman R. The follicular flushing duplicate the pregnancy rate on semi natural cycle IVF. J Gynecol Obstet Biol Reprod (Paris). 2007;36:36–41.
32. von Wolff M, Hua YZ, Santi A, Ocon E, Weiss B. Follicle flushing in monofollicular in vitro fertilization almost doubles the number of transferable embryos. Acta Obstet Gynecol Scand. 2013;92:346–8.
33. Kohl Schwartz AS, Calzaferri I, Roumet M, Limacher A, Fink A, Wueest A, Weidlinger S, Mitter VR, Leeners B, Von Wolff M. Follicular flushing leads to higher oocyte yield in monofollicular IVF: a randomized controlled trial. Hum Reprod. 2020;35:2253–61.
34. van der Linden M, Buckingham K, Farquhar C, Kremer JA, Metwally M. Luteal phase support for assisted reproduction cycles. Cochrane Database Syst Rev. 2015;2015:CD009154.
35. von Wolff M, Kohl Schwartz A, Stute P, Fäh M, Otti G, Schürch R, Rohner S. Follicular flushing in natural cycle IVF does not affect the luteal phase—a prospective controlled study. Reprod Biomed Online. 2017;35:37–41.
36. Domar AD, Rooney K, Hacker MR, Sakkas D, Dodge LE. Burden of care is the primary reason why insured women terminate in vitro fertilization treatment. Fertil Steril. 2018;109:1121–6.
37. Haemmerli Keller K, Alder G, Loewer L, Faeh M, Rohner S, von Wolff M. Treatment-related psychological stress in different in vitro fertilization therapies with and without gonadotropin stimulation. Acta Obstet Gynecol Scand. 2018;97:269–76.
38. Heape W. Preliminary note of the transplantation and growth of mammalian ova within a uterine foster-mother. Proc R Soc Lond. 1891;48:457–9.
39. Edwards RG, Steptoe PC, Purdy JM. Fertilization and cleavage in vitro of preovulator human oocytes. Nature. 1970;227:1307–9.
40. Zhang J, Liu H, Luo S, Lu Z, Chávez-Badiola A, Liu Z, Yang M, Merhi Z, Silber SJ, Munné S, Konstantinidis M, Wells D, Tang JJ, Huang T. Live birth derived from oocyte spindle transfer to prevent mitochondrial disease. Reprod Biomed Online. 2017;34:361–8.

Part II
Physiology

Chapter 5
Folliculogenesis

Michael von Wolff

5.1 Background

In natural cycles, folliculogenesis is regulated by a finely tuned system consisting of the hypothalamic-pituitary-ovarian hormone axis, the pulsatile secretion of these hormones, and the expression pattern of hormone receptors. This system usually leads to the formation of a mature follicle (Fig. 5.1). Ovulation is initiated by the release of luteinizing hormone (LH) from the pituitary gland, triggered by estradiol (E2) concentrations which are high enough to allow the oocyte to mature and the endometrium to proliferate sufficiently.

In conventional gonadotropin stimulated IVF (cIVF), endogenous gonadotropins from the pituitary gland are suppressed by high concentrations of E2 and by the administration of GnRH analogues and are replaced by constantly high doses of exogenous gonadotropins. This makes it possible to break through the natural regulatory mechanisms that are supposed to prevent a polyfollicular ovarian response. However, in cIVF the hormone profile is different, which has an impact on folliculogenesis, follicular steroidogenesis, and thus on the function of the follicles and oocytes.

M. von Wolff (✉)
Division of Gynecological Endocrinology and Reproductive Medicine,
University Women's Hospital, University of Bern, Bern, Switzerland
e-mail: Michael.vonwolff@insel.ch

© The Author(s), under exclusive license to Springer Nature Switzerland AG 2022
M. von Wolff (ed.), *Natural Cycle and Minimal Stimulation IVF*,
https://doi.org/10.1007/978-3-030-97571-5_5

Fig. 5.1 Initiation of
folliculogenesis by the
hypothalamus and the
pituitary gland (Reprinted
with permission from
Michael von Wolff and
Florian Lenz)

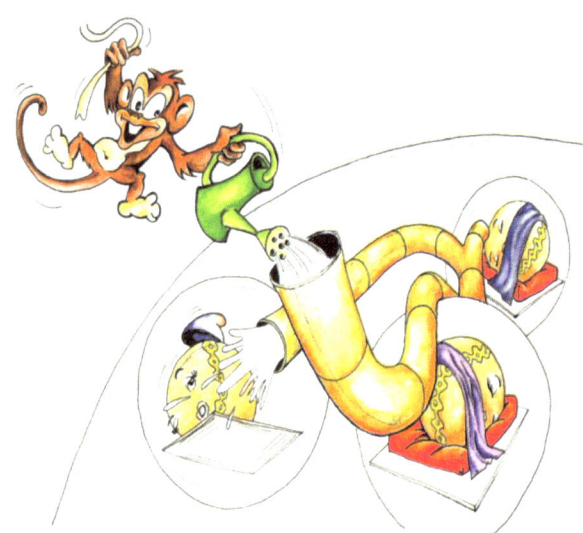

Fig. 5.1 Initiation of folliculogenesis by the hypothalamus and the pituitary gland (Reprinted with permission from Michael von Wolff and Florian Lenz)

5.2   Preantral Folliculogenesis

Primordial follicles develop into primary and then into secondary follicles, which all are defined preantral follicles, with a maximum diameter of 0.1–0.2 mm (reviewed by [1–3]). Secondary follicles consist of several layers of granulosa cells, which are surrounded by a basal lamina. The basal lamina is surrounded by theca cells. Theca cells differentiate into the theca interna and externa cell layer, which synthesize androgens. The theca cell layer becomes increasingly vascularized as the follicle develops, while the granulosa cell layer remains avascular.

Oocyte development is supported by the granulosa cells. However, the oocyte also has a critical role in regulating follicular growth by controlling proliferation and differentiation of granulosa and theca cells [1].

Growth of preantral follicles is gonadotropin independent. It is controlled by bidirectional communication between the oocyte and the surrounding follicular cells. Many of the signalling molecules involved in this dialogue belong to the transforming growth factor β (TGF-β) superfamily. Among these, growth and differentiation factor (GDF) has a central role in the dialogue between the oocyte and the surrounding follicular cells. In GDF9-null mice, folliculogenesis is blocked at the primary stage. GDF9 originating from the oocyte is also responsible for the theca cell differentiation.

Growth of preantral follicles growth is not only controlled by paracrine signalling but also by direct cell-to-cell communication via gap junctions, as evident from mice with deficiencies of connexin43 (CX43) and connexin37 (CX37), two of the core proteins that form the gap junctions in the ovary. In CX43-deficient mice, follicles fail to develop beyond the primary stage [4], whereas CX37-deficient mice fail to develop mature (Graafian) follicles [5].

To control recruitment and growth of preantral follicles, granulosa cells of primary, secondary, preantral, and early antral follicles produce anti-mullerian hormone (AMH). AMH inhibits primordial follicle growth and also decreases (in mice) the sensitivity of follicles to FSH, thereby inhibiting FSH-induced antral follicle growth.

5.3   Antral Folliculogenesis

Late preantral follicles (secondary follicles) develop into early antral (tertiary follicles) with a diameter of at least 0.2–0.4 mm. Gonadotropins such as follicle stimulating hormone (FSH) and luteinizing hormone (LH) stimulate the follicles which form a fluid-filled cavity, the antrum, which separates the granulosa cells into two functional cell types, the mural granulosa cells, adjacent to the basal lamina, which are responsible for steroidogenesis, and the cumulus cells, adjacent to the oocyte [1]. The final stage of the antral follicles is the pre-ovulatory follicle (Graafian follicle).

Around menstruation, a cohort of several follicles grow under the influence of FSH. The largest (dominant) follicle possesses several characteristics to support its growth and to inhibit the growth of the still smaller, so-called subordinate follicles. If it reaches a diameter of 10–12 mm, its granulosa cells produce large amounts of inhibin B (Fig. 5.2) which inhibits pituitary FSH secretion. The dominant follicle is able to further grow in a declining FSH environment, while the subordinate follicles are not.

The dominant follicle contains more granulosa cells and a higher level of FSH receptors compared to the subordinate follicles. It produces more estrogen and thereby mediates the effect of FSH on the expression of LH receptors on its granulosa cells. While subordinate follicles only have LH receptors in theca cells, the dominant follicle becomes less dependent on FSH and acquires further responsiveness to LH by expressing LH receptors in its granulosa cells. It is thereby more effective in eliciting its negative feedback on FSH production, which results in reduced circulation of FSH. Subordinate follicles are more sensitive to FSH decrease which result in the induction of death receptors initiating apoptosis.

The dominant follicle steadily grows until ovulation. Helmer et al. (2022) [7] analyzed the dynamics of follicular growth in 290 women undergoing 606 natural cycle IVF treatments within the last 5 days before follicle aspiration. They found a daily increase of (dominant) follicle size by 1.04 ± 0.64 mm (Fig. 5.3).

Bacrwald et al. (2009) [8] also analyzed the dynamic of follicular growth in 50 ovulatory women, beginning on the day of ultrasonographic detection of the follicles until the day of maximum follicle size. They found a daily increase of (dominant) follicle size by 1.48 ± 0.1 mm.

Based on these two studies, the daily increase of follicle size can expected to be around 1–1.5 mm. This is in line with the following calculation: Assuming that the size of the leading follicle is around 10 mm in the mid follicular phase on cycle day

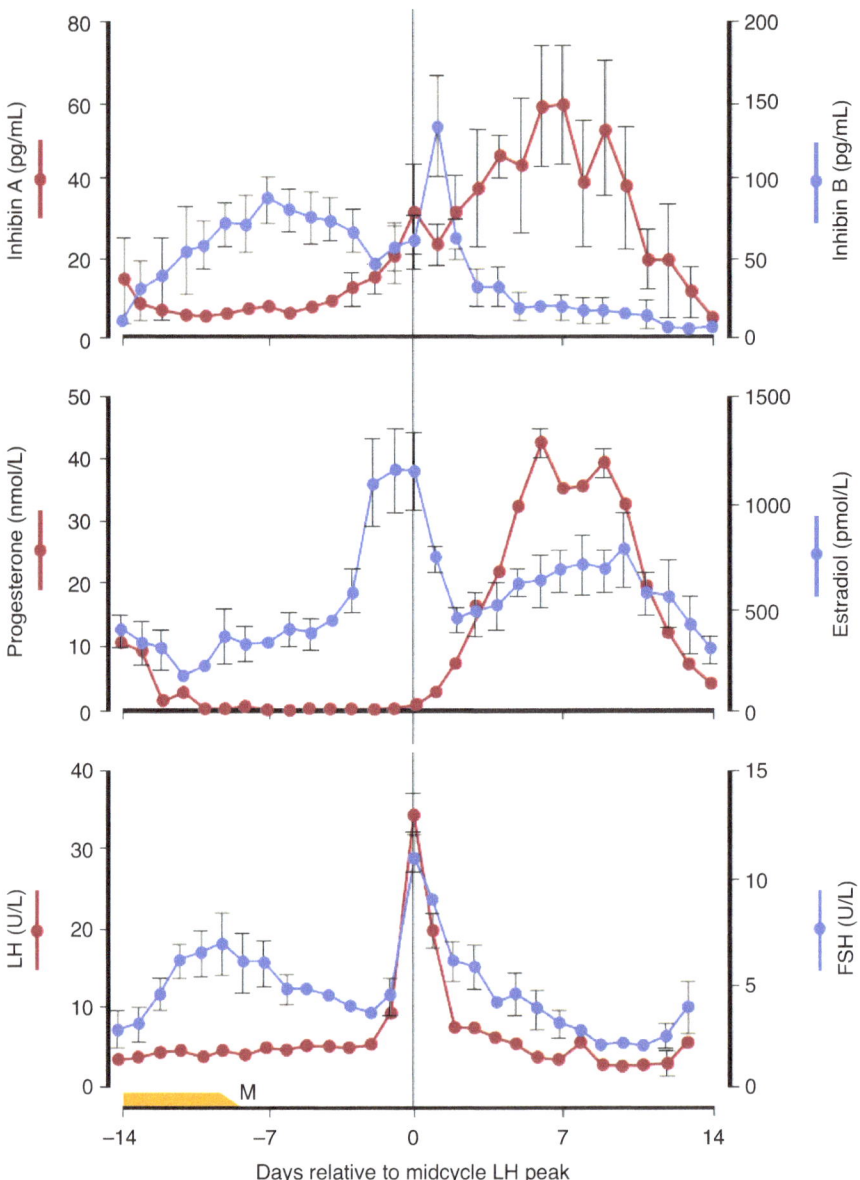

Fig. 5.2 Plasma concentrations of 6 women with daily blood tests during the cycle. Data were aligned with respect to the day of the midcycle LH peak. Mean concentrations are shown ±2 standard errors [6]

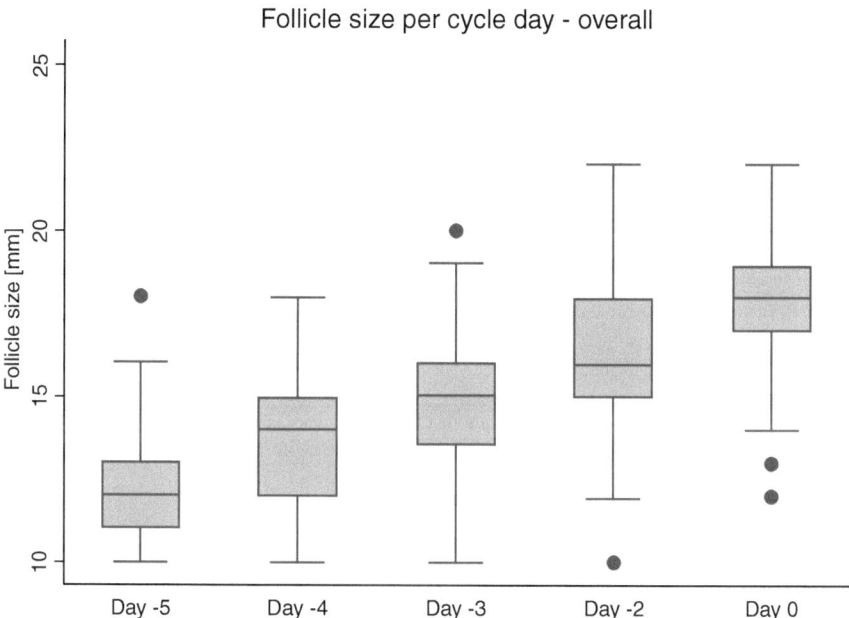

Fig. 5.3 Follicle size per cycle day in natural cycles within the 5 days before follicle aspiration (Day 0 = day of follicle aspiration) (according to [7])

7 and assuming that the follicle ovulates with a diameter of around 20 mm on cycle 14, an average increase of follicle diameter of 1.4 mm per day would be expected.

Helmer et al. (2022) [7] also analyzed the dynamics of E2 increase within the last 3 days before HCG triggering to induce ovulation. They found an increase of E2 concentration by 167.3 ± 76.8 pmol/L per day (Fig. 5.4).

Furthermore, they evaluated in natural cycles if follicle size and E2 concentrations are associated with the maturity (metaphase II) of the oocyte [7]. They found that maturity of oocytes is associated with follicle size (aOR 1.24, 95% CI: 1.01–1.53; $p = 0.037$) and even more with E2 concentration (aOR 1.84, 95% CI: 1.15–2.94; $p = 0.010$). Accordingly, high E2 concentration seems to better reflect the chance to retrive metaphase II oocytes than the size of the follicle.

Overall, a follicle size of ≥ 18 mm seems to be ideal for follicle aspiration (Fig. 5.5). Live birth rate in natural cycle IVF with follicles sized 18–22 mm was 8.5–12.5% and in follicles sized 14–17 mm only 2.2–3.5% per initiated cycle [7].

Interestingly, these findings in natural cycles are similar to gonadotropin stimulated cycles. Dubey et al. (1995) [9] found in gonadotropin stimulated cycles a fertilization rate of 57.9% in oocytes retrieved from follicles sized 10–14 mm, of 69.8% in oocytes from follicles sized 16–20 mm, and 73.9% in oocytes retrieved from follicles sized 22–26 mm. The fertilization rates were significantly higher in follicles ≥ 16 mm compared to follicles ≤ 14 mm. Wirtleitner et al., 2018 [10] compared follicles sized ≥ 24 mm versus 13–23 mm in gonadotropin stimulated cycles.

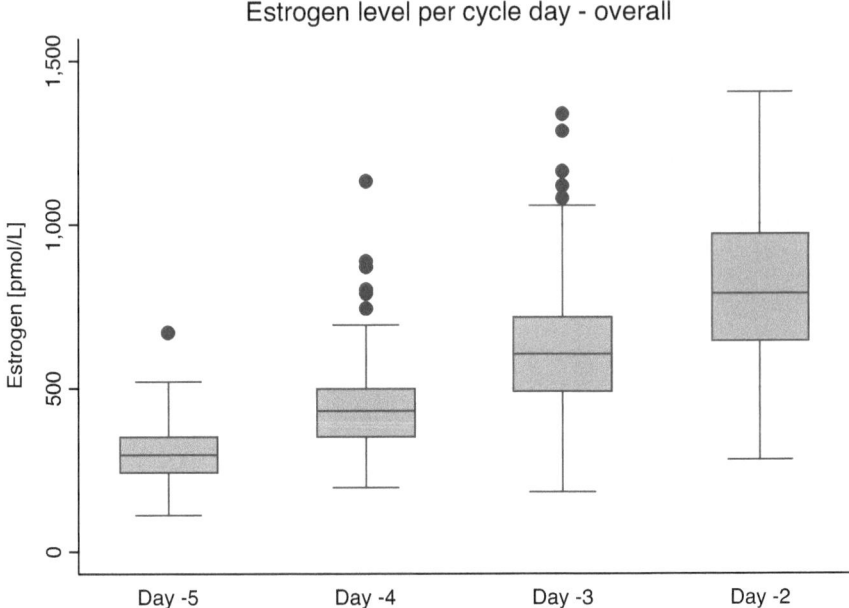

Fig. 5.4 Estrogen (Estradiol) level per cycle day in natural cycles within the 3 days before HCG triggering to induce ovulation (Day-2 = day of HCG triggering) (according to [7])

The oocyte retrieval rate was 81.3% vs. 76.6%, the proportion of metaphase II oocytes per retrieved oocytes was 70.1% vs. 64.0%, and the zygote development rate per metaphase II oocyte was 81.4% vs. 75.3%. However, the differences were not significant. Other parameters such as blastocyst development and implantation rates were not increased for oocytes retrieved from larger follicles.

5.4 Follicular Steroidogenesis

Theca cells are capable of de novo production of androgens from cholesterol. Androgen biosynthesis is modulated in preantral and small antral follicles, granulosa cells modulate androgen synthesis by inhibitory factors such as activin and theca cells by TGF-α and TGF-β [1, 11].

Once the late preantral (secondary follicle) stage is reached, theca cells express LH receptors and androgen biosynthesis is also regulated by LH. LH controls the key enzymes of the synthesis [11], namely StAR (transporter of cholesterol to the inner mitochondrial membrane), CYP11A1 (which converts cholesterol to pregnenolone), CYP17A1 (which converts pregnenolone to dehydroepiandrosterone, DHEA), and 3β-hydroxysteroid dehydrogenase (3β-HSD) (which converts DHEA to androstenedione) (Fig. 5.6).

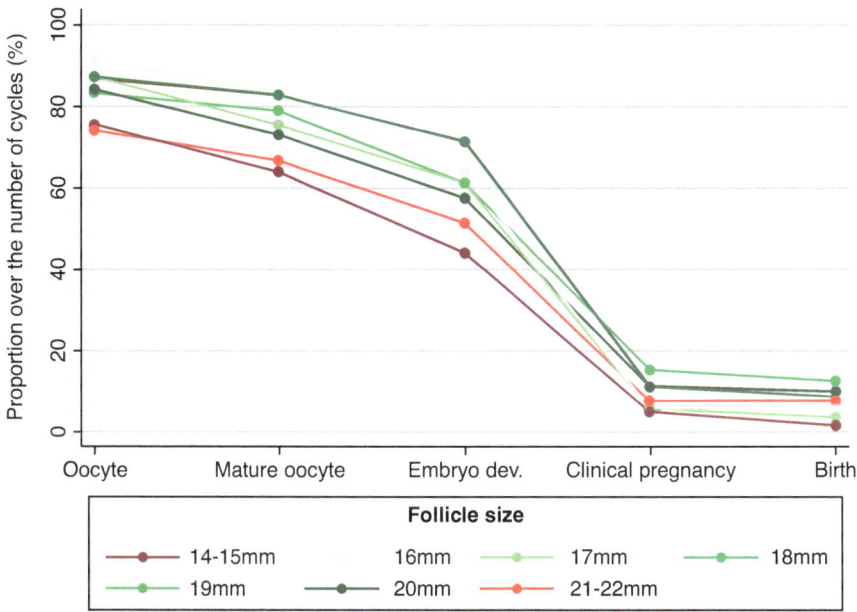

Fig. 5.5 Association of follicle size with outcome parameters such as oocyte collection rate (Oocyte), maturity (metaphase II) of oocytes (Mature oocyte), embryo development rate (Embryo dev.), clinical pregnancy (Clinical pregnancy) and live birth rate (Birth) (according to [7])

Theca cell androgens are transported through the basal lamina into granulosa cells. Under the regulation of FSH, androstenedione and testosterone are converted to estradiol by CYP19A1 (aromatase) and 17β-hydroxysteroid dehydrogenase (17β-HSD).

Granulosa cells also respond to FSH by producing pregnenolone from cholesterol which contributes to the theca cell androgen production.

5.5   Endocrinology of Naturally Matured Follicles Compared to Stimulated Follicles

Ever since gonadotropins were introduced into IVF treatment, it has been discussed whether they have an effect on oocyte quality and which gonadotropin preparations or stimulation regimens are more advantageous.

However, the follicular physiology and endocrinology in naturally matured follicles (as found in natural cycle IVF, NC-IVF) compared to stimulated follicles (as found in gonadotropin stimulated conventional IVF, cIVF) have been poorly studied.

Kollmann et al. 2017 [12] demonstrated that concentrations of immune cells and cytokines are different in follicles from natural cycles and gonadotropin stimulated cycles. Follicular fluid from NC-IVF follicles contain proportionally less CD45+

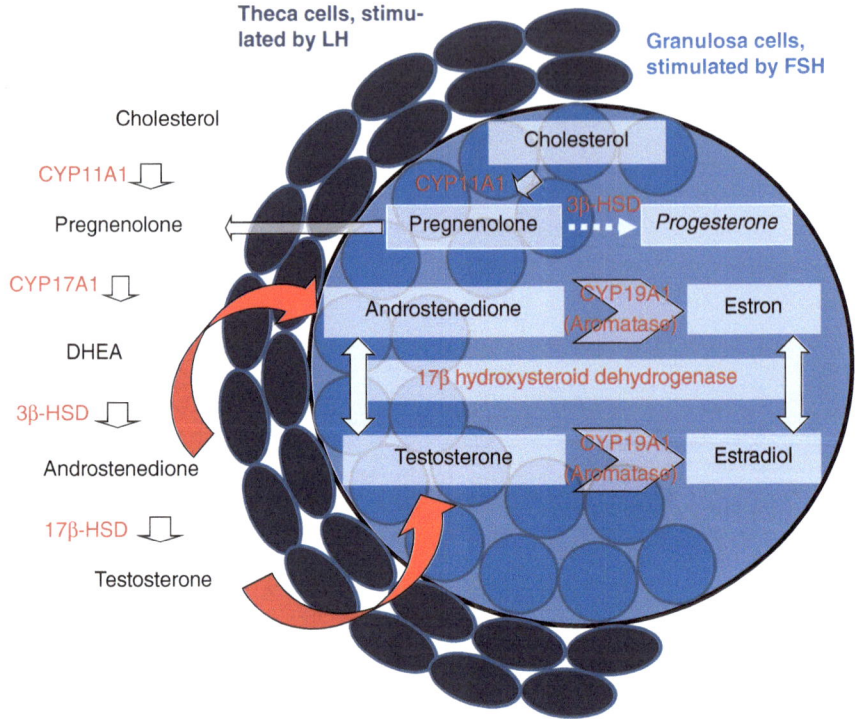

Fig. 5.6 LH driven androgen synthesis in theca cells, FSH driven estrogen production in granulosa cells, and theca and granulosa cell cooperation in estrogen synthesis

leukocytes but more CD8+ cytotoxic T cells than follicular fluid from cIVF. NC-IVF follicles also contain lower levels of vascular endothelial growth factor (VEGF) concentrations and marginally increased concentrations of Interleukin 8.

Furthermore, several follicular hormone concentrations such as LH, testosterone (T), E2 and AMH were significantly reduced in cIVF follicles (Fig. 5.7). Von Wolff et al. [13] drew the conclusion that the suppressed LH release in cIVF, due to the use of GnRH analogues, initiates a cascade of endocrine dysregulations, including follicular androgens, E2, and AMH (Fig. 5.7).

Suppressed LH concentrations in cIVF result in reduced testosterone and E2 concentration and, possibly based on this, also in reduced follicular AMH concentration.

The dysregulation of the follicular endocrine milieu in cIVF follicles is further supported by a recent study by von Wolff et al. [14], in which the association of follicular fluid hormones with RNA in cumulus oophorus complex (COC) cells was studied. In naturally matured (NC-IVF) follicles, they found a significant correlation of follicular fluid hormones with RNA concentration in COC cells. In contrast, in gonadotropin stimulated follicles (cIVF), the hormone and RNA concentrations

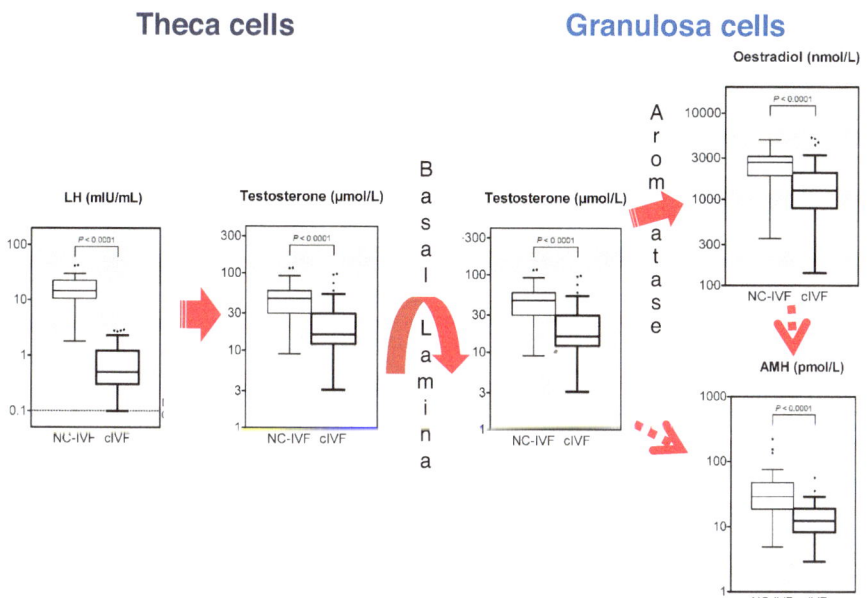

Fig. 5.7 Tukey Box and Whisker plot of hormones in follicular fluid in naturally matured follicles (NC-IVF) and conventional gonadotropin stimulated follicles (cIVF) during the process of steroidogenesis in theca and granulosa cells (adapted from [13, 14])

were not correlated, further supporting the concept of dysfunctional follicular hormone synthesis due to exogenous gonadotropin stimulation (Fig. 5.8).

The dysfunctional endocrine system might be clinically relevant as AMH, which is part of the follicular endocrine milieu is a marker for the implantation potential of oocytes in unstimulated [15] and stimulated IVF [16]. Furthermore, E2 which is part of the steroidogenesis in granulosa cells also seems to be a marker for the oocyte competence, as E2 is correlated with the embryo score in naturally matured (NC-IVF) follicles [15]. If, however, the function of granulosa cells, which produces AMH and E2, is altered by high dose gonadotropin stimulation as in cIVF, these alterations might have an impact on follicular and thereby on oocyte function and quality (Fig. 5.9).

This theory has been supported by recent clinical data which have demonstrated that the potential of the embryos to implant and the live birth rates per transferred embryo are around 1.4-fold higher in NC-IVF than in cIVF. In parous women ($n = 66$) the difference was even more pronounced in which adjusted live birth rates were 2.35-fold higher in NC-IVF (see Chap. 7, Fig. 7.2, Table 7.3).

Gonadotropin stimulation also seems to lead to premature increase of progesterone in around 35% (5–35%) of gonadotropin stimulated cycles [17]. Patients with progesterone concentrations >1.5 ng/mL (>4.8 pmol/L) on the day of the HCG application to trigger ovulation have a lower pregnancy rate (19.1% versus 31.0% in patients with lower progesterone concentration, $p = 0.00006$) [17]. It is speculated

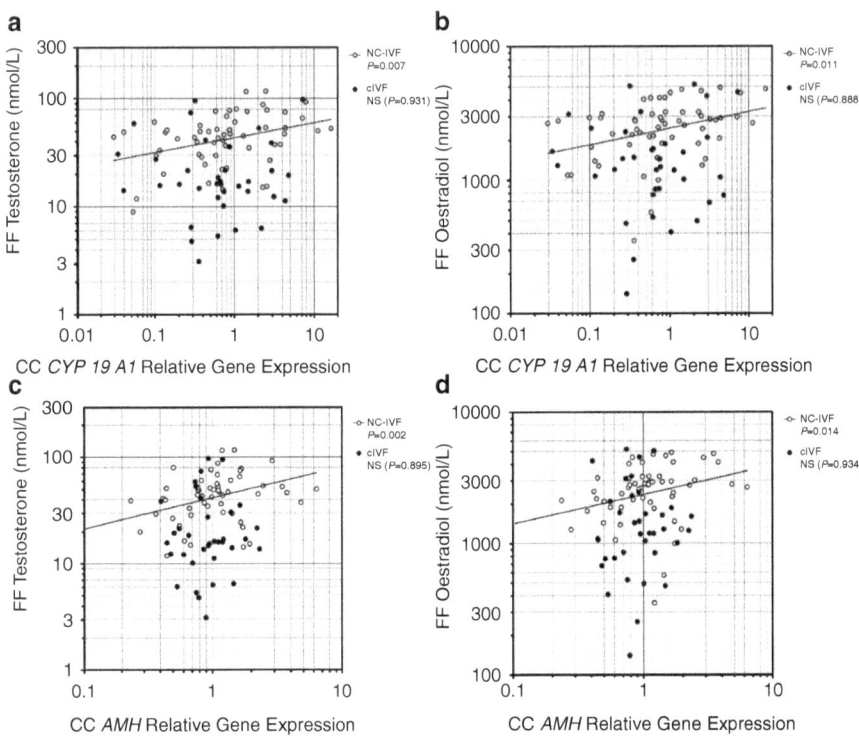

Fig. 5.8 Associations of several follicular hormones (analyzed by immunoassays) with cumulus cell (CC) RNA concentrations (analyzed by RT-PCR) in naturally matured follicles (NC-IVF) and conventional gonadotropin stimulated follicles (cIVF). (**a**) Follicular fluid (FF) Testosterone vs. CC *CYP 19A1* RNA; (**b**) FF Oestradiol vs. CC *CYP 19A1* RNA; (**c**): FF Testosterone vs. CC *AMH* RNA; (**d**) FF Oestradiol vs. *AMH* RNA). Only statistically significant regression lines are shown in the graphs (adapted from [14])

that this effect is due to high FSH concentrations, which stimulate the conversion of cholesterol to pregnenolone in granulosa cells (Fig. 5.6). Pregnenolone is converted to progesterone (Fig. 5.6), especially as the steroidogenesis in theca cells in slowed down due to decreased LH concentration caused by GnRH analogues (Fig. 5.7), which cause a dysbalance of increased FSH action and decreased LH action.

5.6   Dysfunction of Folliculogenesis—Ovarian Cysts

In normal menstrual cycles, follicles grow up to a diameter of around 18–20 mm. The follicles secrete E2 which triggers the LH surge at a concentration of around 800pmol/l (see Chap. 6). The follicle ovulates around cycle day 14–17 and forms the luteal body. The luteal body dissolves due to decreasing LH concentrations and menstruation starts around 12–13 days after ovulation (see Chap. 8).

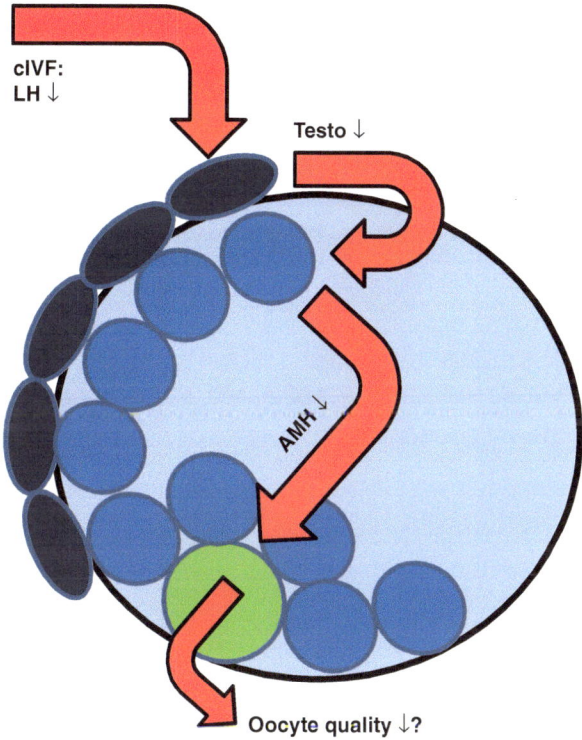

cIVF:
LH ↓

Testo ↓

AMH ↓

Oocyte quality ↓?

Fig. 5.9 Model of pathophysiology of follicular endocrinology in high dose gonadotropin stimulated conventional IVF (cIVF)

However, sometimes a cystic formation is found a few days before the expected ovulation. The cystic formation appears sonographically as a follicle but E2 concentration is lower than expected. The question arises if the cystic formation is a follicle or rather a cyst which should not be aspirated.

Figure 5.10 shows the development of follicles and their regulation leading to a follicle or a cyst. The diagram demonstrates that cysts might by of different origin.

The cyst might be a follicle which has become dysfunctional, forming a follicular cyst (cyst lining composed of granulosa cells and theca cells). In follicular cysts, FSH and LH receptor concentration in granulosa cells is reduced [19], leading to lower estrogen secretion and an unresponsiveness of follicular cells to LH surge.

The cyst might also be a persistent corpus luteum cyst (cyst lining composed of luteinized granulosa cells and theca cells) possibly due to high basal LH concentration as in women treated with high dosages of clomiphene citrate. Clomiphene citrate has a long biological half-life, leading to increased LH concentrations in the luteal phase (see Chap. 11).

It is hardly possible to differentiate between these different cysts by ultrasound examination. Analysis of hormone concentration can be helpful as follicular cysts

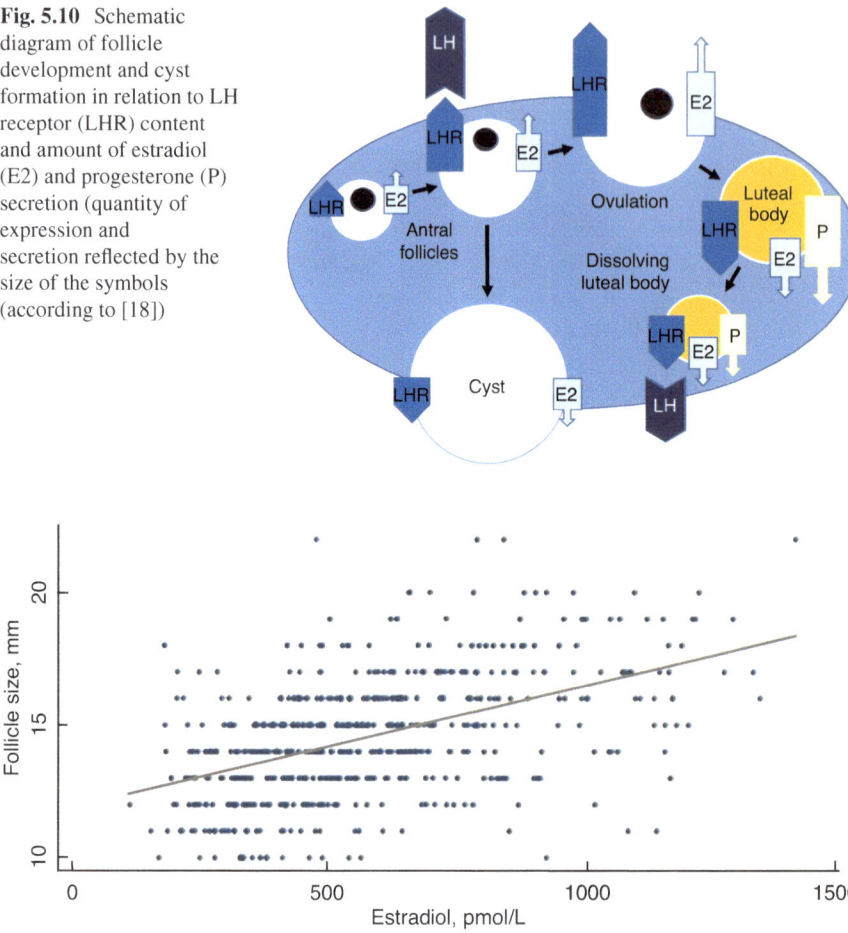

Fig. 5.10 Schematic diagram of follicle development and cyst formation in relation to LH receptor (LHR) content and amount of estradiol (E2) and progesterone (P) secretion (quantity of expression and secretion reflected by the size of the symbols (according to [18])

Fig. 5.11 Association between follicle size and estradiol concentration and fitted values in women undergoing natural cycle IVF (Infertility center Bern, Switzerland)

produce E2, corpus luteum cysts produce progesterone but some cysts do not produce any steroid hormones.

In clinical practice, any cyst formation with E2 serum concentration which is lower than expected in relation to its size or which produces low amounts of progesterone should not be aspirated as the chance to collect an oocyte is almost zero.

However, it needs to be noted that the association of follicle size and E2 concentration is not high. Figure 5.11 demonstrates this association in women undergoing NC-IVF. Follicle size is statistically associated with E2 concentration after adjustment for age, cause of infertility, and previous embryo transfers without pregnancy (Coefficient: 0.47; 95% CI: 0.40–0.54). An increase of follicle size of 0.47 mm is associated with an E2 increase of 100 pmol/L (27.3 ng/mL). However, even though the association is statistically strong, the scatter diagram demonstrates the great variability between follicle size and E2 concentration. This is probably due to some degree of inaccuracy in the calculation of follicle diameter due to the often ellipsoid shape of the follicle. It might also be due to the additional growth of a second E2 producing follicle and due to individual differences. Therefore, it is advisable to start NC-IVF treatment with a diagnostic cycle to learn about the individual association of follicle size and E2 concentration as well as the level at which the LH surge starts.

If cysts are repeatedly be detected, it might be advisable to perform the first sonographic assessment around menstruation. If a cyst is detected, E2 and progesterone concentrations are analyzed. The IVF treatment cycle can be started if E2 and progesterone concentrations are low.

5.7 Dysfunction of Folliculogenesis—LOOP (Luteal Out-of-Phase) Syndrome

If ovarian reserve is very low, FSH blood concentrations tend to be slightly increased to stimulate follicular growth. As a result, follicular growth can already start prematurely in the luteal phase. As a result, the follicle is already very large in the early follicular phase, whereas the endometrium is still thin. This desynchronization of follicular and endometrial growth can lead to decreased pregnancy rates.

The prevalence of the so-called LOOP syndrome is 20–37% of the ovulatory cycles in women in their menopausal transition [20] (around 40–49 years of age [21]).

In case of frequent LOOPs, treatment options are inhibition of follicular growth in the luteal phase.

One option is to give a combined oral contraceptive pill (i.e., 30 µg ethinyl estradiol plus levenorgestrel) for around 10–20 days to inhibit follicular growth. However, this option is associated with an increased risk of thrombosis and every second cycle is lost.

Another option is to add transdermal estradiol in the luteal phase (i.e. estradiol patches a 50–100 µg per day) to suppress premature FSH increase.

It should be noted that these options have not been proven in clinical studies.

References

1. Edson MA, Nagaraja AK, Matzuk MM. The mammalian ovary from genesis to revelation. Endocr Rev. 2009;30:624–712.
2. Rimon-Dahari N, Yerushalmi-Heinemann L, Alyagor L, Dekel N. Ovarian folliculogenesis. Results Probl Cell Differ. 2016;58:167–90.
3. Holesh JE, Bass AN, Lord M. Physiology, ovulation. In: StatPearls [Internet]. Treasure Island, FL: StatPearls Publishing; 2020.

4. Ackert CL, Gittens JE, O'Brien MJ, Eppig JJ, Kidder GM. Intercellular communication via connexin43 gap junctions is required for ovarian folliculogenesis in the mouse. Dev Biol. 2001;233:258–70.
5. Simon AM, Goodenough DA, Li E, Paul DL. Female infertility in mice lacking connexin 37. Nature. 1997;385:525–9.
6. Groome NP, Illingworth PJ, O'Brien M, Pai R, Rodger FE, Mather JP, McNeilly AS. Measurement of dimeric inhibin B throughout the human menstrual cycle. J Clin Endocrinol Metab. 1996;81:1401–5.
7. Helmer A, Magaton IM, Stalder O, Surbek D, Stute P, von Wolff M. Otimal timing of ovulation triggering to achieve highest success rates in natural cycles - an analysis based on follicle size and estradiol concentration in natural cycle IVF. Front Endocrinol. 2022, May 26.
8. Baerwald AR, Walker RA, Pierson RA. Growth rates of ovarian follicles during natural menstrual cycles, oral contraception cycles, and ovarian stimulation cycles. Fertil Steril. 2009;91:440–9.
9. Dubey AK, Wang HA, Duffy P, Penzias AS. The correlation between follicular measurements, oocyte morphology, and fertilization rates in an in vitro fertilization program. Fertil Steril. 1995;64:787–90.
10. Wirleitner B, Okhowat J, Vištejnová L, Králíčková M, Karlíková M, Vanderzwalmen P, Ectors F, Hradecký L, Schuff M, Murtinger M. Relationship between follicular volume and oocyte competence, blastocyst development and live-birth rate: optimal follicle size for oocyte retrieval. Ultrasound Obstet Gynecol. 2018;51:118–25.
11. Magoffin DA. Ovarian theca cell. Int J Biochem Cell Biol. 2005;37:1344–9.
12. Kollmann Z, Schneider S, Fux M, Bersinger NA, von Wolff M. Gonadotrophin stimulation in IVF alters the immune cell profile in follicular fluid and the cytokine concentrations in follicular fluid and serum. Hum Reprod. 2017;32:820–31.
13. von Wolff M, Kollmann Z, Flück CE, Stute P, Marti U, Weiss B, Bersinger NA. Gonadotrophin stimulation for in vitro fertilization significantly alters the hormone milieu in follicular fluid: a comparative study between natural cycle IVF and conventional IVF. Hum Reprod. 2014;29:1049–57.
14. von Wolff M, Eisenhut M, Stute P, Bersinger NA. Gonadotropin stimulation in In vitro Fertilisation (IVF) reduces follicular fluid hormone levels and disrupts their quantitative association with cumulus cell mRNA. Reprod Biomed Online. 2022;44:193–9.
15. von Wolff M, Mitter VR, Jamir N, Stute P, Eisenhut M, Bersinger NA. The endocrine milieu in naturally matured follicles is different in women with high serum anti-Müllerian hormone concentrations. Reprod Biomed Online. 2021;43:329–37.
16. Ciepiela P, Dulęba AJ, Kario A, Chełstowski K, Branecka-Woźniak D, Kurzawa R. Oocyte matched follicular fluid anti-Müllerian hormone is an excellent predictor of live birth after fresh single embryo transfer. Hum Reprod. 2019;34:2244–53.
17. Bosch E, Labarta E, Crespo J, Simón C, Remohí J, Jenkins J, Pellicer A. Circulating progesterone levels and ongoing pregnancy rates in controlled ovarian stimulation cycles for in vitro fertilization: analysis of over 4000 cycles. Hum Reprod. 2010;25:2092–100.
18. Kawate N. Studies on the regulation of expression of luteinizing hormone receptor in the ovary and the mechanism of follicular cyst formation in ruminants. J Reprod Dev. 2004;50:1–8.
19. Ortega HH, Marelli BE, Rey F, Amweg AN, Díaz PU, Stangaferro ML, Salvetti NR. Molecular aspects of bovine cystic ovarian disease pathogenesis. Reproduction. 2015;149:R251–64.
20. Harlow SD, Gass M, Hall JE, Lobo R, Maki P, Rebar RW, Sherman S, Sluss PM, de Villiers TJ, STRAW + 10 Collaborative Group. Executive summary of the Stages of Reproductive Aging Workshop + 10: addressing the unfinished agenda of staging reproductive aging. J Clin Endocrinol Metab. 2012;97:1159–68.
21. Hale GE, Hughes CL, Burger HG, Robertson DM, Fraser IS. Atypical estradiol secretion and ovulation patterns caused by luteal out-of-phase (LOOP) events underlying irregular ovulatory menstrual cycles in the menopausal transition. Menopause. 2009;16:50–9.

Chapter 6
Ovulation

Michael von Wolff

6.1 Background

Ovulation occurs as a result of positive feedback from rising estrogen concentrations on gonadotropin releasing hormone (GnRH) release from the hypothalamus. GnRH stimulates secretion of luteinizing hormone (LH) which, by binding to its receptor in the follicular theca and granulosa cells, induces a cascade of molecular changes leading to resumption of meiosis, cumulus expansion, and finally to rupture of the follicle (Fig. 6.1). The implementation of natural cycle IVF (NC-IVF) requires an understanding of the endocrinology and physiology of ovulation. This understanding is also necessary to define the optimal time for follicular aspiration (see Chap. 5).

6.2 Regulation of the LH Surge

GnRH neurons release GnRH into the pituitary portal circulation to generate distinct pulses of LH and follicle-stimulating hormone (FSH) throughout the ovarian cycle (Fig. 6.2).

GnRH is released with one pulse generated every 1–1.5 h during the follicular phase of the cycle, and a slower rate of one pulse every 3–4 h in the luteal phase [1, 2]. This release pattern is substantially changed in the late follicular phase, when an abrupt and massive release of GnRH generates a preovulatory LH, and to some extent also a FSH surge, which leads to ovulation.

M. von Wolff (✉)
Division of Gynecological Endocrinology and Reproductive Medicine, University Women's Hospital, University of Bern, Bern, Switzerland
e-mail: Michael.vonwolff@insel.ch

© The Author(s), under exclusive license to Springer Nature Switzerland AG 2022   45
M. von Wolff (ed.), *Natural Cycle and Minimal Stimulation IVF*,
https://doi.org/10.1007/978-3-030-97571-5_6

Fig. 6.1 Ovulation
requires a complex system
of hormones, mediators,
and proteases, which
finally releases the oocyte
into the fallopian tube
(Reprinted with the
permission from Michael
von Wolff and Florian
Lenz)

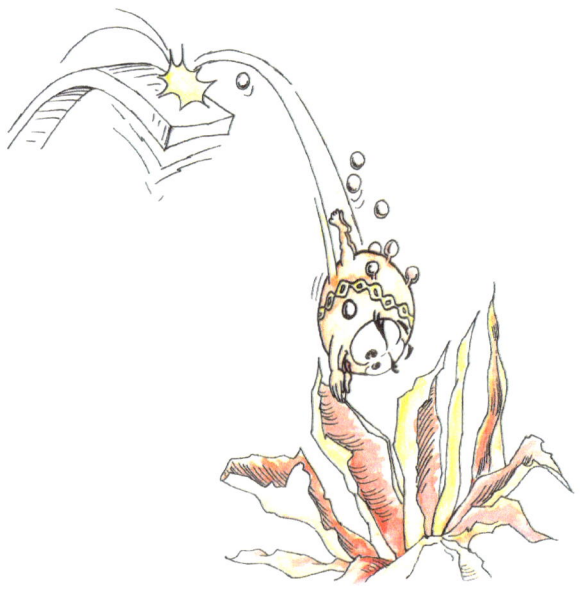

Fig. 6.2 The preoptic area
seems to be a direct target
of ovarian estrogen
positive (green) feedback
and thereby functions as
the central ovulation
regulator

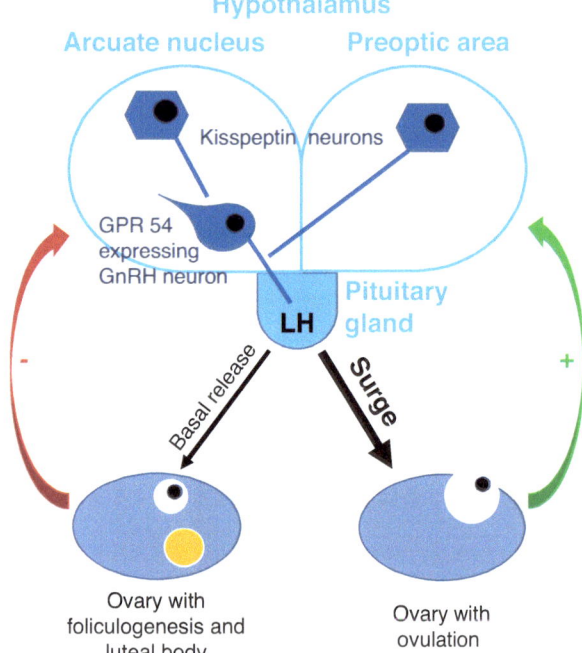

The changes in GnRH/LH/FSH releases result primarily from the modulatory effects of estradiol (E2) and progesterone on the brain and pituitary gland. Depending on its concentration, E2 exerts both negative and positive feedback on the hypothalamus (Fig. 6.2).

The negative estrogen feedback can be observed in the early- and mid-follicular phase, when moderately increased E2 concentrations keep LH concentrations rather low.

Positive estrogen feedback can be observed in the late follicular phase. Due to the gradual rise in E2, the feedback system switches from negative to positive feedback, leading to the LH surge [1, 3]. Apparently, a gradual rise in E2 and a physiological concentrations of E2 seem to be essential for this switch. If E2 concentration rises sharply, as in gonadotropin stimulated IVF with a polyfollicular ovarian response, LH surge is blocked or occurs at E2 levels much higher than in natural cycles.

The regulation of these opposite feedback effects of estrogen is still not fully understood.

They seem to be due to a neural "switch," where different levels of estrogen have opposite effects on LH secretion. This switch seems to be regulated by different kisspeptin releasing neurons. Kisspeptin stimulates the GnRH release from kisspeptin receptor (a gene product of the Kiss 1 receptor gene, also known as GPR 54 gene) expressing GnRH neurons.

The arcuate nucleus of the hypothalamus is a target of estrogen negative feedback and regulates a basal release of LH required for folliculogenesis and to prevent luteolysis. The preoptic area is a target of estrogen positive feedback. The neurons are stimulated by increasing estrogen concentrations, releasing kisspeptin which binds to GnRH neurons, and inducing the release of large amounts of LH to trigger ovulation (according to [4]).

Kisspeptin neurons are located in two hypothalamic regions: the preoptic area of the anterior hypothalamus and the arcuate nucleus of the mediobasal hypothalamus. Kisspeptin expression in the kisspeptin neurons of the arcuate nucleus is negatively regulated, whereas kisspeptin neurons in the preoptic area are positively regulated by estrogen via estrogen receptor α. Therefore, the preoptic area seems to be a direct target of estrogen positive feedback and thereby functions as the central ovulation regulator [4].

Accordingly, Kiss 1 knock out rats never showed puberty onset and estrogen induced LH surge. [5]. Furthermore, GPR 54 gene mutation caused infertility in humans due to hypogonadotropic hypogonadism [6].

6.3 Regulation of Ovulation

Ovulation is regulated by complex signalling pathways, as reviewed by Richards and Ascoli (2018) [7].

Preovulatory follicles contain an oocyte and two phenotypically distinct somatic cells, the mural granulosa cells (lining the follicle) and the cumulus granulosa cells (embedding the oocyte). The gap junctions connecting the cumulus cells and the oocyte contain mostly connexin 37 protein, whereas those connecting the cumulus cells and those between the cumulus and mural cells contain mostly connexin 43 [8].

Theca cells, surrounding the follicle and separated from the granulosa cells by a basal lamina, are in contact with the vasculature and are readily exposed to circulating endocrine stimuli such as LH, whereas the cells inside the basal lamina, the granulosa cells and the oocyte, receive endocrine stimuli with some delay.

The LH/choriogonadotropin (LHCG) receptor is expressed in theca and mural granulosa cells and, according to von Wolff et al. [9], also in mature preovulatory cumulus granulosa cells. The LHCG receptor present in mural granulosa cells is responsible for generating the signals which trigger the paracrine and autocrine pathways that lead to ovulation.

Ovulation can be divided into three steps: resumption of meiosis, expansion of cumulus cells, and finally rupture of the follicle.

6.3.1 Resumption of Meiosis

The meiosis is initiated in the 12th to 16th week of the pregnancy before birth. It is arrested in the diplotän stage of the meiotic prophase I. The four chromatids are formed, a crossing over takes place but the spindle is not yet formed. High concentrations of cyclic adenosine monophosphate, cAMP, keep it arrested. The high concentration is due to a high rate of cAMP synthesis and a low rate of cAMP degradation. Activation of the LHCG receptor (= LH surge) leads to reduction of cAMP and thereby to resumption of the meiosis.

Synthesis of cAMP is stimulated in mice by activation of the G-protein coupled receptor 3 (GPR3), which is located on the membrane of the oocyte. Accordingly, GPR3-null mice which have low cAMP concentrations undergo meiosis even without activation of LHCG receptor (= LH surge) as cAMP concentration is too low to keep meiosis arrested [10].

Degradation of cAMP is inhibited by high concentration of cyclic guanosine monophosphate, cGMP, which is produced in granulosa cells and is transported into the oocyte through gap junctions (Connexin 37) connecting the cumulus cells and the oocyte. cGMP inhibits in the oocyte phosphodiesterase 3A, PDE3A, which catalyzes cAMP degradation in the oocyte. Therefore, high levels of cGMP concentration keep cAMP concentration high. Accordingly, PDE3A null mice ovulate with meiotically arrested oocytes as meiosis cannot resume due to high (non-degraded) cAMP concentration [11].

If the dominant follicle reaches a diameter of around 12 mm, FSH induces the expression of LHCG receptor in granulosa cells. This allows the dominant follicle to further grow, despite falling FSH concentrations induced by inhibin B which is released from the dominant follicle and inhibits pituitary FSH release (see Chap. 5). It also prepares the follicle to respond to the LH surge.

When the LH surge occurs, LH bind to the LHCG receptor of granulosa cells which leads to a decrease of cGMP concentration in granulosa cells. cGMP concentration also decreases in the oocyte (through connexin gap junctions) and thereby PDEA3 is activated in the oocyte. Activated PDEA3 catalyzes cAMP degradation and concentration of cAMP drops in the oocyte. As a result cAMP concentration is too low to keep the meiosis arrested and the meiosis resumes.

6.3.2   Cumulus Expansion

During meiotic maturation of the oocyte, cumulus cells change their morphology and metabolic activity resulting morphologically in expansion of the cumulus cells.

Cumulus expansion is based on increased concentration of glycosaminoglycan in the extracellular space, where it plays a role as the structural component of expanded cumuli as well as signal molecule regulating oocyte maturation.

Therefore, expansion of the cumulus oocyte complex is necessary for meiotic maturation and for acquiring developmental competence.

In vitro experiments show that cumulus expansion involves the LHCGR-promoted increase of prostaglandin-endoperoxide synthase 2, Ptgs2, in cumulus cells which increases the synthesis of prostaglandins such as prostaglandin E2 (PGE2) [12].

Cumulus expansion can therefore be restored by adding PGE2 to follicles of Ptgs2-null mice [13].

6.3.3   Rupture of the Follicle

The rupture of the ovulating follicle requires induction and activation of the progesterone receptor, Pgr, in mural granulosa cells [14, 15].

Pgr expression is low or absent in mural granulosa cells of preovulatory follicles but increases several hours before ovulation on activation of the LHCG receptor [16].

The activated Pgr mediates the enhanced expression of a number of LHCG receptor-inducible ovarian genes including endothelin 2. Endothelin 2 encodes proteases [14, 17], which leads to the rupture of the follicle.

Accordingly, Pgr null mice are anovulatory due to the lack of proteases and thereby lack of follicular rupture. Furthermore, ovulation in Pgr wild type mice can be prevented with ulipristal, a selective progesterone receptor modulator that acts as an antagonist of the ovarian progesterone receptor [15].

6.4   Inflammatory Mediators in Ovulation

Activation of LHCGR by the LH surge initiates a cascade of mediators which resemble an inflammatory response (Fig. 6.3).

Fig. 6.3 Activation of LH/
choriogonadotropin receptor
(LHCGR), which is expressed
in theca cells and mural
granulosa cells, initiates a
cascade of mediators such as
prostaglandins (PG),
cytokines, and matrix
metalloproteases (MMP)
which resemble an
inflammatory response. As a
result, the cumulus oophorus
complex detaches and the
follicle ruptures

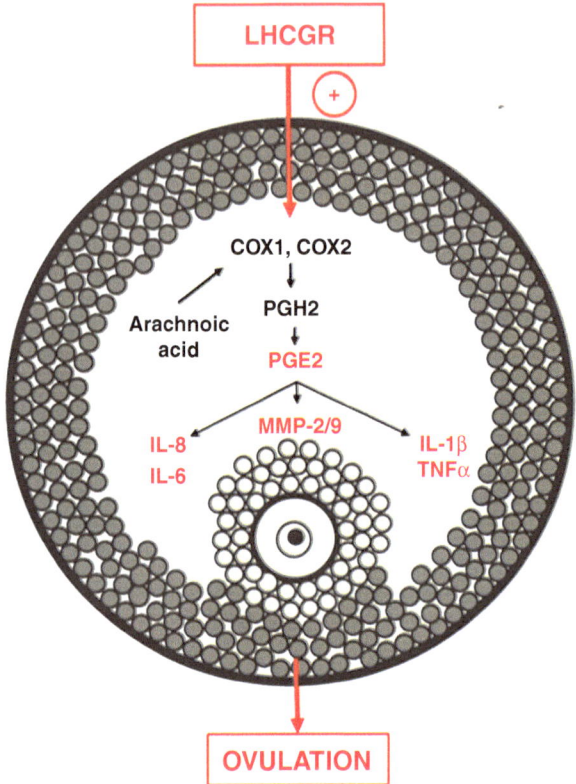

First responders to the LH surge are theca and mural granulosa cells, which produce inflammatory associated mediators such as steroids, prostaglandins, chemokines, and cytokines.

The LH-induced mediators initiate cumulus expansion and cumulus oocyte complex detachment, whereas the follicular apex, the granulosa cells opposite to the cumulus oocyte complex, undergoes extensive extracellular matrix remodelling and loss of its surface epithelium [18] leading to rupture of the follicle.

These mediators also activate follicular nonimmune cells, resident immune cells and attract non-resident immune cells which contribute to this process.

Prostaglandins reach the highest concentration around the time of ovulation [19]. PGE2 in particular is elevated following the LH surge and controls the timing of key ovulatory events [20]. PGE2 regulates ovulation by promoting local attraction and activation of neutrophils, macrophages, and mast cells like at the early stage of inflammation [21].

Within the ovary, these immune cells produce different cytokines, i.e., neutrophils produce interleukin (IL)-8, IL-1β, tumor necrosis factor (TNF)-α, monocytes release IL-6, IL-8, TNF-α, granulocyte-macrophage colony-stimulating factor

(GM-CSF), whereas mast cells potentially produce TNF-α and vascular endothelial growth factor (VEGF) [22]. Additionally, PGE2 is involved in regulating the balance between different forms of T helper cells, including an antagonistic activity of IL-12 (reviewed by Kalinski (2012) [21]).

Prostaglandins act also on the granulosa and theca cells to induce matrix metalloproteases, MMPs, allowing cumulus oocyte complex detachment, follicular apex degradation, follicle rupture and thereby oocyte release [23].

The remainder of the follicle undergoes rapid angiogenesis and functional differentiation of granulosa and theca cells to form the luteal body (see Chap. 8).

6.5   Cycle Day of the Ovulation

Length of the follicular phase and the day of ovulation were analyzed by Bull et al. (2019) [24], in natural cycles, based on App recordings of more than 600,000 cycles. The average length was 16.9 ± 5.3 days (mean ± SD) (Fig. 6.4). The length of the follicular phase and thereby the time of ovulation can vary substantially. The follicular phase shortens with increasing age.

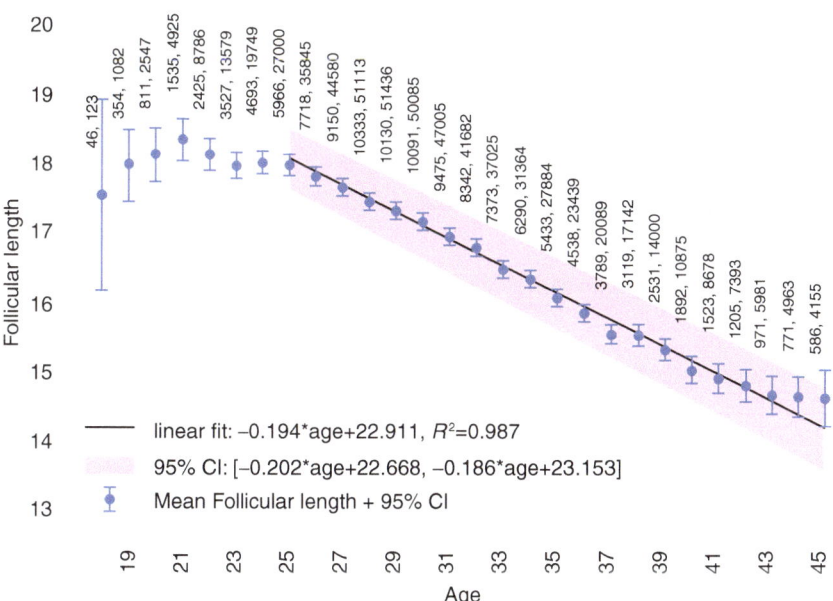

Fig. 6.4 Age versus mean follicular phase length ±2 standard errors of the mean (blue). Linear regression (black) fitted in the range 25–45 with 95% confidence intervall (CI) (pink). Points are labelled with the number of users followed by the number of cycles (Reprinted with the permission from [24])

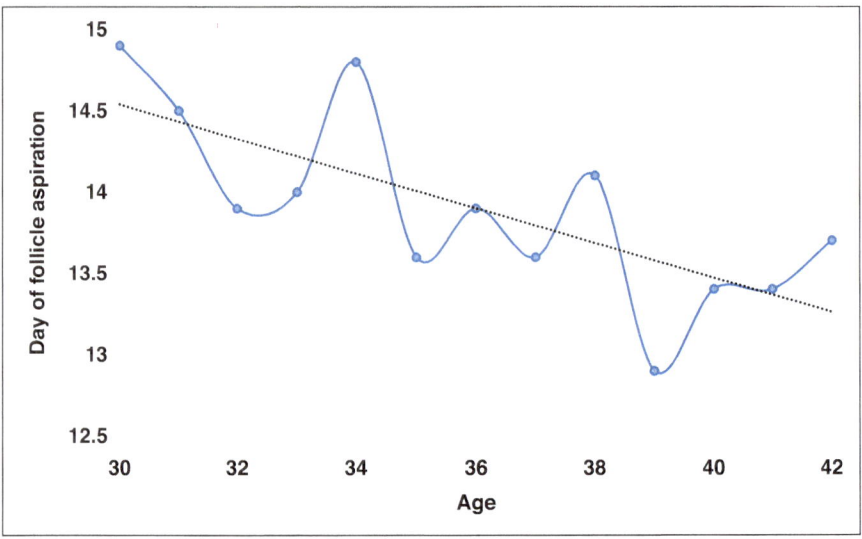

Fig. 6.5 Age versus mean cycle day of follicle aspiration in natural cycle IVF cycles (Infertility center Bern, Switzerland)

The shortening of the follicular phase can also be observed in natural cycle IVF (NC-IVF), leading to follicle aspiration at early stages. An evaluation from our own center based on 475 NC-IVF cycles shows the time of follicle aspiration depending on the woman' age (Fig. 6.5).

6.6   Ovulation Triggered by Estrogen-Dependent LH Surge

Ovulation is initiated by the LH surge after a sufficiently long stimulation of the hypothalamus by a sufficiently high E2 concentration in blood.

Most studies give the impression that the LH surge occurs at a largely precisely defined E2 concentration. These studies are based on hormone levels which were measured in a small number of subjects every day. Accordingly, the hormone fluctuations are low (Chap. 5, Fig. 5.2).

In practice, however, it has been shown that the increase in LH can occur at very different E2 concentrations. Figure 6.6 shows that, based on an analysis of 606 NC-IVF cycles in 290 women [25], LH increase occurs in 50% of women at E2 concentrations of ≤854 pmol/L.

However, the figure also clearly shows that the E2 concentration at which LH increases can vary considerably. Calculations per quantile revealed that it can be expected that LH increase occurs in 25% of cases at E2 concentrations as low as ≤545 pmol/L and in 75% of cases LH increase can be expected at E2 concentrations as high as ≤1531 pmol/L.

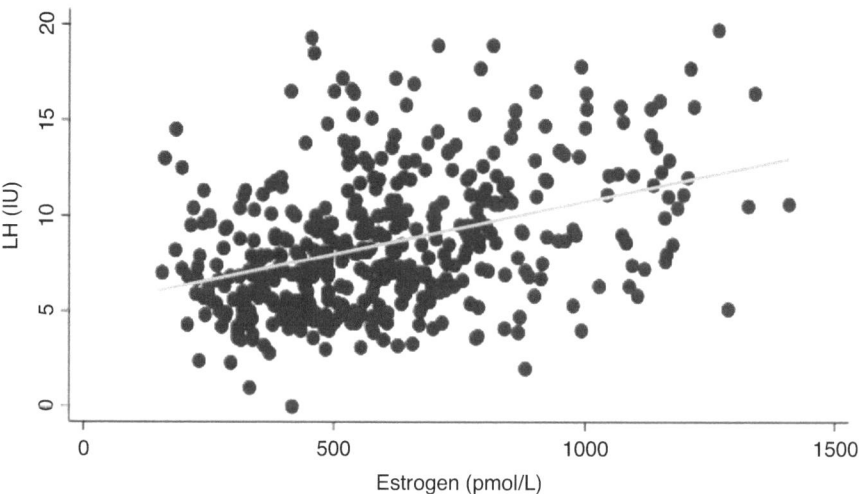

Fig. 6.6 Association of estrogen (estradiol, E2) and LH concentration of 606 natural cycle IVF cycles with a follicle size of ≥15 mm with a beginning LH surge (LH 10–20 IU) and fitted values. In 50% of women, LH surge started (= LH 10 - <20 IU) at an E2 concentration of ≤854 pmol/L. Calculations per quantile revealed that LH increases in 25% of cases at E2 concentrations ≤545 pmol/L and in 75% of cases at E2 concentrations ≤1531 pmol/L [25]

6.7   Time Interval Between Ovulation Triggering and Aspiration

With conventional IVF therapies, follicle aspiration is usually performed approx. 34–36 h after hCG administration. According to a study by Nargund et al. (2001) [26], in which 533 women were treated with a long agonist protocol and underwent follicle aspiration after a time interval of 33–41 h after administration of 10,000 IU hCG the proportion of oocytes per follicle was independent of the length of the time interval. No premature ovulation was documented in the case of a short or a long time interval (Table 6.1).

Hardly any studies have been carried out to date on how long the time interval between hCG administration and follicle aspiration in NC-IVF should be.

A control group of 18 women was included in a study in the infertility center in Bern on the effect of ibuprofen on delaying ovulation (see Chap. 11). The women completed a natural cycle without follicle aspiration. Ovulation was induced with 5000 IU hCG administered subcutaneously and vaginal sonography was performed after 42 h. Follicles were still found in 4 out of 18 (22%) women, indicating that the ovulation can also occur in NC-IVF much later than commonly expected.

Although it can be assumed that ovulation may occur later than 36 h after the ovulation trigger, aspiration should not be performed too late. This is particularly true if antagonists or clomiphene citrate are not given to delay the LH surge. The

Table 6.1 Outcome of conventional IVF therapies with different time intervals (33–41 hours) between oocyte triggering with 10,000 IU hCG and follicle aspiration (mod. according to Nargund et al. (2001) [26])

	33–<34	34–<35	35–<36	36–<37	37–<38	38–<39	39–<40	40–<41
No. of patients	23	101	134	108	56	53	37	21
Oocytes/follicle, %	50.0	63.6	66.7	62.5	54.6	58.8	62.5	66.7
Zygotes/oocytes, %	60.0	50.0	57.1	59.4	50.0	65.4	66.7	66.7
Pregnancies, n (%)	1 (4.3%)	7 (6.9%)	19 (14.2%)	16 (14.8%)	5 (8.9%)	9 (17.0%)	7 (18.0%)	4 (19.0%)
Patients without oocytes, n (%)	1 (4.3%)	2 (2.0%)	1 (0.7%)	0 (0.0)	0 (0.0)	1 (1.9%)	0 (0.0)	1 (4.8%)

Table 6.2 Time interval between ovulation trigger and aspiration in three large centers specialized in NC-IVF and/or minimal stimulation IVF

Center	Time interval between triggering and aspiration[a]
University Women's Hospital, Bern, Switzerland.	36 h
Kato Ladies Clinic, Tokyo, Japan	34–35 h
New Hope Fertility center, New York, U.S.	34–36 h

[a] See also Chap. 15

reason for this is that in most cases, follicle monitoring is carried out in the morning, but hCG is not administered until the evening. It is therefore possible that an hCG increase already occurs during the interval between follicle monitoring and hCG administration. Therefore, the interval between ovulation trigger and aspiration should not be too long. Table 6.2 shows the interval between ovulation trigger and follicle aspiration in three centers specialized in NC-IVF and/or minimal stimulation IVF.

6.8   Dysfunction of Ovulation: Empty Follicle Syndrome, EFS

For NC-IVF to be successful, it is not only crucial to have the lowest possible rate of premature ovulation (see Chap. 11). It is also important to have a high oocyte collection rate (see Chap. 13) to achieve the highest possible transfer rate.

Follicle flushing can be performed to increase the oocyte collection rate. Nevertheless, despite follicle flushing, oocytes can be aspirated in only about 85% of follicular aspirations [27–29]. This raises the question of whether there are pathophysiological reasons for the reduced oocyte aspiration rate.

One pathophysiological concept is the "Empty follicle syndrome", EFS. In conventional gonadotropin stimulated IVF, in which a large number of follicles are aspirated, EFS rarely occurs. Incidences of 0.1–7% of IVF cycles are found in the literature [30]. According to Zreik et al. (2000) [31], the risk of recurrence is age dependant. In women aged 35–39 years the risk of recurrence of EFS was 27% lower than in women aged >40 years with a risk of 57%. Since the risk of recurrence is not very high, it is obvious that EFS seems to be more of a temporary event [32]. Furthermore, in most cases, EFS seems to be due to technical errors such as inadequate ovulation triggering.

However, clinical practice suggests that although EFS is rare, there are women with a repeatedly high or low egg retrieval rate.

The infertility center in Bern, Switzerland performed an analysis to find out how likely egg retrieval is in a second NC-IVF cycle (Table 6.3). The probability of aspirating an oocyte was the same in women with or without an oocyte in the first cycle. This does not exclude that EFS can repeatedly occur in NC-IVF but it suggests that an empty follicle is rather a single incident but not a systematic error of oocyte release.

In addition to the above-mentioned increase in the risk of EFS, disturbed folliculogenesis and rare genetic causes such as a mutation of the LHCG receptor are also discussed [33].

Therapeutically, an increase in the hCG dose, as well as an extension of the time interval between hCG administration and aspiration, e.g., from 36 to 37 hours can be considered.

Another option might be the so-called dual triggering. Haas et al. (2020) [34] published a randomized controlled trial in which uhCG 10,000 IU versus uhCG 10,000 IU plus 0.5 mg buserelin was administered subcutaneously in conventional gonadotropin stimulated IVF cycles with normal responders. The number of oocytes obtained was 11.1 without versus 13.4 with dual triggering ($p = 0.002$) and the number of blastocytes 2.9 versus 3.9 ($p = 0.01$). Thus, this procedure could increase the chance of retrieving oocytes, even with repeated EFS. The physiological concept of the better oocyte recovery rate is the GnRH-induced release of not only LH, but also FSH.

It remains to be seen whether this procedure could also be successful with NC-IVF. It must be noted that the luteal phase could be insufficient after dual triggering because of GnRH administration. Therefore, luteal phase support should be administered after dual triggering.

Table 6.3 Probability of retrieving an oocyte in a 2nd NC-IVF cycle following a 1st NC-IVF cycle with or without an oocyte (Infertility center Berne, Switzerland)

	Number of women analyzed, n	Proportion of women with retrieval of an oocyte in the 2nd natural cycle IVF cycle
Women with retrieval of an oocyte in the 1st natural cycle IVF cycle	87	78.2%
Women without retrieval of an oocyte in the 1st natural cycle IVF cycle	39	76.9%

References

1. Herbison AE. Control of puberty onset and fertility by gonadotropin-releasing hormone neurons. Nat Rev Endocrinol. 2016;12:452–66.
2. Herbison AE. The gonadotropin-releasing hormone pulse generator. Endocrinology. 2018;159:3723–36.
3. Plant TM. A comparison of the neuroendocrine mechanisms underlying the initiation of the preovulatory LH surge in the human, Old World monkey and rodent. Front Neuroendocrinol. 2012;33:160–8.
4. Matsuda F, Ohkura S, Magata F, Munetomo A, Chen J, Sato M, Inoue N, Uenoyama Y, Tsukamura H. Role of kisspeptin neurons as a GnRH surge generator: comparative aspects in rodents and non-rodent mammals. J Obstet Gynaecol Res. 2019;45:2318–29.
5. Uenoyama Y, Nakamura S, Hayakawa Y, Ikegami K, Watanabe Y, Deura C, Minabe S, Tomikawa J, Goto T, Ieda N, Inoue N, Sanbo M, Tamura C, Hirabayashi M, Maeda KI, Tsukamura H. Lack of pulse and surge modes and glutamatergic stimulation of luteinising hormone release in Kiss1 knockout rats. J Neuroendocrinol. 2015;27:187–97.
6. de Roux N, Genin E, Carel JC, Matsuda F, Chaussain JL, Milgrom E. Hypogonadotropic hypogonadism due to loss of function of the KiSS1-derived peptide receptor GPR54. Proc Natl Acad Sci U S A. 2003;100:10972–6.
7. Richards JS, Ascoli M. Endocrine, paracrine, and autocrine signaling pathways that regulate ovulation. Trends Endocrinol Metab. 2018;29:313–25.
8. Richard S, Baltz JM. Prophase I arrest of mouse oocytes mediated by natriuretic peptide precursor C requires GJA1 (connexin-43) and GJA4 (connexin-37) gap junctions in the antral follicle and cumulus-oocyte complex. Biol Reprod. 2014;90:137.
9. von Wolff M, Eisenhut M, Stute P, Bersinger NA. Gonadotropin stimulation in In vitro Fertilisation (IVF) reduces follicular fluid hormone levels and disrupts their quantitative association with cumulus cell mRNA. Reprod Biomed Online. 2022;44(1):193–9. https://doi.org/10.1016/j.rbmo.2021.08.018.
10. Ledent C, Demeestere I, Blum D, Petermans J, Hämäläinen T, Smits G, Vassart G. Premature ovarian aging in mice deficient for Gpr3. Proc Natl Acad Sci U S A. 2005;102:8922–6.
11. Masciarelli S, Horner K, Liu C, Park SH, Hinckley M, Hockman S, Nedachi T, Jin C, Conti M, Manganiello V. Cyclic nucleotide phosphodiesterase 3A-deficient mice as a model of female infertility. J Clin Invest. 2004;114:196–205.
12. Richards JS, Russell DL, Ochsner S, Espey LL. Ovulation: new dimensions and new regulators of the inflammatory-like response. Annu Rev Physiol. 2002;64:69–92.
13. Blaha M, Prochazka R, Adamkova K, Nevoral J, Nemcova L. Prostaglandin E2 stimulates the expression of cumulus expansion-related genes in pigs: the role of protein kinase B. Prostaglandins Other Lipid Mediat. 2017;130:38–46.
14. Robker RL, Russell DL, Espey LL, Lydon JP, O'Malley BW, Richards JS. Progesterone-regulated genes in the ovulation process: ADAMTS-1 and cathepsin L proteases. Proc Natl Acad Sci U S A. 2000;97:4689–94.
15. Nallasamy S, Kim J, Sitruk-Ware R, Bagchi M, Bagchi I. Ulipristal blocks ovulation by inhibiting progesterone receptor-dependent pathways intrinsic to the ovary. Reprod Sci. 2013;20:371–81.
16. Natraj U, Richards JS. Hormonal regulation, localization, and functional activity of the progesterone receptor in granulosa cells of rat preovulatory follicles. Endocrinology. 1993;133:761–9.
17. Sriraman V, Eichenlaub-Ritter U, Bartsch JW, Rittger A, Mulders SM, Richards JS. Regulated expression of ADAM8 (a disintegrin and metalloprotease domain 8) in the mouse ovary: evidence for a regulatory role of luteinizing hormone, progesterone receptor, and epidermal growth factor-like growth factors. Biol Reprod. 2008;78:1038–48.
18. Duffy DM, Ko C, Jo M, Brannstrom M, Curry TE. Ovulation: parallels with inflammatory processes. Endocr Rev. 2019;40:369–416.

19. Espey LL. Current status of the hypothesis that mammalian ovulation is comparable to an inflammatory reaction. Biol Reprod. 1994;50:233–8.
20. Richards JAS. Sounding the alarm-does induction of prostaglandin endoperoxide synthase-2 control the mammalian ovulatory clock? Endocrinology. 1997;138:4047–8.
21. Kalinski P. Regulation of immune responses by prostaglandin E2. J Immunol. 2012;188:21–8.
22. Field SL, Dasgupta T, Cummings M, Orsi NM. Cytokines in ovarian folliculogenesis, oocyte maturation and luteinisation. Mol Reprod Dev. 2014;81:284–314.
23. Curry TE Jr, Osteen KG. The matrix metalloproteinase system: changes, regulation, and impact throughout the ovarian and uterine reproductive cycle. Endocrinol Rev. 2003;24:428–65.
24. Bull JR, Rowland SP, Scherwitzl EB, Scherwitzl R, Danielsson KG, Harper J. Real-world menstrual cycle characteristics of more than 600,000 menstrual cycles. NPJ Digit Med. 2019;2:83. https://doi.org/10.1038/s41746-019-0152-7.
25. Helmer A, Magaton I, Stalder O, Surbek D, Stute P, von Wolff M. Optimal timing of ovulation triggering to achieve highest success rates in natural cycles - an analysis based on follicle size and estradiol concentration in natural cycle IVF. Front Endocrinol, 2022, 26 May.
26. Nargund G, Reid F, Parsons J. Human chorionic gonadotropin-to-oocyte collection interval in a superovulation IVF program. A prospective study. J Assist Reprod Genet. 2001;18:87–90.
27. Aanesen A, Nygren KG, Nylund L. Modified natural cycle IVF and mild IVF: a 10 year Swedish experience. Reprod Biomed Online. 2010;20:156–62.
28. von Wolff M, Hua YZ, Santi A, Ocon E, Weiss B. Follicle flushing in monofollicular in vitro fertilization almost doubles the number of transferable embryos. Acta Obstet Gynecol Scand. 2013;92:346–8.
29. Kohl Schwartz AS, Calzaferri I, Roumet M, Limacher A, Fink A, Wueest A, Weidlinger S, Mitter VR, Leeners B, Von Wolff M. Follicular flushing leads to higher oocyte yield in mono-follicular IVF: a randomized controlled trial. Hum Reprod. 2020;35:2253–61.
30. Revelli A, Carosso A, Grassi G, Gennarelli G, Canosa S, Benedetto C. Empty follicle syndrome revisited: definition, incidence, aetiology, early diagnosis and treatment. Reprod Biomed Online. 2017;35:132–8.
31. Zreik TG, Garcia-Velasco JA, Vergara TM, Arici A, Olive D, Jones EE. Empty follicle syndrome: evidence for recurrence. Hum Reprod. 2000;15:999–1002.
32. Ben-Shlomo I, Schiff E, Levran D, Ben-Rafael Z, Mashiach S, Dor J. Failure of oocyte retrieval during in vitro fertilization: a sporadic event rather than a syndrome. Fertil Steril. 1991;55:324–7.
33. Yariz KO, Walsh T, Uzak A, Spiliopoulos M, Duman D, Onalan G, King MC, Tekin M. Inherited mutation of the luteinizing hormone/choriogonadotropin receptor (LHCGR) in empty follicle syndrome. Fertil Steril. 2011;96:e125–30.
34. Haas J, Bassil R, Samara N, Zilberberg E, Mehta C, Orvieto R, Casper RF. GnRH agonist and hCG (dual trigger) versus hCG trigger for final follicular maturation: a double-blinded, randomized controlled study. Hum Reprod. 2020;35:1648–54.

Chapter 7
Oocytes

Michael von Wolff

7.1 Background

In natural cycles, a cohort of follicles is recruited at the beginning of the cycle by the increasing concentration of follicle stimulation hormone (FSH). The recruited follicles all grow until the first follicle reaches a size of about 12 mm [1]. Induced by FSH, the follicle secretes large amounts of inhibin B from follicular granulosa cells, thereby inhibiting pituitary FSH release [2]. The smaller follicles become apoptotic due to the decrease in FSH. The large inhibin B-secreting leading follicle develops further due to the FSH-induced increase in its luteinizing hormone (LH) receptor expression and the associated higher LH sensitivity and releases the oocyte during ovulation (see Chap. 5).

In the case of high-dose gonadotropin stimulation, this natural selection of the leading follicle is omitted. With gonadotropin stimulation, more follicles are usually recruited at the beginning of the cycle, and most of the recruited follicles continue to grow due to the constantly high FSH concentrations and do not become apoptotic.

Because of this, it can be assumed that the oocytes from naturally selected follicles are better in terms of a higher development potential. But is this actually true?

Three questions arise in this context:

- Does ovarian gonadotropin stimulation affect the ploidy status of blastocysts?
- Does the in vitro culture affect the ploidy status of the blastocysts?
- Does ovarian gonadotropin stimulation affect oocyte development potential and thus the live birth rate? (Fig. 7.1)

M. von Wolff (✉)
Division of Gynecological Endocrinology and Reproductive Medicine, University Women's Hospital, University of Bern, Bern, Switzerland
e-mail: Michael.vonwolff@insel.ch

© The Author(s), under exclusive license to Springer Nature Switzerland AG 2022
M. von Wolff (ed.), *Natural Cycle and Minimal Stimulation IVF*,
https://doi.org/10.1007/978-3-030-97571-5_7

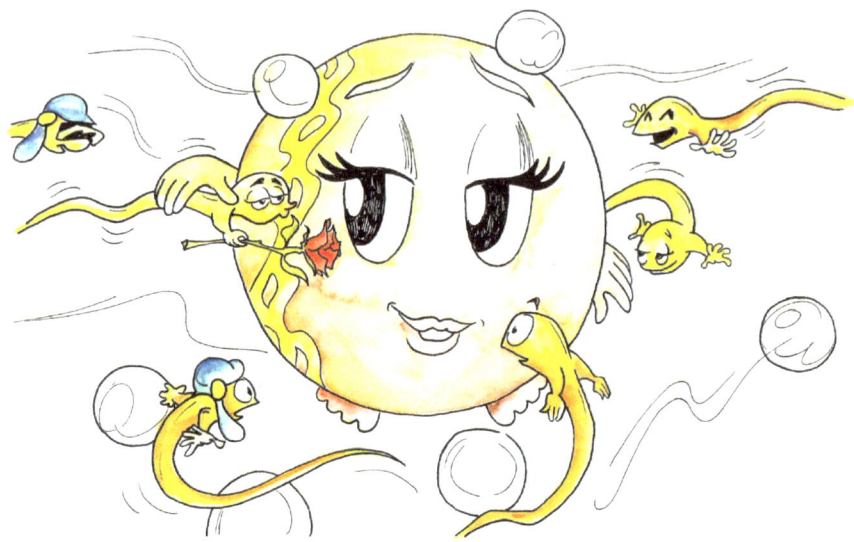

Fig. 7.1 The oocyte, arrested in prophase of meiosis, is activated after the LH surge and fertilized (Reprinted with permission from Michael von Wolff and Florian Lenz)

Table 7.1 Ploidy status of blastocysts developed after natural cycle IVF versus conventional IVF [3]

	Natural cycle IVF (without gonadotropin stimulation)	Conventional IVF (with gonadotropin stimulation)	p-value
Women, n	431	2846	
Age, years ±SD	36.9 ± 5.2	36.1 ± 4.4	
Oocytes/woman, n ±SD	0.9 ± 0.6	14.7 ± 9.9	
Blastocysts/woman, n ±SD	0.4 ± 0.5	4.8 ± 3.9	
Euploid blastocysts, %	56.5%	63.3%	$p > 0.05$
Aneuploid blastocysts, %	43.5%	36.7%	
Clinical implantation rate, n, (%); (only frozen cycles)	48/79 (60.8%)	986/1567 (62.9%)	$p > 0.05$

7.2 Influence of Ovarian Gonadotropin Stimulation on the Ploidy Status of Blastocysts

Hong et al. (2019) [3] used comprehensive chromosome screening (CCS) to investigate the ploidy status of blastocysts obtained after natural cycle IVF (NC-IVF) and conventional high-dose gonadotropin stimulated IVF (cIVF). Table 7.1 shows that the rate of euploid embryos is independent of gonadotropin stimulation. The odds ratio after adjustment for female age for the development of euploid embryos in NC-IVF versus cIVF was OR 0.908 (95% CI: 0.636, 1.182; $p > 0.05$).

This is in line with a large study by Barash et al. (2017) [4], in which the ploidy status was investigated as a function of the total gonadotropin dose used (<3000, 3000–5000, >5000 IU) and the number of oocytes obtained (1–5, 5–10, 10–15, >15 oocytes) in 4034 blastocysts. The rate of euploid embryos was not significantly different in the groups studied.

Thus, gonadotropin stimulation does not seem to increase the risk of embryonic aneuploidy.

7.3 Influence of In Vitro Culture on the Ploidy Status of Blastocysts

Munne et al. (2019) [5], stimulated 81 women (26.3 ± 5.3 years) with gonadotropins for subsequent intrauterine insemination (IUI). Uterine lavage was performed 4–6 days after ovulation induction. The blastocysts developed in vivo and obtained by uterine lavage were subjected to aneuploidy screening using Next Generation Sequencing (NGS).

cIVF therapy was later carried out in 20 of these women. The 163 blastocysts generated by cIVF were also subjected to aneuploidy screening. Both groups of patients were similarly stimulated.

In the in vivo lavage group 8.5 (2–18) follicles ≥16 mm developed with a mean E2 concentration of 2388 pg/mL (352–8538 pg/mL).

In the in vitro cIVF group 9.7 (0–19) follicles ≥16 mm developed with a mean E2 concentration of 2628 pg/mL (339–5931 pg/mL).

Table 7.2 compares the data of women who had both an in vivo cycle and an in vitro cycle. The rate of aneuploidy and the rate of mosaicism were the same in both groups.

Thus, in vitro culture does not seem to increase the risk of embryonic aneuploidy.

7.4 Influence of Ovarian Gonadotropin Stimulation on Oocyte Development Potential

The studies presented above have shown that neither gonadotropin stimulation nor embryo culture over several days seems to increase the risk of aneuploidy.

This leads to the question of whether the pregnancy and birth potential of oocytes obtained in natural cycle IVF and cIVF treatments is the same or different due to other reasons?

Magaton et al. [6] analyzed 2110 oocytes from natural cycle IVF and conventional IVF (cIVF) cycles and compared the development of the oocytes retrieved. The analysis was based on data of 783 cycles without embryo selection to allow the comparison of both therapies.

Table 7.2 Ploidy status of blastocysts developed after gonadotropin stimulation in vivo (uterine lavage of blastocysts developed in gonadotropin stimulated intrauterine insemination cycles) and in vitro (blastocysts developed after gonadotropin stimulated IVF) [5]

	In vivo blastocysts (Gonadotropin stimulation without IVF)	In vitro blastocysts (Gonadotropin stimulation with IVF)	p-value
Women, n	20	20	
Cycles with oocytes, n	28	20	
Analyzed blastocysts, n	65	163	
Euploid blastocysts, n	35 (54%)	83 (51%)	
Low-grade mosaic (≤40%), n	6 (9%)	22 (13%)	
High-grade mosaic (>40%), n	3 (5%)	14 (9%)	>0.05
Aneuploid blastocysts, n	13 (20%)	28 (17%)	
Complex abnormal, triploid, n	8 (12%)	16 (10%)	

Fig. 7.2 Percentages of developmental stages per retrieved oocytes in natural cycle IVF (NC-IVF) (green) and conventional IVF (cIVF) (blue) (adapted from [6])

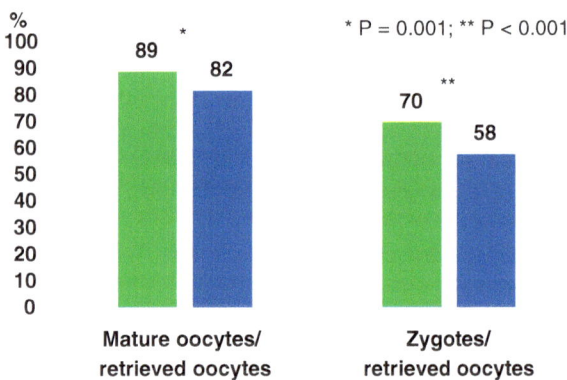

As shown in Fig. 7.2, the percentage of mature (metaphase II) and fertilized oocytes is significantly higher in natural cycle IVF oocytes compared to cIVF oocytes. The adjusted odds ratios for the proportion of mature/retrieved oocytes were aOR 1.79 (95% CI: 1.26–2.53) and for the proportion of zygotes/retrieved oocytes were aOR 1.76 (95% CI: 1.37–2.26).

Magaton et al. [6] also analyzed the morphology of 390 cleavage stage embryos derived from 783 NC-IVF cycles two days after aspiration. The study was based on the ASEBIR criteria [7], indicating that embryos with 4 blastomeres and with low fragmentation rate have the highest potential to further develop into a pregnancy and live birth. As shown in Fig. 7.2, the percentages of embryos with 4 blastomeres and of embryos with fragmentation <10% are significantly higher in NC-IVF embryos compared to cIVF embryos. The adjusted Odds ratios for the development of a cleavage stage embryo in NC-IVF with 4 blastomeres and not less or more blastomeres were aOR 1.85 (95% CI: 1.13-3.02). The aOR for the development of a cleavage stage embryo with fragmentation <10% was aOR 2.44 (95% CI: 1.45-4.05).

Figure 7.3 Mitter et al. (2021) [8] evaluated the potential of transferred embryos to generate a pregnancy and a live birth by comparing 1447embryos derived from NC-IVF and cIVF.

NC-IVF was defined as IVF without any stimulation of follicular growth and cIVF as IVF with gonadotropin stimulation ≥75 IE/d and >3 retrieved oocytes. As zygote, but not embryo selection was performed, both treatments were comparable regarding the potential of the transferred embryos to generate a pregnancy. Embryos were transferred on day 2–3. Figure 7.4 gives an overview of the outcome numbers (Table 7.3).

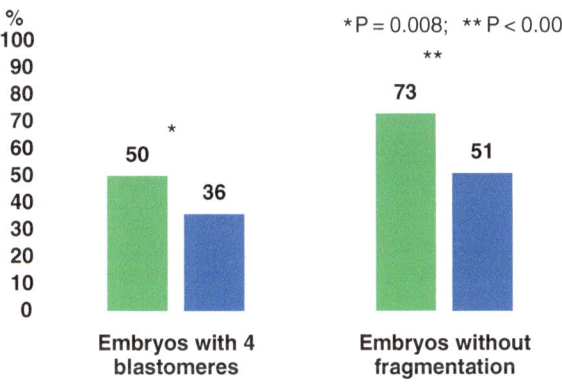

Fig. 7.3 Percentages of cleavage stage embryos with 4 versus <4 and >4 blastomeres and embryos without versus with fragmentation in natural cycle IVF (NC-IVF) (green) and conventional IVF (cIVF) (blue) (adapted from [6])

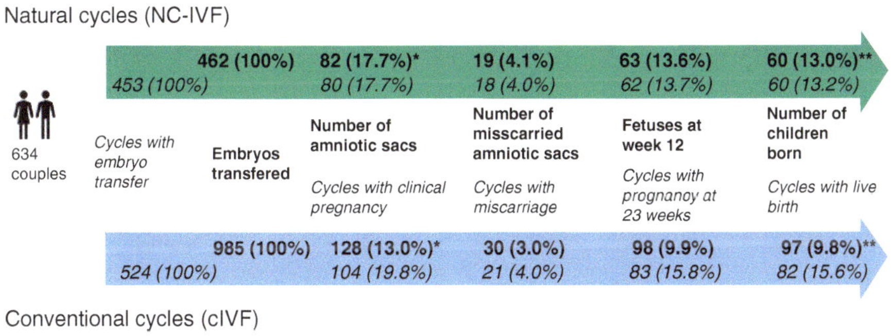

Natural cycles (NC-IVF)

634 couples	Cycles with embryo transfer	Embryos transfered	Number of amniotic sacs / Cycles with clinical pregnancy	Number of misscarried amniotic sacs / Cycles with miscarriage	Fetuses at week 12 / Cycles with prognanoy at 23 weeks	Number of children born / Cycles with live birth
NC-IVF		462 (100%)	82 (17.7%)*	19 (4.1%)	63 (13.6%)	60 (13.0%)**
	453 (100%)		80 (17.7%)	18 (4.0%)	62 (13.7%)	60 (13.2%)
cIVF		985 (100%)	128 (13.0%)*	30 (3.0%)	98 (9.9%)	97 (9.8%)**
	524 (100%)		104 (19.8%)	21 (4.0%)	83 (15.8%)	82 (15.6%)

Conventional cycles (cIVF)

Fig. 7.4 Success rates per transferred embryo in natural cycle IVF (NC-IVF) versus conventional gonadotropin stimulated IVF (cIVF) (*significantly different, **significantly different after adjustment) (according to [8])

Table 7.3 Implantation, miscarriage, and live birth rates in natural cycle IVF versus conventional gonadotropin stimulated IVF (cIVF), adjusted for female age, parity, and infertility characteristics (primary or secondary infertility, indication for IVF) [8]

	Implantation rate, risk ratio (95% CI)	p-value	Miscarriage rate per amniotic sac, risk ratio (95% CI)	p-value	Live birth rate per transferred embryo, rRisk ratio (95% CI)	p-value
All women						
cIVF	1.00 (ref.)		1.00 (ref.)		1.00 (ref.)	
Natural cycle IVF	1.42 (1.10–1.84)	0.008	0.90 (0.52–1.53)	0.698	1.38 (1.01–1.88)	0.044
Parous women						
cIVF	1.00 (ref.)		1.00 (ref.)		1.00 (ref.)	
Natural cycle IVF	2.23 (1.38–3.61)	0.001	n.a. (numbers too low for calculation)		2.35 (1.35–4.10)	0.003

Implantation (aRR 1.42, 95% CI: 1.10–1.84) and live birth rates (aRR 1.38, 95% CI: 1.01–1.88) were higher in embryos derived from NC-IVF, whereas miscarriages rates (aRR 0.90, 95% CI: 0.52–1.53) were not different.

The reasons for the higher implantation and pregnancy rates are not clear. One reason might be the better oocyte quality in NC-IVF, leading to better embryo quality as shown above [6] (Fig. 7.3).

However, another reason might be the endometrial quality. Endometrium in cIVF is functionally affected by high E2 concentration. Furthermore, it can be affected by pre-ovulatory progesterone increase due to supraphysiological FSH stimulation of granulosa cells and suppression of steroidogenesis in theca cells (see Chap. 9).

Overall, summarizing the data from Magaton et al. [6] and Mitter et al. [8], the potential of an oocyte retrieved from a natural cycle follicle might be up to two times higher to generate a live birth compared to oocytes retrieved from cIVF follicles.

References

1. Yding AC. Inhibin-B secretion and FSH isoform distribution may play an integral part of follicular selection in the natural menstrual cycle. Mol Hum Reprod. 2017;23:16–24.
2. Groome NP, Illingworth PJ, O'Brien M, Pai R, Rodger FE, Mather JP, McNeilly AS. Measurement of dimeric inhibin B throughout the human menstrual cycle. J Clin Endocrinol Metab. 1996;81:1401–5.
3. Hong KH, Franasiak JM, Werner MM, Patounakis G, Juneau CR, Forman EJ, Scott RT Jr. Embryonic aneuploidy rates are equivalent in natural cycles and gonadotropin-stimulated cycles. Fertil Steril. 2019;112:670–6.

4. Barash OO, Hinckley MD, Rosenbluth EM, Ivani KA, Weckstein LN. High gonadotropin dosage does not affect euploidy and pregnancy rates in IVF PGS cycles with single embryo transfer. Hum Reprod. 2017;32:2209–17.
5. Munné S, Nakajima ST, Najmabadi S, Sauer MV, Angle MJ, Rivas JL, Mendieta LV, Macaso TM, Sawarkar S, Nadal A, Choudhary K, Nezhat C, Carson SA, Buster JE. First PGT-A using human in vivo blastocysts recovered by uterine lavage: comparison with matched IVF embryo controls†. Hum Reprod. 2020;35:70–80.
6. Magaton IM, Helmer A, Eisenhut M, Roumet M, Stute P, von Wolff M. Oocyte maturity, fertilization rate and cleavage stage embryo morphology are better in natural compared to high dose gonadotropin stimulated cycles. Submitted.
7. de los Santos MJ, Arroyo G, Busquet A, Calderón G, Cuadros J, Hurtado de Mendoza MV, Moragas M, Herrer R, Ortiz A, Pons C, Ten J, Vilches MA, Figueroa MJ, ASEBIR Interest Group in Embryology. A multicenter prospective study to assess the effect of early cleavage on embryo quality, implantation, and live-birth rate. Fertil Steril. 2014;101:981–7.
8. Mitter VR, Grädel F, Kohl Schwartz AS, von Wolff M. Gonadotropin stimulation reduces the implantation and live birth but not the miscarriage rate a study based on the comparison of gonadotropin stimulated and unstimulated IVF. Hum Reprod. 2021 (Suppl 1), i452.

Chapter 8
Luteal Phase

Michael von Wolff

8.1 Background

Ovulation, followed by the transformation of the follicle into the corpus luteum, marks the beginning of the luteal phase. Luteal progesterone transforms the endometrium and enables the implantation of the embryo or, if pregnancy does not occur, its regulated shedding (Fig. 8.1). The function of the corpus luteum and its maintenance is controlled by luteinizing hormone, LH, and, if pregnancy occurs, by the trophoblastic human chorionic gonadotropin, hCG. The function of the corpus luteum, the luteolysis, and its maintenance at the onset of pregnancy require a sensitive interaction between pituitary gonadotropin secretion, luteinizing steroid hormone synthesis, and the expression of luteinizing and luteolytic factors.

8.2 Follicular Luteinization

The LH surge induces final oocyte maturation, dissociation of the cumulus oophorus complex (COC) from the follicular wall, rupture of the follicle, and finally formation of the corpus luteum.

Morphologically localized hemorrhage occurs at the site of ovulation and fills the former follicle. The wall of the follicle collapses, and some granulosa and thecal cell layers are pushed into the ruptured follicle. The protrusion of the cell layers and ruptured blood vessels form the corpus hemorrhagicum. The theca interna and granulosa cells subsequently differentiate into small and large luteal cells, respectively.

M. von Wolff (✉)

Division of Gynecological Endocrinology and Reproductive Medicine, University Women's Hospital, University of Bern, Bern, Switzerland
e-mail: Michael.vonwolff@insel.ch

© The Author(s), under exclusive license to Springer Nature Switzerland AG 2022   67
M. von Wolff (ed.), *Natural Cycle and Minimal Stimulation IVF*,
https://doi.org/10.1007/978-3-030-97571-5_8

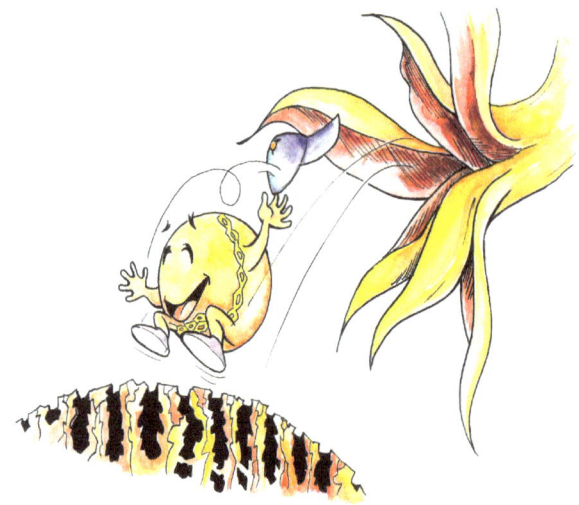

On the molecular level, granulosa cell expression of LH receptors and progesterone receptors increases. Furthermore, several molecular processes are initiated such as binding of activating transcription factors to the promoter of the steroidogenic acute regulatory protein (StAR) gene and increased production of cytochrome P450 sidechain cleavage enzyme (P450scc), cyclo-oxygenase-2, and members of the matrix metalloproteinase (MMP) family, which are critical determinants of progesterone synthesis [1]. As a result, progesterone and 17α-hydroxyprogesterone (17α-OHP) plasma concentrations increase rapidly, indicating the beginning of granulosa and theca cell luteinization.

Small luteal cells are presumably derived from the theca interna, while large luteal cells from the granulosa cell lineage. Basal production of progesterone is generally greater in granulosa luteal cells, which are also the main site of luteal estradiol (E2) production because they express aromatase. Theca luteal cells produce the androgen precursors that are aromatized by granulosa luteal cells and are also the site of 17α-OHP synthesis. These findings indicate that the follicular two-cell model of theca cell androgen and granulosa cell E2 biosynthesis is also preserved in the corpus luteum [2].

The luteal vasculature is regulated by vascular endothelial growth factor (VEGF) which is localized in human granulosa luteal cells. VEGF also has an impact on luteal steroidogenesis [3].

8.3   Luteal Progesterone Biosynthesis

The first step in progesterone biosynthesis is to take up lipoprotein-carried cholesterol by endocytosis and to maintain stores of esterified cholesterol. High-density lipoproteins may also contribute as precursors for steroidogenesis [4].

Upon gonadotropin stimulation, cholesterol is conveyed to the inner membrane of the mitochondria to serve as a substrate for steroid production (see Chap. 5, Fig. 5.6). It is thought that the rate-limiting step in progesterone synthesis is the translocation of cholesterol from the outer mitochondrial membrane to the inner membrane, where the P450scc complex is located which catalyses conversion of cholesterol to pregnenolone. Steroidogenic acute regulatory protein (StAR) is essential to this sterol translocation process in response to tropic hormones, including LH and hCG [5].

Subsequently, pregnenolone, the first compound of the steroidogenic pathways, is converted to progesterone by 3β-hydroxysteroid dehydrogenase (3β-HSD) present in the smooth endoplasmic reticulum. Prior to the LH surge, StAR is virtually absent from the human granulosa cells, which are unable to synthesize progesterone from cholesterol precursors. Conversely, StAR is found in high concentrations in the periovulatory human theca cells that are able to synthesize androgens from cholesterol [6]. Thus, the rapid increase in progesterone at the time of the LH surge suggests that luteinizing theca cells are the possible source of progesterone. In the luteal phase, the expression of StAR transcripts and proteins is greatest in the early and mid-luteal phase corpus luteum and has a positive correlation with progesterone concentrations. Accordingly, mid-luteal progesterone concentrations are highest (Fig. 8.2).

In the human corpus luteum, StAR concentrations appear to be greater in theca luteal cells than in granulosa luteal cells, irrespective of the stage of the luteal phase [7]. A decline in StAR mRNA and protein expression heralds the initiation of functional luteolysis.

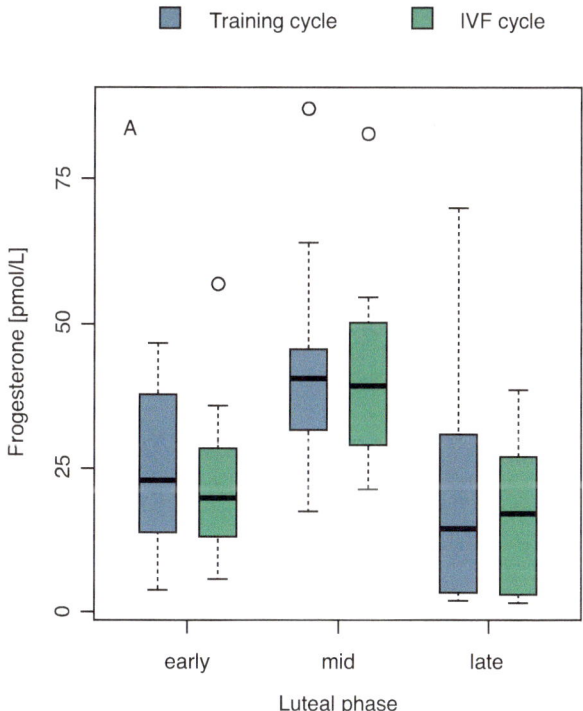

Fig. 8.2 Progesterone concentration in natural IVF cycles (IVF cycle, green) compared to natural non-IVF cycles (Training cycles, grey) of 23 women, both triggered with 5000 IU hCG. Follicles in IVF cycles were aspirated and flushed 3 times (according to [8]). Early luteal phase: day 2–3, mid-luteal phase day 6–7, and late luteal phase day 10–11 after ovulation/aspiration. Presentation of median with interquartile ranges and whiskers with maximum length of 1.5 interquartile ranges (according to [8])

8.4   Luteal Estradiol Biosynthesis

The corpus luteum also produces estrogen. As stated before, the two-cell model of E2 biosynthesis is preserved in the corpus luteum. Accordingly, theca luteal cells produce the androgen precursors that are aromatized to estrogen by granulosa luteal cells.

It is well established that E2 synthesis by follicular granulosa cells is stimulated by follicle stimulating hormone (FSH). However, FSH does not directly stimulate E2 synthesis in luteal cells [9]. The steroidogenic action of FSH in luteal cells is promoted by LH and insulin-like growth factor-1 [7].

Interestingly, E2 secretion by the human luteal body does not appear to be essential for pregnancy, as progesterone replacement alone in luteectomized women maintains pregnancy [10]. However, this does not mean that E2 is not required for the maintenance of the pregnancy at all. It can be assumed that the luteal phase ovary secretes a substantial amount of estrogen independent from the luteal body. The high mid-luteal phase estrogen concentrations (Fig. 8.3) are due to the luteal body which aromatizes luteal androgens to estrogen, but they might also be due to the corpus luteum recruitment of estrogen producing follicles due to the physiological mid-luteal increase of FSH levels [11].

Luteal phase estrogen might also play a role in luteolysis and the following follicle recruitment. Owing to the demise of the corpus luteum during the late luteal phase of the menstrual cycle, E2, inhibin A (which is, in contrast to inhibin B, mainly produced by the luteal body), and progesterone concentrations fall, which results in an increased frequency of pulsatile GnRH hormone secretion. This in turn induces FSH secretion and the recruitment of early antral follicles at the end of the luteal phase [12].

8.5   Luteolysis

In non-fertile cycles, the corpus luteum undergoes a process of regression, known as luteolysis, that encompasses a loss of functional and structural integrity of the luteal body. The functional regression is associated with a decrease in progesterone production, while structural regression is associated with different forms of cell death.

These changes are induced by a reduced effect of LH on the luteal cells. In the early luteal phase, LH pulse frequency [13] and luteal LH sensitivity are highest. Both decrease in the mid-luteal phase.

However, the reduced LH sensitivity probably results from LH-receptor desensitization and not receptor downregulation, since LH-receptor expression only decreases with declining progesterone secretion in the late luteal phase [14].

As a consequence of the LH receptor desensitization and receptor downregulation, the levels of local luteotropic factors decline and the level of luteolytic factors increases (Fig. 8.4).

Fig. 8.3 Estradiol (E2) concentration in natural IVF cycles (IVF cycle, green) compared to natural non-IVF cycles (Training cycles, grey) of 23 women, both triggered with 5000 IU hCG. Follicles in IVF cycles were aspirated and flushed 3 times (according to [8]). Early luteal phase: day 2–3, mid-luteal phase day 6–7, and late luteal phase day 10–11 after ovulation/aspiration. Presentation of median with interquartile ranges and whiskers with maximum length of 1.5 interquartile ranges (according to [8])

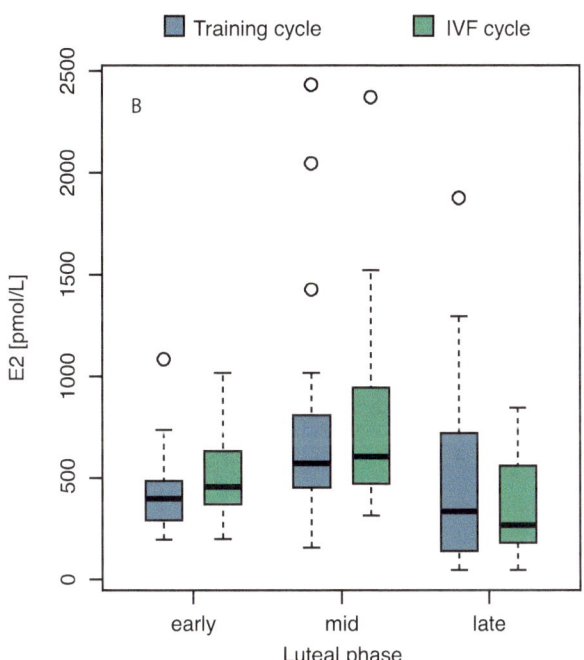

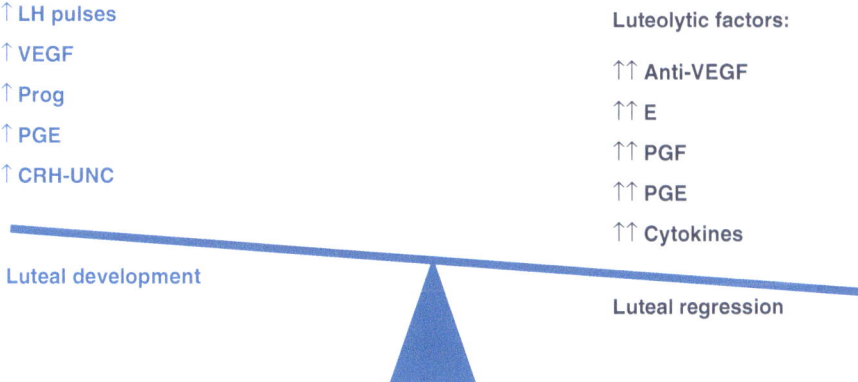

Fig. 8.4 Proposed changes in the balance between luteotropic and luteolytic signals in the corpus luteum during its lifespan in the non-fecund menstrual cycle. Increased production/concentration of luteolytic factors lead to luteal regression. *VEGF* Vascular endothelial growth factor, *Prog* Progesterone, *PGE* Prostaglandin E, *CRH-UCN* Corticotropin-releasing hormone/urocortin, *E* Estrogen, *PGF* Prostaglandin F (according to [17])

For example, the levels of vascular endothelial growth factor (VEGF) are markedly reduced by mid-late luteal phase at the onset of luteal regression [15]. Given the role of VEGF in maintaining the luteal vasculature and perhaps non-vascular actions, it can be speculated that the level of VEGF receptor signalling is no longer sufficient by mid-luteal phase to meet its luteotropic role.

Likewise, by mid-late luteal phase, progesterone secretion is entrained to the intermittent LH pulses such that the corpus luteum is producing a milieu of sequential intervals of progesterone repletion and depletion [13]. Moreover, the number of progesterone receptor-positive cells [16] diminish with age.

8.6 Length of the Luteal Phase

In contrast to the follicular phase, the length of the luteal phase is quite stable.

In a study with 23 women (age 33 ± 3.4 years, range 27–40 years) with natural cycles with ovulation triggered with 5000 IU hCG, median duration of the luteal phase was 13 days (interquartile range 12d, 14.5d). The length of cycles stayed stable and was not affected by aspiration and flushing of the follicles (Fig. 8.5).

Length of the luteal phase was also analyzed by Bull et al. (2019) [18] in natural cycles, based on App recordings of more than 600,000 cycles. The average length was 12.4 ± 2.4 days (mean ± SD) (Fig. 8.6) which is roughly in line the above shown natural cycles (Fig. 8.5) triggered with 5000IU hCG [8].

Bull et al. (2019) also analyzed the length of the luteal phase in relation to age and found shorter luteal phases in young women and a subtle increase in women

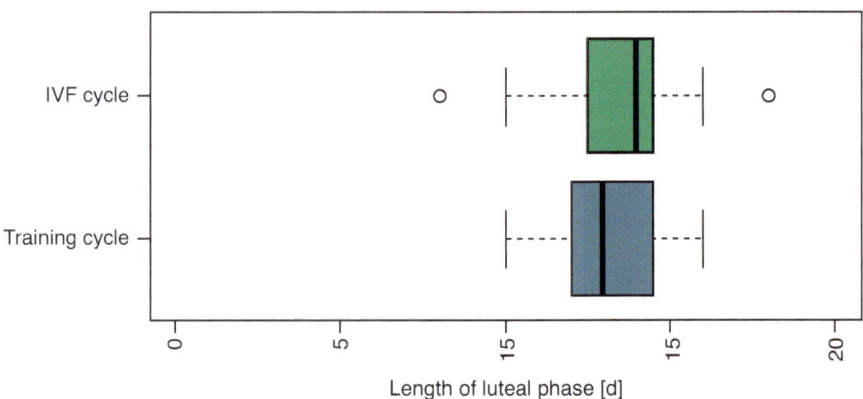

Fig. 8.5 Length of the luteal phases in natural IVF cycles (IVF cycle) compared to natural non-IVF cycles (Training cycles) of 23 women, both triggered with 5000 IU hCG. Follicles in IVF cycles were aspirated and flushed 3 times (according to [8])

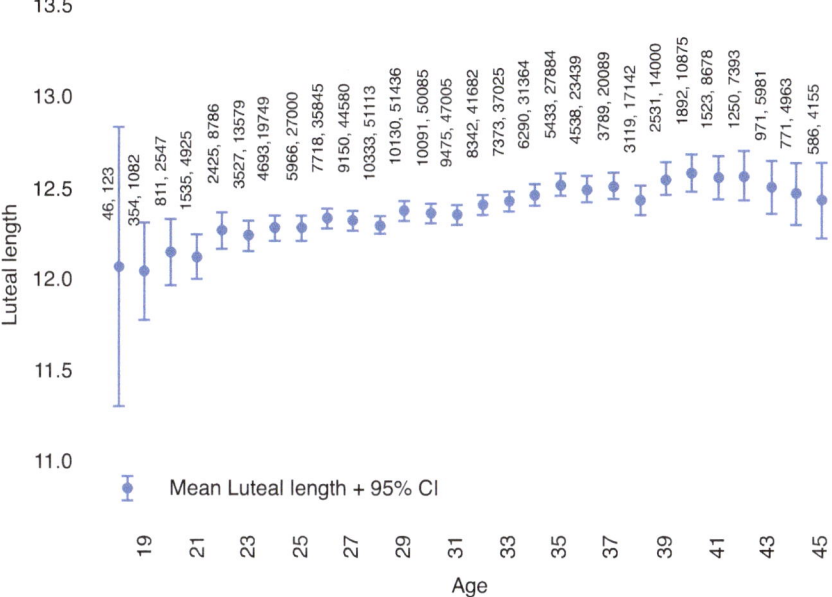

Fig. 8.6 Age versus mean luteal phase length ±2 standard errors of the mean. Points are labelled with the number of users followed by the number of cycles (Reprinted with the permission from [18])

above age 30 years (Fig. 8.5). At the age of 25–30 years, the length of the luteal phase was 12.4 ± 2.2 days and at the age of 31–35 years 12.9 ± 2.3 days.

References

1. Richards JS. Genetics of ovulation. Semin Reprod Med. 2007;25:235–42.
2. Kohen P, Castro O, Palomino A, Muñoz A, Christenson LK, Sierralta W, Carvallo P, Strauss JF 3rd, Devoto L. The steroidogenic response and corpus luteum expression of the steroidogenic acute regulatory protein after human chorionic gonadotropin administration at different times in the human luteal phase. J Clin Endocrinol Metab. 2003;88:3421–30.
3. Fraser HM, Dickson SE, Lunn SF, Wulff C, Morris KD, Carroll VA, Bicknell R. Suppression of luteal angiogenesis in the primate after neutralization of vascular endothelial growth factor. Endocrinology. 2000;141:995–1000.
4. Devoto L, Kohen P, Muñoz A, Strauss JF 3rd. Human corpus luteum physiology and the luteal-phase dysfunction associated with ovarian stimulation. Reprod Biomed Online. 2009;18(Suppl 2):19–24.
5. Strauss JF 3rd, Kallen CB, Christenson LK, Watari H, Devoto L, Arakane F, Kiriakidou M, Sugawara T. The steroidogenic acute regulatory protein (StAR): a window into the complexities of intracellular cholesterol trafficking. Recent Prog Horm Res. 1999;54:369–94.

6. Kiriakidou M, McAllister JM, Sugawara T, Strauss JF 3rd. Expression of steroidogenic acute regulatory protein (StAR) in the human ovary. J Clin Endocrinol Metab. 1996;81:4122–8.
7. Devoto L, Kohen P, Vega M, Castro O, González RR, Retamales I, Carvallo P, Christenson LK, Strauss JF. Control of human luteal steroidogenesis. Mol Cell Endocrinol. 2002;186:137–41.
8. von Wolff M, Kohl Schwartz A, Stute P, Fäh M, Otti G, Schürch R, Rohner S. Follicular flushing in natural cycle IVF does not affect the luteal phase—a prospective controlled study. Reprod Biomed Online. 2017;35:37–41.
9. Devoto L, Vega M, Navarro V, Sir T, Alba F, Castro O. Regulation of steroid hormone synthesis by human corpora lutea: failure of follicle-stimulating hormone to support steroidogenesis in vivo and in vitro. Fertil Steril. 1989;51:628–33.
10. Csapo AI, Pulkkinen MO, Wiest WG. Effects of luteectomy and progesterone replacement therapy in early pregnant patients. Am J Obstet Gynecol. 1973;115:759–65.
11. Baerwald AR, Adams GP, Pierson RA. Characterization of ovarian follicular wave dynamics in women. Biol Reprod. 2003;69:1023–31.
12. le Nestour E, Marraoui J, Lahlou N, Roger M, de Ziegler D, Bouchard P. Role of estradiol in the rise in follicle-stimulating hormone levels during the luteal-follicular transition. J Clin Endocrinol Metab. 1993;77:439–42.
13. Ellinwood WE, Norman RL, Spies HG. Changing frequency of pulsatile luteinizing hormone and progesterone secretion during the luteal phase of the menstrual cycle of rhesus monkeys. Biol Reprod. 1984;31:714–22.
14. Cameron JL, Stouffer RL. Gonadotropin receptors of the primate corpus luteum. II. Changes in available luteinizing hormone- and chorionic gonadotropin-binding sites in macaque luteal membranes during the nonfertile menstrual cycle. Endocrinology. 1982;110:2068–73.
15. Tesone M, Stouffer RL, Borman SM, Hennebold JD, Molskness TA. Vascular endothelial growth factor (VEGF) production by the monkey corpus luteum during the menstrual cycle: isoform-selective messenger RNA expression in vivo and hypoxia-regulated protein secretion in vitro. Biol Reprod. 2005;73:927–34.
16. Hild-Petito S, Stouffer RL, Brenner RM. Immunocytochemical localization of estradiol and progesterone receptors in the monkey ovary throughout the menstrual cycle. Endocrinology. 1988;123:2896–905.
17. Stouffer RL, Bishop CV, Bogan RL, Xu F, Hennebold JD. Endocrine and local control of the primate corpus luteum. Reprod Biol. 2013;13:259–71.
18. Bull JR, Rowland SP, Scherwitzl EB, Scherwitzl R, Danielsson KG, Harper J. Real-world menstrual cycle characteristics of more than 600,000 menstrual cycles. NPJ Digit Med. 2019;2:83. https://doi.org/10.1038/s41746-019-0152-7.

Chapter 9
Endometrium

Michael von Wolff

9.1 Background

In a natural cycle, the endometrium proliferates under the influence of slowly increasing physiological estrogen concentrations and is transformed by progesterone. A complex interplay of endometrial glandular and stromal cells, immune cells, and endocrine, paracrine, and autocrine regulatory mechanisms leads to the development of an endometrial functional state that allows the implantation of the semi-allogenic embryo and enables the development of the placenta (Fig. 9.1). If the function of the endometrium is impaired, e.g., by supraphysiological estrogen concentrations or by a disturbance of the corpus luteum function, lower implantation rates, increased miscarriage rates, and pregnancy disorders such as pre-eclampsia may result. For conventional high-dose gonadotropin stimulation IVF, a variety of adjuvants are discussed which are intended to improve endometrial function. Ultimately, this is an attempt to reduce the collateral damage of high-dose gonadotropin stimulation. It can be assumed that such treatments are not effective in natural cycle IVF, since a naturally proliferated and transformed endometrium is not or is hardly impaired in its function, or at least cannot be improved.

M. von Wolff (✉)
Division of Gynecological Endocrinology and Reproductive Medicine,
University Women's Hospital, University of Bern, Bern, Switzerland
e-mail: Michael.vonwolff@insel.ch

Fig. 9.1 The endometrium is a unique tissue to allow implantation of the semi-allogenic embryo (Reprinted with permission from Michael von Wolff and Florian Lenz)

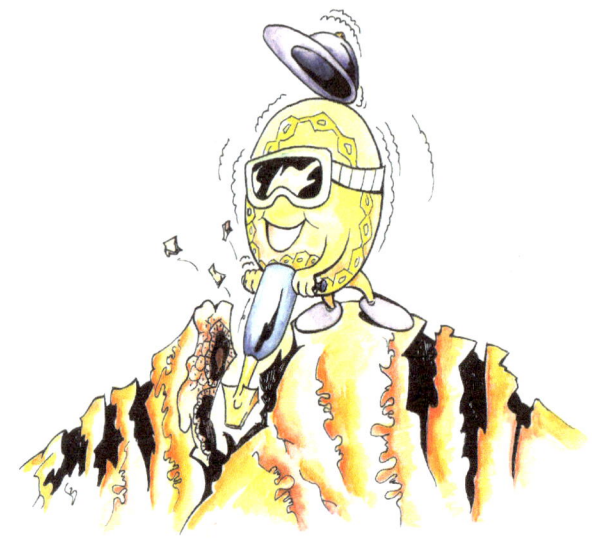

9.2   Physiology of the Endometrium

The endometrium is a unique tissue, as

- it proliferates, transforms, and is shed every 4 weeks,
- it creates a rather implantation preventing environment, but opens the so-called window of implantation, lasting just a few days, during which the embryo can implant,
- recognizes and immunologically accepts the embryo as a semi-allogenic graft.

These unique characteristics require a complex and well-orchestrated set of endometrial cells, local immune regulators, adhesion proteins, and mediators (reviewed by Strowitzki et al. (2006) [1] and Ochoa-Bernal and Fazleabas (2020) [2]).

9.2.1   The Proliferative Phase

The main feature of the endometrial tissue during the proliferative phase is active proliferation and angiogenesis to ensure nutrition of the developing new tissue while suppressing apoptotic factors. Adequate development of endometrial tissue during this phase is crucial for synchronization of the maturation process necessary for implantation during the secretory phase.

One of the key players during the proliferative phase is the rising estrogen. Estrogen induces the proliferation of cells and demonstrates an indirect effect by stimulating the expression of steroid receptors such as estrogen receptor α and β, androgen receptor, and progesterone receptor, which is crucial for progesterone action during the secretory phase.

9.2.2   The Secretory Phase

Progesterone, which suppresses proliferation and induces cell differentiation, is the major player during this second half of the menstrual cycle and acts at least partially via the progesterone receptor type A (PR A).

PR A acts as a repressor of PR B, which is the most transcriptionally active receptor. PR B is diminished in the glandular epithelial cells but is still present in the stroma. Therefore, the action of progesterone during the implantation window is most likely through stromal PR B.

Epithelial cells are characterized by their glandular secretory transformation. Stromal cell are characterized by their decidualization which is accompanied by the production and secretion of distinct decidual proteins such as prolactin and insulin-like growth factor binding protein 1 (IGFBP-1).

The endometrium in the mid- to late-secretory phase, as well as the decidua, is also infiltrated by a variety of bone marrow-derived immune cells. The predominant population constitutes decidual natural killer (NK) cells as well as T cells and macrophages. During the secretory phase, vascular remodelling occurs, with the main angiogenic mechanism being coiling and intussusception of the spiral arteries.

With these distinct morphological and biochemical changes, the endometrium is prepared for the implantation of the blastocyst. The embryo apposes and attaches to the endometrial epithelial cells and invades the endometrial stroma (Fig. 9.2).

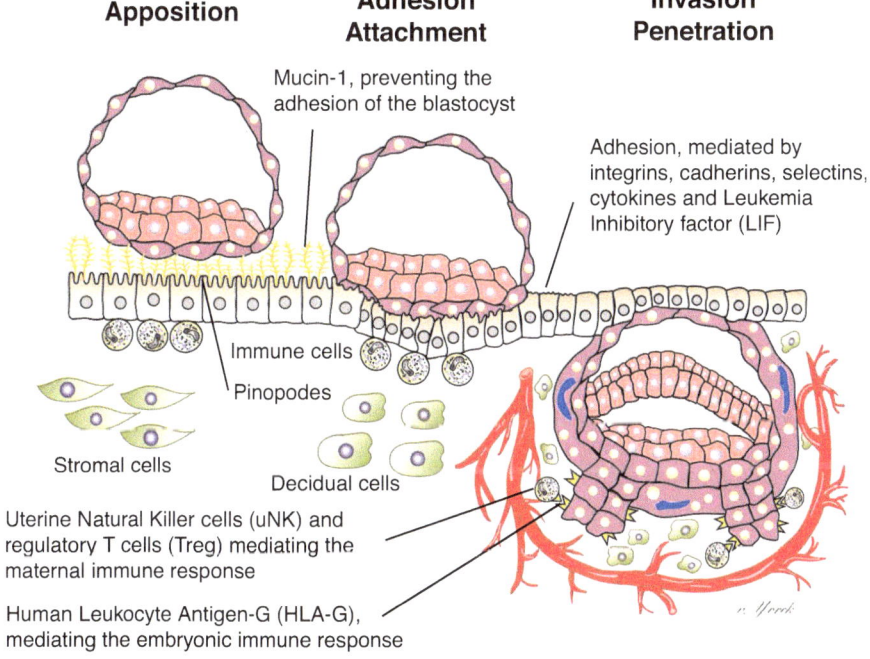

Fig. 9.2 Stages and regulation of implantation (according to [1])

9.2.3   Decidualization

Decidualization is the transformation of endometrial stromal into decidual cells. This process is initiated in the mid-secretory phase of each menstrual cycle as a result of elevated levels of progesterone.

Stromal differentiation and angiogenesis during decidualization are essential for the establishment and maintenance of pregnancy. Apart from the decidual stromal cells, the endometrium hosts a dynamic population of cells, including hematopoietic cells that can play a role in implantation, but also in the absence of pregnancy and menstruation. Macrophages, lymphocytes, and decidual leukocytes are also involved in decidualization.

Decidual leukocytes not only play a role in providing maternal immune tolerance but also contribute to decidual remodelling during pregnancy. Among these leukocytes, the uterine natural killer (uNK) cells are the most involved in the maternal immune tolerance. They are present in the human endometrium across the cycle and become activated and substantially increase during decidualization. They are abundant around spiral arteries, endometrial glands and adjacent to the growing conceptus to support the maternal blood supply. Monocytes are the second largest component of the leukocyte population in the decidua.

9.3   Implantation

Implantation can be divided into three different stages: Apposition, in which a first loose contact of the hatched blastocyst to the endometrium is established; adhesion/attachment, in which the blastocyst binds firmly to the luminal epithelium; and invasion/penetration, when the trophoblast cells invade the endometrium and when the placenta is formed (reviewed by Strowitzki et al. (2006) [1] and Ochoa-Bernal and Fazleabas (2020) [2]).

9.3.1   Apposition

The embryo arrives in the uterine cavity in the morula stage around 4 days after ovulation and develops into a blastocyst on day 5–6. The endometrium becomes receptive and thereby the window of implantation opens (around 6–9 days after ovulation).

Implantation starts with apposition (Fig. 9.2). Communication between the blastocyst and the endometrium is established, and the blastocyst connects loosely to the luminal endometrial epithelium.

The blastocyst is still not tightly connected with the endometrium. It encounters a glycocalyx associated with the luminal epithelium that contains different adhesion molecules. Part of the glycocalyx is the mucin MUC-1, an anti-adhesion molecule.

The purpose of MUC-1 at this stage is to prevent the blastocyst from binding to an area with poor chances of implantation.

The human embryo needs to align to the endometrium with the inner cell mass, the embryoblast, facing the endometrium to ensure a proper apposition. The apposition of the blastocyst is mediated by several molecules including the adhesion protein, L-selectin. Selectins interact with L-selectin ligands, which are mainly detected on pinopodes where blastocyst adhesion is initiated.

9.3.2   Adhesion/Attachment

Adhesion of the blastocyst is initiated by removal of the pre-existing endometrial layer of mucins. During the apposition stage, the presence of the blastocyst promotes the increase in MUC-1 levels in the luminal epithelium, but, at the beginning of the adhesion phase, the blastocyst induces the cleavage of MUC-1 at the implantation site to promote successful attachment (Fig. 9.2).

Several chemokines and cytokines are essential during the process of adhesion. One of their functions is to attract the blastocyst to the location of implantation. The most relevant is leukemia inhibitory factor, LIF. It is expressed by uterine luminal epithelium and epithelial pinopodes which also mediate implantation. In the human endometrium, expression of LIF reaches maximal levels during the mid-secretory phase. Adhesion molecules such as integrins are also necessary to attach the blastocyst to the pinopodes to ensure firm implantation. Among these integrins, $\alpha V\beta 3$ integrin is crucial for endometrial recognition. It is expressed in the human trophoblast cells and uterine luminal epithelium during implantation and participates in endometrial recognition.

9.3.3   Invasion/Penetration

Trophoblast cells infiltrate the luminal epithelium by developing invadopodia, which grow between adjacent endometrial epithelial cells. They degrade the basement membrane, allowing the trophoblast cells to spread into the endometrial stroma (Fig. 9.2).

The invasion of the semi-allogenic trophoblast requires a complex interaction of trophoblast cells and the maternal immune system at the feto-maternal interphase. One of the fetal key players in this interaction is human leukocyte antigen-G (HLA-G) which is expressed on invading extravillous trophoblast cells. The maternal immune response is mediated by T regulatory cells (Treg) which regulate alloreactive T helper 1 (Th1) cell subsets and a broad spectrum of immune response-associated mediators.

In humans, the embedding of the blastocyst within the stroma is completed around 8 days after ovulation. The implantation site is covered with fibrin.

Trophoblast cells from the implanting embryo further invade the endometrial stroma. The invasive trophoblast cells create the cytotrophoblast which produces high amounts of hCG, released into the blood 10 days after ovulation, and forms the placenta.

9.4   Dynamics of Endometrial Growth in Natural Cycles

Magaton et al. [3] analyzed the endometrial growth in 616 natural cycle IVF (NC-IVF) cycles within the last 5 days before follicle aspiration. They found that endometrium thickness increases by 0.58 mm per day (95% CI: 0.43–0.73) (Fig. 9.3).

Magaton et al. also analyzed the association of endometrial thickness and estrogen concentration. After multiple adjustments, linear regression analysis revealed a significant ($P < 0.01$) association between endometrial thickness and estradiol (E2) concentration (Coef. 0.19; 95% CI: 0.14, 0.24). Endometrium thickness increased by 0.19 mm per 100 pmol/L E2 (unpublished data).

However, even though the association of endometrial thickness and E2 concentration was highly significant, Fig. 9.4 demonstrates the high variability of endometrial thickness in relation to E2 concentration.

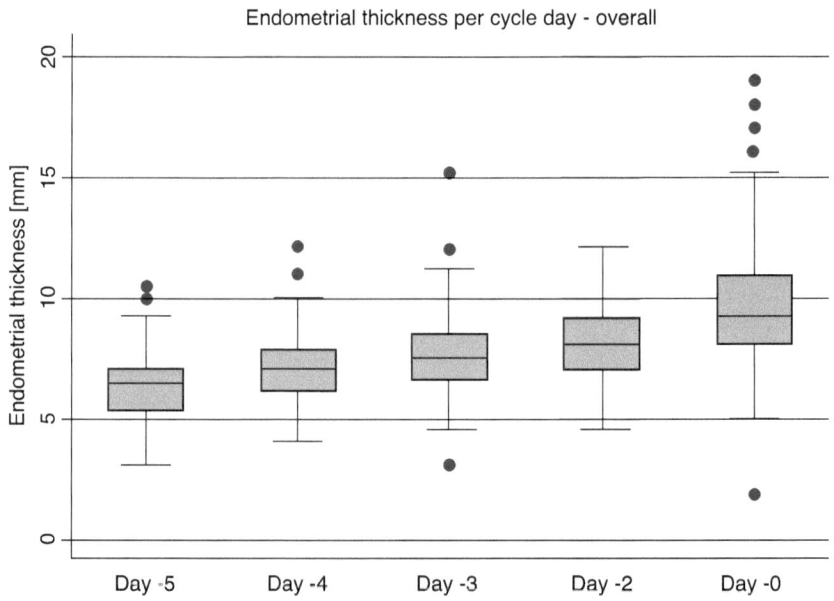

Fig. 9.3 Endometrial thickness per cycle day in natural cycles within the 5 days before follicle aspiration (Day 0 = day of follicle aspiration) (according to [3])

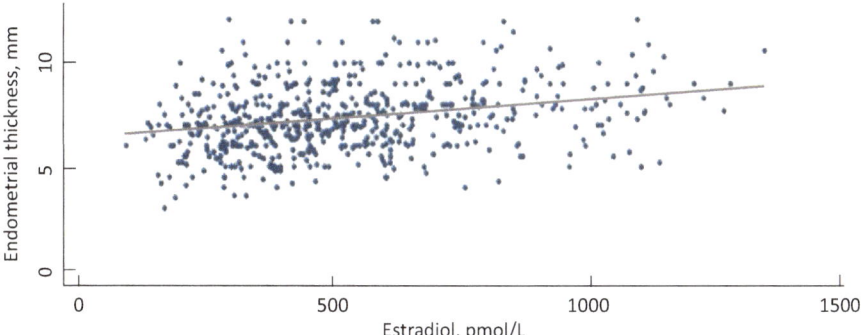

Fig. 9.4 Association of endometrial thickness and estradiol concentration and fitted values in women undergoing natural cycle IVF (according to [3])

Dynamics of endometrial growth is different in high-dose gonadotropin stimulation cycles (as in conventional IVF, cIVF) from natural cycles (as in NC-IVF). In cIVF, endometrial growth is accelerated at the beginning of the follicular phase due to the sharp gonadotropin induced increase of E2 concentration. However, in the last 5 days before follicle aspiration, endometrial growth is slower in cIVF (0.22 mm/day; 95% CI: −0.12, 0.55) compared to NC-IVF (0.58 mm/day; 95% CI: 0.43, 0.73) ($p = 0.034$). On day 2, when ovulation was triggered, mean endometrial thickness is slightly thicker in cIVF (9.75 ± 2.05 mm) compared to NC-IVF (8.12 ± 1.66 mm) [3].

9.5 Impact of Endometrial Thickness on Pregnancy Rate

The significance of the endometrial thickness has been investigated in numerous studies, mainly in high-dose gonadotropin stimulation (cIVF) and intrauterine insemination (IUI) treatments with different ovarian stimulation regimes.

In cIVF treatments, a thin endometrium is associated with lower pregnancy rates. The clinical pregnancy rate is clearly reduced at an endometrial thickness of ≤7 mm (OR 0.42, 95% CI: 0.27, 0.67) [4].

In women undergoing IUI with low-dose gonadotropin stimulation, such a relationship does not appear to exist. In a meta-analysis with IUI treatments combined with gonadotropin, clomiphene citrate, or aromatase inhibitor stimulation, there was no evidence of a difference in endometrial thickness between women who conceived and women who did not conceive (MDrandom: 0.51; 95% CI: −0.05, 1.07) [5].

Von Wolff et al. 2018 [6] analyzed the association of endometrial thickness with pregnancy rate in NC-IVF. 105 women with regular menstrual cycles undergoing their first NC-IVF cycle with embryo transfer were studied (Fig. 9.5). Clinical pregnancy and live birth rates were calculated, and data was adjusted for women's age, cycle day of follicle aspiration, and body mass index (BMI).

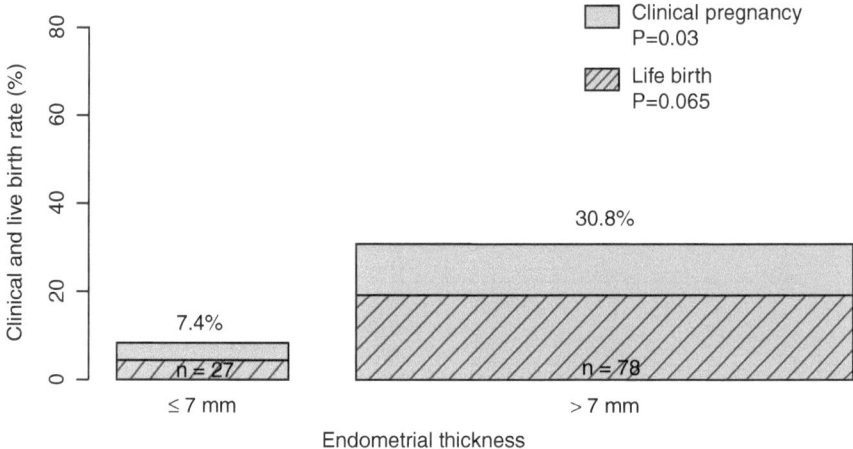

Fig. 9.5 Clinical pregnancy rate (not hatched) and live birth rate (hatched) in women with endometrial thickness ≤7 mm versus >7 mm undergoing natural cycle IVF. The bar width is proportional to the number of women in each category. Clinical pregnancy rate was significantly lower in women with endometrial thickness ≤7 mm (Reprint with permission from [6])

Pregnancy rate in women with endometrial thickness ≤7 mm ($n = 27$) was 7.4% and 30.8% in women >7 mm ($n = 78$) (OR 5.56; 95% CI: 1.22, 25.36) ($p = 0.03$). Live birth rates were not significantly different. Quadratic regression analysis revealed lower pregnancy rates in women with thin as well as with thick endometria. P-value after crude quadratic analysis was 0.028 and after adjustment for age, day of aspiration, and BMI was 0.039. Significance was not reached for live birth rates.

9.6   Impact of Clomiphene and Letrozole Stimulation on Endometrial Thickness

Several minimal stimulation IVF protocols involve clomiphene citrate and letrozole stimulation (see Chap. 15). The advantage of both medications is the increased oocyte yield compared to NC-IVF [7], without requiring expensive gonadotropin injections. However, both medications can also reduce endometrial thickness [8] which might be a matter of concern as thin endometrium is associated with lower pregnancy rates as described above.

Clomiphene citrate is a selective estrogen receptor modulator, SERM. SERMs bind to endometrial estrogen receptors and have tissue-specific effects that allow them to function as estrogen agonists in some tissues and estrogen antagonists in other tissues. In human endometrium, clomiphene reduces its thickness [7, 8], has an effect on estrogen regulated molecular pathways [9], and apparently delays its maturation [10].

Letrozole reduces estrogen concentration by reducing the activity of aromatase in endometrium and in follicles.

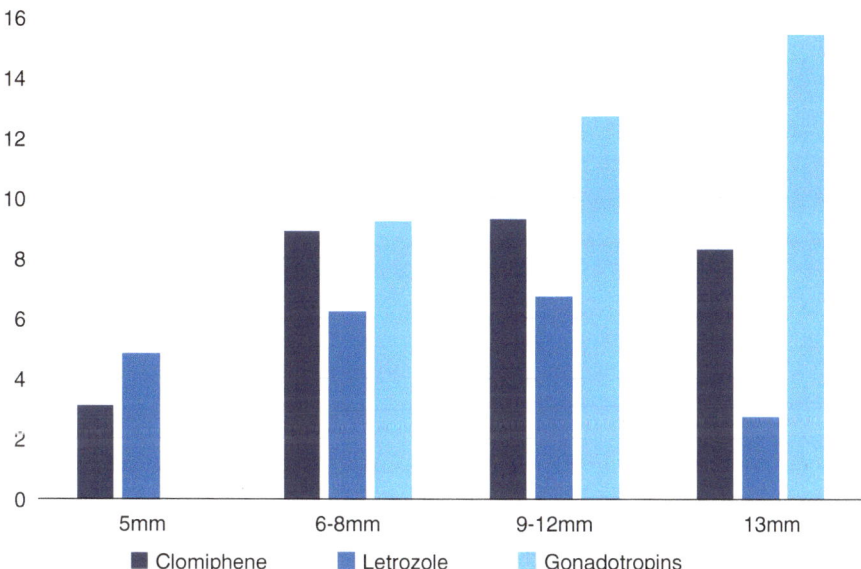

Fig. 9.6 Live birth rates (y-axis, %) in relation to endometrial thickness in 2459 treatment cycles, in which patients were treated with gonadotropins, clomiphene citrate, or letrozole, followed by intrauterine insemination (AMIGOS clinical trial) (according to [8])

According to a meta-analysis [11], endometrium thinning is more pronounced in clomiphene citrate stimulations than in letrozole stimulations (weighted mean difference −1.39; 95% CI: −2.27 to −0.51).

Absolute numbers were prepared by a subanalysis of the AMIGOS clinical trial. 2459 treatment cycles, in which patients were treated with gonadotropins, clomiphene citrate, or letrozole, followed by intrauterine insemination, were compared [8] (Fig. 9.6). The mean endometrium thickness was 10.6 mm (95% CI: 10.4–10.9) in gonadotropin stimulated cycles, 8.0 mm (95% CI: 7.7–8.2) in clomiphene citrate stimulated cycles, and 8.5 mm (95% CI: 8.3–8.7) in letrozole stimulated cycles ($P < 0.0001$ for the pairwise comparison of clomiphene versus gonadotropin, $p < 0.0001$ for letrozole versus gonadotropin, $p = 0.002$ for clomiphene versus letrozole).

Quaas et al. (2020) [8] revealed a reduced live birth rate in women with a thin endometrium for all different treatments (Fig. 9.6). However, this difference was not significant.

Von Wolff et al. (2014) [7] compared endometrial thickness in natural cycle IVF cycles without versus natural cycle IVF cycles with low doses (25 mg) of clomiphene citrate per day until the day of ovulation triggering. They also found a reduced endometrial thickness (8.4 ± 1.7 mm versus 7.9 ± 1.6 mm) but the difference was rather small and not significant (Table 9.1).

What are the consequences of these findings in clinical practice? Even though not based on solid statistical evaluations, it seems clinically plausible in minimal stimulation IVF therapies

Table 9.1 Clinical pregnancies per transferred embryo in women undergoing NC-IVF without and with clomiphene citrate (CC) at a dosage of 25 mg per day, starting on day 5–7 of the cycle and given until the day of ovulation trigger (according to [12])

NC-IVF protocol	RR	p-value	95% CI
NC-IVF	1		
NC-IVF +CC (crude)	1.19	0.21	0.90–1.58
NC-IVF +CC (adjusted[a])	1.16	0.27	0.90–1.50

[a] Adjusted for age, parity, duration of subfertility, primary/secondary infertility, cause of infertility

- to start the treatment with a diagnostic cycle or a NC-IVF cycle to define the physiological endometrial thickness,
- not to treat women with a physiologically thin endometrium with clomiphene citrate or letrozole but rather with low dose gonadotropins,
- to change the treatment regime from clomiphene citrate to letrozole or gonadotropins in women who develop a thin endometrium under clomiphene treatment, and
- to avoid high dosages of clomiphene citrate.

These principles are part of the indications for specific IVF treatments as described in the Chap. 15.

9.7 Impact of Clomiphene on Implantation

In the above chapters, it was stated that thin endometrium is associated with lower pregnancy and live birth rates. It was also stated that clomiphene, especially at higher dosages, reduces endometrial thickness and has tissue-specific effects which might negatively affect implantation.

To analyze if clomiphene, at a low dosage of 25 mg clomiphene citrate per day, starting on day 5–7 of the cycle and given until the day of ovulation trigger [7] reduces implantation rates, Grädel et al. [12] performed the following study:

499 couples underwent a total of 1043 NC-IVF cycles, 453 without and 590 with clomiphene. A total of 1175 embryos were transferred. Both groups were not different regarding female age and infertility characteristics. No statistically significant difference between the cycles treated without and with clomiphene could be observed, demonstrating that clomiphene at low dosages does not negatively affect embryo implantation (Table 9.1).

9.8 Impact of Supraphysiological Estradiol Concentration on Endometrial Function

Several studies have revealed that children born after IVF treatments with supraphysiological estradiol (E2) concentration have a lower birth weight [13, 14] (see Chap. 21). It is assumed that supraphysiological E2 concentrations have an effect on endometrial function and placentation, creating some degree of placental dysfunction and insufficiency.

Indeed, Bonagura et al. (2008) [15], showed a negative effect of high E2 on placental extravillous trophoblast (EVT) invasion and remodelling of the uterine spiral arteries in baboons. Bonagura et al. (2012) [16] also revealed a suppression of uterine artery remodelling and expression of extravillous placental vascular endothelial growth factor (VEGF) as well as of $\alpha 1\beta 1$ and $\alpha 5\beta 1$ integrins in baboons. A negatively affected trophoblast differentiation distribution of cell types in the placenta was also shown in mice [17].

In humans, in vitro experiments provided evidence of a negative impact of this supraphysiological E2 effect. Chou et al. (2020) [18] found mitochondrial dysfunction in endometrial epithelial cells, and Cottrell et al. (2019) [19] described effects of supraphysiologic levels of E2 on endometrial decidualization, sFlt1, and HOXA10 expression.

Assisted reproductive technologies, ART (IVF and IUI) have also been associated with an increased risk of pregnancy-induced hypertension (RR 1.30, 95% CI: 1.04–1.62) [20] which is supposed to be due to endometrial and placental dysfunction. It has been speculated that these disorders are also induced by supraphysiological E2 concentration [21]. However, it cannot be excluded that the above shown increased risk of pregnancy-induced hypertension in ART therapies is not only due to supraphysiological E2 concentration, but also due to the transfer of frozen embryos in HRT substituted (HRT = hormone replacement treatment) cycles. Such thawing cycles, which are included in the meta-analysis by Quin et al., 2016 [20], have clearly been shown to be a clinically relevant risk factor for hypertensive disorders, preeclampsia, and other pregnancy related risks [22]. The increased risk of hypertensive disorders seems to be due to the missing luteal body in HRT thawing cycles. The luteal body apparently has some still unknown effects on the function of the endometrium and the placenta.

Even though several studies indicate a negative effect of supraphysiological E2 concentration on endometrial and placental function, it is not known if this effect also has an impact on the health of the children (see Chap. 21).

9.9 Impact of Pre-ovulatory Progesterone Increase on Endometrial Function

As described in Chapter "Endocrinology of naturally matured follicles compared to stimulated follicles" in Chap. 5, high-dose gonadotropin stimulation can lead to preovulatory progesterone increase in around 35% (5–35%) of gonadotropin stimulated cycles. Patients with serum progesterone concentrations >1.5 ng/mL (>4.8 pmol/L) versus lower progesterone concentrations on the day of the hCG trigger have a lower pregnancy rate (19.1 versus 31.0%, $p = 0.00006$) according to a large study published by Bosch et al. (2010) [23]. It is speculated that this effect is due to an FSH induced overproduction of pregnenolone in granulosa cells, which is converted to progesterone as the steroidogenesis in theca cells in slowed down by GnRH analogues induced LH decrease.

As a result, endometrium is transformed too early resulting in a dys-synchronization of the endometrial and the embryo development and thereby to lower pregnancy rates.

It can be assumed that such an effect does not occur in NC-IVF and minimal stimulation IVF. Therefore, the recently published data revealing a higher implantation potential of embryos derived from NC-IVF compared to conventional IVF leading to 1.4-fold higher live birth rates (see Chap. 7, Table 7.3) might not only be a result of better oocyte quality due to natural follicle selection or better functioning endometrium due to physiological E2 concentrations but also due to cycles without such a detrimental pre-ovulatory progesterone increase.

9.10   Increasing Estrogen Concentration to Increase Endometrial Thickness?

As described above, in gonadotropin stimulated IVF and in NC-IVF cycles, an endometrial thickness of ≤ 7 mm is associated with a lower pregnancy rate. It has also been shown that endometrial thickness is reduced by clomiphene citrate and by letrozole, both of which are used in minimal stimulation IVF therapies (see Chap. 15).

This raises the question of whether endometrial thickness can be increased by higher estrogen concentrations, thereby improving pregnancy and live birth rates. In a natural cycle, supplementation with estrogens, e.g., with estrogen patches is not possible because of the feedback effect of estrogen on LH release (see Chap. 6). However, additional gonadotropin stimulation would be possible. With gonadotropin stimulation, it should be noted that higher E2 concentrations can lead to premature LH peaks, and additional GnRH antagonists may have to be administered. As GnRH antagonists also reduce the pituitary FSH release, gonadotropins need to be added if GnRH antagonists are given for more than one day.

Magaton et al. performed retrospective, cross-sectional studies and compared inter- and intraindividually the endometrial thickness,

firstly in women undergoing NC-IVF and conventional high-dose gonadotropin stimulated IVF (cIVF) (Magaton et al. [3]), and

secondly in minimal stimulation IVF with clomiphene citrate (clomiphene-IVF) and minimal stimulation IVF with clomiphene citrate plus low dose human menopausal gonadotropins (HMG) (Clomiphene+HMG-IVF) (Magaton et al. (2022) [24]).

The analysis revealed that endometrium was thicker in women undergoing IVF with high E2 concentrations. They found on the day of hCG triggering:

- In NC-IVF, endometrium thickness was 8.12 ± 1.66 mm with E2 concentration of 814 ± 220 pmol/L. In contrast, in cIVF thickness increased to

9.75 ± 2.05 mm with E2 concentration of 8.094 ± 5.366 pmol/L (both $p < 0.001$) [3].

- In clomiphene-IVF, endometrium thickness was 9.20 ± 2.52 mm with E2 concentration of 1.705 ± 643 pmol/L. In clomiphene+HMG-IVF, thickness increased to 10.5 ± 2.47 mm with E2 concentration of 2.527 ± 1431 pmol/L (both $p < 0.001$) [24].

Pregnancy and birth rates were also compared to analyze if the increased thickness is also associated with higher success rates. To allow comparison with cIVF treatments, only those cycles were considered which were performed before embryo selection was introduced in Switzerland in 2017.

- In NC-IVF, clinical implantation rate per embryo, transferred on day 2/3, was 15.4%. In cIVF, clinical implantation rate was 19.1% ($p > 0.05$) [3].
- In clomiphene-IVF, clinical implantation rate per embryo, transferred on day 2/3, was 13.7%. In clomiphene +HMG-IVF, clinical implantation rate was 12.7% ($p > 0.05$) [23].

Accordingly, clinical pregnancy rates were not different, indicating that artificially thickened endometrium by additional gonadotropin stimulation leads to thicker endometrium but without any effects on implantation rates.

This confirms that naturally proliferated and transformed endometrium can be seen as the optimum and cannot be improved.

9.11 Relevance of Adjuvants to Improve Implantation

Many adjuvants such as immune therapies, endometrial scratching, endometrial receptivity array, uterine artery vasodilation, and installation of hCG into the uterine cavity, etc. have been suggested and studied to improve implantation. These adjuvants were studied in the context of cIVF treatments [25]. As shown above, the endometrium is altered in cIVF, so these adjuvants are an attempt to reduce the collateral damage of high-dose gonadotropin stimulation.

It can be assumed that such treatments are not effective in a NC-IVF, since a naturally proliferated and transformed endometrium is not or is hardly impaired in its function or at least cannot be improved. Because of this, such adjuvants have not yet been investigated in NC-IVF.

References

1. Strowitzki T, Germeyer A, Popovici R, von Wolff M. The human endometrium as a fertility-determining factor. Hum Reprod Update. 2006;12:617–30.
2. Ochoa-Bernal MA, Fazleabas AT. Physiologic Events of Embryo Implantation and Decidualization in Human and Non-Human Primates. Int J Mol Sci. 2020;21:1973.

3. Magaton IM, Helmer A, Roumet M, Stute P, von Wolff M. High dose gonadotropin stimulation increases endometrial thickness but this gonadotropin stimulation induced thickening does not have an effect on implantation. J Gynecol Obstet Hum Reprod. in press.

4. Kasius A, Smit JG, Torrance HL, Eijkemans MJ, Mol BW, Opmeer BC, Broekmans FJ. Endometrial thickness and pregnancy rates after IVF: a systematic review and meta-analysis. Hum Reprod Update. 2014;20:530–41.

5. Weiss NS, van Vliet MN, Limpens J, Hompes PGA, Lambalk CB. Endometrial thickness in women undergoing IUI with ovarian stimulation. How thick is too thin? A systematic review and meta-analysis. Hum Reprod. 2017;32:1009–18.

6. von Wolff M, Fäh M, Roumet M, Mitter V, Stute P, Griesinger G, Kohl SA. Thin endometrium is also associated with lower clinical pregnancy rate in unstimulated menstrual cycles: a study based on natural cycle IVF. Front Endocrinol (Lausanne). 2018;9:776. https://doi.org/10.3389/fendo.2018.00776.

7. von Wolff M, Nitzschke M, Stute P, Bitterlich N, Rohner S. Low-dosage clomiphene reduces premature ovulation rates and increases transfer rates in natural-cycle IVF. Reprod Biomed Online. 2014;29:209–15.

8. Quaas AM, Gavrizi SZ, Peck JD, Diamond MP, Legro RS, Robinson RD, Casson P, Christman GM, Zhang H, Hansen KR, Eunice Kennedy Shriver National Institute of Child Health and Human Development Reproductive Medicine Network. Endometrial thickness after ovarian stimulation with gonadotropin, clomiphene, or letrozole for unexplained infertility, and association with treatment outcomes. Fertil Steril. 2021;115:213–20.

9. Mehdinejadiani S, Amidi F, Mehdizadeh M, Barati M, Safdarian L, Aflatoonian R, Alyasin A, Aghahosseini M, Pazhohan A, Hayat P, Mohammadzadeh Kazorgah F, Sobhani A. The effects of letrozole and clomiphene citrate on ligands expression of Wnt3, Wnt7a, and Wnt8b in proliferative endometrium of women with Polycystic ovarian syndrome. Gynecol Endocrinol. 2018;34:775–80.

10. Montenegro IS, Kuhl CP, Schneider RA, Zachia SA, Durli ICLO, Terraciano PB, Rivero RC, Passos EP. Use of clomiphene citrate protocol for controlled ovarian stimulation impairs endometrial maturity. JBRA Assist Reprod. 2021;25:90–6.

11. Gadalla MA, Huang S, Wang R, Norman RJ, Abdullah SA, El Saman AM, Ismail AM, van Wely M, Mol BWJ. Effect of clomiphene citrate on endometrial thickness, ovulation, pregnancy and live birth in anovulatory women: systematic review and meta-analysis. Ultrasound Obstet Gynecol. 2018;51:64–76.

12. Grädel F, Mitter VR, Kohl Schwartz AS, von Wolff M. Low dose clomiphene citrate does not reduce implantation rates - a cohort study based on modified Natural Cycle IVF. Hum Reprod. 2022 (Suppl 1), in press.

13. Kamath MS, Kirubakaran R, Mascarenhas M, Sunkara SK. Perinatal outcomes after stimulated versus natural cycle IVF: a systematic review and meta-analysis. Reprod Biomed Online. 2018;36:94–101.

14. Kohl Schwartz AS, Mitter VR, Amylidi-Mohr S, Fasel P, Minger MA, Limoni C, Zwahlen M, von Wolff M. The greater incidence of small-for-gestational-age newborns after gonadotropin-stimulated in vitro fertilization with a supraphysiological estradiol level on ovulation trigger day. Acta Obstet Gynecol Scand. 2019;98:1575–84.

15. Bonagura TW, Pepe GJ, Enders AC, Albrecht ED. Suppression of extravillous trophoblast vascular endothelial growth factor expression and uterine spiral artery invasion by estrogen during early baboon pregnancy. Endocrinology. 2008;149:5078–87.

16. Bonagura TW, Babischkin JS, Aberdeen GW, Pepe GJ, Albrecht ED. Prematurely elevating estradiol in early baboon pregnancy suppresses uterine artery remodeling and expression of extravillous placental vascular endothelial growth factor and $\alpha 1 \beta 1$ and $\alpha 5 \beta 1$ integrins. Endocrinology. 2012;153:2897–906.

17. Mainigi MA, Olalere D, Burd I, Sapienza C, Bartolomei M, Coutifaris C. Peri-implantation hormonal milieu: elucidating mechanisms of abnormal placentation and fetal growth. Biol Reprod. 2014;90:26.

18. Chou CH, Chen SU, Chen CD, Shun CT, Wen WF, Tu YA, Yang JH. Mitochondrial dysfunction induced by high estradiol concentrations in endometrial epithelial cells. J Clin Endocrinol Metab. 2020;105:dgz015.
19. Cottrell HN, Deepak V, Spencer JB, Sidell N, Rajakumar A. Effects of supraphysiologic levels of estradiol on endometrial decidualization, sFlt1, and HOXA10 expression. Reprod Sci. 2019;26:1626–32.
20. Qin J, Liu X, Sheng X, Wang H, Gao S. Assisted reproductive technology and the risk of pregnancy-related complications and adverse pregnancy outcomes in singleton pregnancies: a meta-analysis of cohort studies. Fertil Steril. 2016;105:73–85.e1-6.
21. Imudia AN, Awonuga AO, Doyle JO, Kaimal AJ, Wright DL, Toth TL, Styer AK. Peak serum estradiol level during controlled ovarian hyperstimulation is associated with increased risk of small for gestational age and preeclampsia in singleton pregnancies after in vitro fertilization. Fertil Steril. 2012;97:1374–9.
22. Moreno-Sepulveda J, Espinós JJ, Checa MA. Lower risk of adverse perinatal outcomes in natural versus artificial frozen-thawed embryo transfer cycles: a systematic review and meta-analysis. Reprod Biomed Online. 2021;42.1131–45.
23. Bosch E, Labarta E, Crespo J, Simón C, Remohí J, Jenkins J, Pellicer A. Circulating progesterone levels and ongoing pregnancy rates in controlled ovarian stimulation cycles for in vitro fertilization: analysis of over 4000 cycles. Hum Reprod. 2010;25:2092–100.
24. Magaton I, Helmer A, Roumet M, Stute P, von Wolff M. Clomiphene citrate stimulated cycles - additional gonadotrophin stimulation increases endometrial thickness without increasing implantation rate. Facts Views Vis Obgyn. 2022;14:77–81.
25. Lensen S, Shreeve N, Barnhart KT, Gibreel A, Ng EHY, Moffett A. In vitro fertilization add-ons for the endometrium: it doesn't add-up. Fertil Steril. 2019;112:987–93.

Part III
Clinical Practice

Chapter 10
Timing of Aspiration in Natural Cycle and Minimal Stimulation IVF

Michael von Wolff

10.1 Background

Timing of aspiration is essential in IVF treatments. If follicular aspiration is performed too early, the oocytes will be immature. If the follicular aspiration is performed too late, the follicles might already have ovulated or have become too large. Therefore, in natural cycle IVF (NC-IVF), aspiration should be timed just before the expected time of natural ovulation, and in minimal stimulation, aspiration should be timed when the size of the follicles provides the highest chance to retrieve as many mature oocytes as possible.

10.2 Timing According to Follicle Size

The follicle size plays the most important role in the timing of the follicular aspiration. It is equally important for all IVF therapies.

10.2.1 Follicle Size in Conventional IVF

A large number of studies have investigated the relevance of follicle size in conventional IVF with high-dose gonadotropin stimulation. Although the data from these studies can only be transferred to NC-IVF and minimal stimulation IVF to a limited

M. von Wolff (✉)
Division of Gynecological Endocrinology and Reproductive Medicine, University Women's Hospital, University of Bern, Bern, Switzerland
e-mail: Michael.vonwolff@insel.ch

© The Author(s), under exclusive license to Springer Nature Switzerland AG 2022   93
M. von Wolff (ed.), *Natural Cycle and Minimal Stimulation IVF*,
https://doi.org/10.1007/978-3-030-97571-5_10

Table 10.1 Overview of the relevance of follicle size for success rates in different IVF therapies

	Conventional IVF	Natural cycle IVF	Minimal stimulation IVF
Small follicles	Follicles <13 mm: Oocyte retrieval rate reduced. Oocyte maturity rate reduced. Embryo development rate and IVF pregnancy rate per fertilized oocyte not reduced. [1, 2]	Follicles <16 mm: Oocyte retrieval rate reduced.[a] Oocyte maturity rate reduced.[a] Embryo development rate and pregnancy rate per fertilized oocyte not reduced. [3]	
Large follicles	Follicles >23 mm: Oocyte retrieval rate not reduced. Oocyte maturity rate not reduced. Embryo development rate and IVF pregnancy rate not reduced. [1, 7, 8]	Follicles >20 mm: Oocyte retrieval rate slightly reduced.[a] Oocyte maturity rate not reduced.[a] Embryo development rate and IVF pregnancy rate not reduced. [3]	Data only available for clomiphene-stimulated intrauterine inseminations: Follicles > ca. 20 mm: Pregnancy rate higher. [4–6]

[a] Further information regarding significance of data see text

extent, the studies nevertheless provide important information for all kind of IVF therapies.

The studies show that mature (metaphase II, MII) and functioning oocytes can also be retrieved from rather small follicles (Table 10.1).

However, the chance of aspirating mature oocytes from small follicles is reduced. According to Wirtleitner et al. (2018) [1], cumulus oophorus complexes (COC) can be obtained from 63.8% of follicles with a size of 8–12 mm, 59.2% of these COCs contain mature oocytes. This means that mature oocytes can only be obtained from 38% of follicles <13 mm. In follicles of 13–23 mm, mature oocytes can be obtained in 64.0% and in follicles of >23 mm in 70.1%.

It can be assumed that the lower limit of follicle size to obtain mature oocytes is approx. 12 mm since LH receptors are expressed on granulosa cells in follicles ≥12 mm (see Chap. 6). Only then resumption of meiosis and cumulus expansion can be induced by the LH surge.

In monofollicular cycles such as NC-IVF, aspiration of small follicles can possibly lead to luteal phase insufficiency. If the follicle in small, the luteal body will also be small and therefore progesterone production will possibly be insufficient. Because of this, pregnancy rate could be reduced after the aspiration of a small follicle in a monofollicular cycles. Therefore, luteal phase supplementation is recommended in such cases.

The chance of aspirating mature oocytes from large follicles, however, does not seem to be reduced (Table 10.1). According to Ectors et al. (1997) [7], Wirtleitner et al. (2018) [1], and Orvieto et al. (2020) [8], the pregnancy potential of oocytes retrieved from follicles > 23 mm is not reduced.

However, it need to be noted that in monofollicular cycles such as in NC-IVF, large follicles might either be dysfunctional follicles or cysts (see Chap. 5). As dysfunctional follicles produce less estradiol (E2), LH surge is delayed, and dysfunctional follicles can become quite large.

10.2.2 Follicle Size in NC-IVF

Helmer et al. [3] have investigated the relevance of follicle size in NC-IVF and have thus been able to show which parameters are associated with higher pregnancy rate.

In a first step they calculated whether there is an association of follicle size with oocyte retrieval rate. It was shown that for every 1 mm increase in follicle size, the chance of retrieving an oocyte increases (non-significantly) by 10% (Table 10.2). The chance to retrieve oocytes is reduced for follicles <16 mm. The chance to retrieve an oocyte is approx. 75% for follicles of 14–15 mm in size compared to approx. 85% for 18–20 mm follicles (Fig. 10.1, Table 10.2).

In a second step, they calculated whether there is an association between follicle size and the probability of obtaining mature oocytes (metaphase II, MII). It was calculated that with an increase in follicle size of 1 mm, the chance of obtaining a mature oocyte significantly increased by 24% (Table 10.2). The chance of an aspirated oocyte being mature was found to be approx. 85% for follicles of 14–15 mm in size, compared to approx. 95% for 18–20 mm follicles (Table 10.3).

Overall, this means that the chance of retrieving a mature oocyte is 63% for follicles 14–15 mm in size, and approx. 80% for 18–20 mm follicles (Fig. 10.1).

Table 10.2 Natural cycle IVF: Association of outcome parameters with follicle size and estradiol (E2) concentration within the last 5 days before follicular aspiration. Adjusted for age, cause of infertility, and number of previous embryo transfers without pregnancy [3]

Per cycle	Per 1 mm increase of follicle size (95% CI)	p-value	Per 100 pmol/L (27.4 ng/mL) increase of E2 concentration (95% CI)	p-value	Interaction of both parameters	p-value
Number of oocytes	1.10 (0.87;1.38)	0.424	1.80 (1.05;3.11)	0.034	0.97 (0.94;1.00)	0.060
Number of mature (MII) oocytes	1.24 (1.01;1.53)	0.037	1.84 (1.15;2.94)	0.012	0.96 (0.94;0.99)	0.017
Number of clinical pregnancies	1.14 (0.80;1.62)	0.456	1.10 (0.47;2.60)	0.826	0.99 (0.95;1.04)	0.827
Number of live births	1.15 (0.76;1.74)	0.495	1.17 (0.47;2.94)	0.730	0.99 (0.94;1.05)	0.763

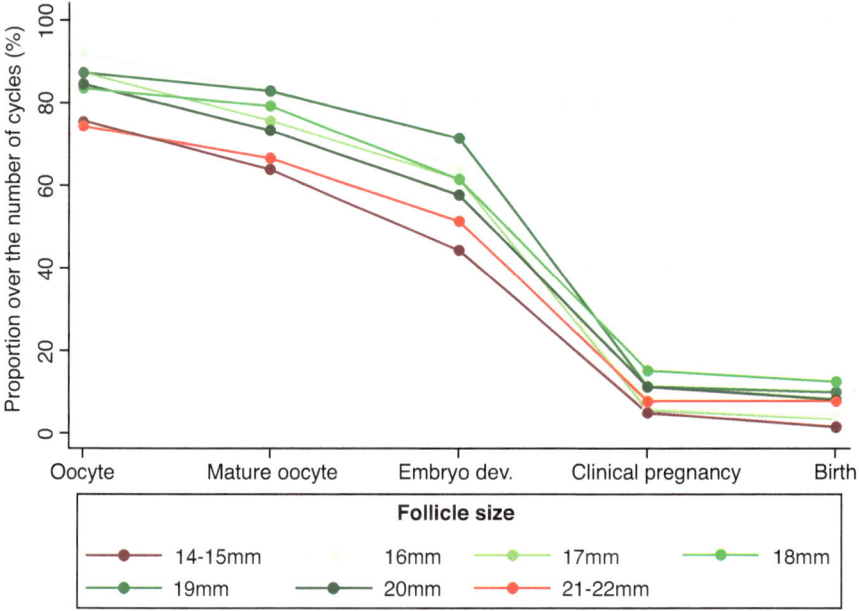

Fig. 10.1 Association of follicle size with outcome parameters such as oocyte collection rate (Oocyte) maturity of oocytes (Mature oocyte), embryo development rate (Embryo dev.), and clinical pregnancy (Clinical pregnancy) and live birth rate (Birth) (according to [3])

Table 10.3 Natural cycle IVF: Outcome in relation to follicles size (according to [3])

Follicle diameter (day of aspiration)	Number of analysed cycles	Oocyte collection rate per aspiration (95% CI)	Oocyte MII rate per aspirated oocyte	Embryo development rate per MII oocyte	Clinical pregnancy rate per transferred embryo	Live birth rate per transferred embryo
14–15 mm	61	75.4% (63.3;84.5)	84.8% (71.8;92.4)	69.2% (53.6;81.4)	12.5% (4.3;31.0)	4.2% (0.7;20.2)
16 mm	47	91.5% (80.1;96.6)	90.7% (78.4;96.3)	76.9% (61.7;87.4)	10.3% (3.6;26.4)	6.9% (1.9;22.0)
17 mm	86	87.2% (78.5;92.7)	86.7% (77.2;92.6)	80.0% (68.7;87.9)	9.6% (4.2;20.6)	5.8% 2.0;15.6)
18 mm	72	83.3% (73,1;90.2)	95.0% (86.3;98.3)	77.2% (64.8;86.2)	25.0% (14.6;39.4)	20.5% (11.2;34.5)
19 mm	70	87.1% (77.3;93.1)	95.1% (86.5;98.3)	84.5% (73.1;91.6)	16.3% (8.5;29.0)	14.3% (7.1;26.7)
20 mm	71	84.5% (74.3;91.1)	86.7% (75.8;93.1)	78.8% (66.0;87.8)	20.0% (10.4;34.8)	15.0% (7.1;29.1)
21–22 mm	39	74.4% (58.9;85.4)	89.7% (73.6;96.4)	76.9% (57.9;89.0)	15.8% (5.5;37.6)	15.8% (5.3;37.6)

Overall, the chance of generating a clinical pregnancy when aspirating a 14–15 mm follicle is only about 5% compared to 10–15% when aspirating a 18–20 mm follicle (Table 10.3).

Helmer et al. [3] also evaluated the outcome of aspiration of larger follicles. Since the follicles in NC-IVF cannot become as large as in conventional IVF, only follicles with a maximum size of 21–22 mm were analysed. The evaluation showed that the oocyte retrieval rate is slightly reduced, but not the rate of mature oocytes and embryos (Fig. 10.1, Table 10.3).

10.2.3   Follicle Size in Minimal Stimulation IVF

Detailed data on the relevance of follicle size in minimal stimulation IVF is not available. It can be assumed that in the case of a monofollicular ovarian response, the data from NC-IVF and, in the case of an oligofollicular response, the data from conventional IVF apply.

However, there are studies that have investigated the importance of follicle size in clomiphene-stimulated intrauterine insemination treatments [4–6]. This data is also relevant for the use of clomiphene in NC-IVF or minimal stimulation IVF (see Chap. 15).

The studies show that clinical pregnancy rate is increased if the leading follicle at the time of ovulation induction is approx. >20 mm in size (Fig. 10.2). It was speculated that this is due to higher E2 concentration leading to better endometrial proliferation. Hancock et al. (2020) [6] showed, however, that endometrial thickness is only a poor predictor for clinical pregnancy in intrauterine inseminations. Indeed, a meta-analysis [9] found no evidence for an association between endometrial thickness and clinical pregnancy rate in clomiphene-stimulated intrauterine insemination cycles.

This is in line with a study which showed that implantation rate could not be increased in clomiphene-stimulated IVF therapies by additional gonadotropin stimulation with higher E2 concentrations [10].

In summary,

pregnancy rate is highest when follicles ≥ 16 mm are aspirated. However, the chance to retrieve mature oocytes and to achieve a pregnancy is also given if smaller follicles are aspirated.

10.3   Timing According to E2 Level

The estradiol (E2) concentration plays an important role as a parameter for the timing of follicular aspiration in both NC-IVF and minimal stimulation IVF therapy. In conventional IVF, however, the E2 concentration is mainly used as a marker for the ovarian response.

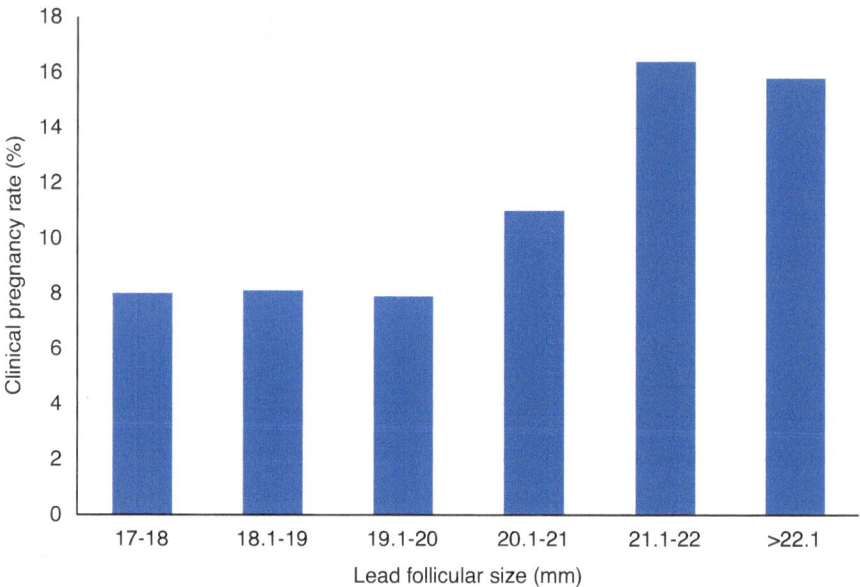

Fig. 10.2 Clinical pregnancy rate stratified by lead follicular size in clomiphene citrate-stimulated intrauterine inseminations (according to [6])

10.3.1 E2 Level in Conventional IVF

In conventional IVF, it has been shown that with >15–20 oocytes retrieved, the cumulative pregnancy rate does not increase further and the pregnancy rate per fresh transfer even decreases [11]. One of the causes could be a dysfunctional endometrium due to very high E2 concentrations. This theory is in line with studies which showed lower birth weight of children born after IVF therapies with high E2 concentrations, probably due to dysfunctional endometrium (see Chaps. 20 and 21). However, no conclusions can be drawn from these studies regarding the timing of follicular aspiration in NC-IVF and minimal stimulation IVF.

10.3.2 E2 Level in NC-IVF

The relevance of the E2 concentration was examined by Helmer et al. [3]. They analysed if the E2 concentration is associated with the probability of obtaining an oocyte. Helmer et al. [3] showed that, within the last 5 days before follicle aspiration, for every 100 pmol increased E2 concentration, the probability of retrieving an oocyte increases significantly by 80% (Table 10.2). The probability of obtaining a mature oocyte also increases with increasing E2 concentration by 84% per 100 pmol increased E2 concentration.

This data shows that in natural cycles, the level of E2 concentration seems to be more relevant than the follicle size. The study also showed that both parameters, follicle size and E2 concentration, interact with one another in terms of the likelihood of obtaining a mature oocyte.

In clinical practice, this means that follicles as small as 13-14mm can be considered to be aspirated if E2 concentration is high enough.

10.3.3   E2 Level in Minimal Stimulation IVF

Detailed data on the relevance of the E2 concentration in minimal stimulation IVF is not available. It can be assumed that in the case of a monofollicular ovarian response, the data from NC-IVF and, in the case of an oligo or polyfollicular response, the data from conventional IVF apply.

In summary,

E2 concentration plays an important role in the timing of follicular aspiration in NC-IVF, but probably not so much in minimal stimulation IVF. In NC-IVF the relevance of E2 concentration seems to be higher than follicle size.

10.4   Timing According to Endometrial Thickness

Endometrial thickness plays a less important role in the timing of follicular aspiration.

Postponing follicular aspiration to allow the endometrium to become thicker may be considered if the endometrium is thin; however, the benefit of this strategy is doubtful.

10.4.1   Endometrial Thickness in Conventional IVF

In conventional IVF treatments, a thin endometrium is associated with lower pregnancy rates. The clinical pregnancy rate is clearly reduced at an endometrial thickness of ≤ 7 mm (OR 0.42, 95% CI: 0.27–0.67) [12]. However, postponing the follicle aspiration to allow the endometrium to become thicker is not a feasible option in conventional IVF.

10.4.2   Endometrial Thickness in NC-IVF

In NC-IVF, a thin endometrium is also associated with lower pregnancy rates. According to a study by von Wolff et al. (2018) [13], pregnancy rate was 7.4% in women with endometrial thickness ≤ 7 mm and 30.8% in women with endometrial

Table 10.4 Increase in follicle diameter, serum E2 concentration and endometrial thickness per day within in the 4–5 days before follicle aspiration in NC-IVF [3], minimal stimulation IVF [10], and conventional IVF [14]

	NC-IVF	NC-IVF	NC-IVF	Minimal stimulation IVF[a]	Conventional IVF
	Follicle diameter, mm ± SD	E2 concentration, pmol/L ± SD (ng/mL ± SD)	Endometrial thickness, mm (95% CI)	Endometrial thickness, mm (95% CI)	Endometrial thickness, mm (95% CI)
Increase per day	1.04 ± 0.64	167 ± 77 (46 ± 21)	0.58 (0.43–0.73)	0.69 mm (−0.07 to 0.19)	0.22 (−0.12 to 0.55)

[a] 25 mg clomiphene citrate and 75 IU gonadotropin per day

thickness >7 mm (OR 5.56, 95% CI: 1.22–25.36). Live birth rates were not significantly different.

Theoretically, it could be deduced from this that if the endometrium is thin, it could be beneficial to delay follicular aspiration, i.e. by administering single doses of GnRH antagonist (see Chap. 11). In NC-IVF cycles, endometrial thickness increases by about 0.58 mm per day during the last 5 days before follicle aspiration (Table 10.4).

However, it is unclear whether a delay would also lead to an increase in pregnancy rate. Even though a thick endometrium is associated with higher pregnancy rates [13], it is not known if an increase in endometrial thickness due to a delay in aspiration also increases the pregnancy rate. Magaton et al. [14], showed that higher E2 concentrations due to additional gonadotropin stimulation led to a thicker endometrium (Table 10.4). However, the increased endometrial thickness was not associated with higher implantation rates.

10.4.3 Endometrial Thickness in Minimal Stimulation IVF

It can be assumed that the above information on NC-IVF applies to any minimal stimulation IVF cycles with monofollicular response and that the information on conventional IVF applies to minimal stimulation IVF with oligofollicular response.

However, if clomiphene citrate is used at standard dosages, endometrial thickness can be expected to be significantly reduced (mean reduction: 1.4 mm; 95% CI: 2.3–0.5 mm) [15]. If very low dosages such as 25 mg per day are used for modified NC-IVF or minimal stimulation IVF (see Chap. 15), endometrial thickness is only reduced (non-significantly) by approx. 0.5 mm [16].

Magaton et al. [10] investigated whether additional gonadotropin stimulation and the accompanying higher E2 concentration led to a thicker endometrium in women stimulated with 25 mg clomiphene citrate per day. Endometrial thickness increased by 0.69 mm but this did not lead to higher implantation rates per retrieved oocyte.

Table 10.5 Natural cycle IVF: Percentage of cases with the given E2 concentration at which LH surge can be expected to be induced [3]

Percentage of cases	E2, pmol/L	E2, ng/mL
25%	≤545	≤149
50%	≤854	≤232
75%	≤1531	≤417

In summary,

endometrial thickness plays only a minor role in the timing of follicular aspiration. It is doubtful whether delaying follicular aspiration in women with a thin endometrium leads to a relevant improvement in pregnancy rate.

10.5 Timing According to Expected LH Increase

Timing of follicle aspiration according to the time of expected luteinizing hormone (LH) surge only plays a role in NC-IVF, since in conventional IVF and often also in minimal stimulation IVF, GnRH antagonists are administered to prevent an LH surge.

Table 10.5 shows at which E2 concentrations an LH surge can be expected [3]. The data shows that the level of E2 concentration at which an LH surge is induced varies greatly between individuals. The reasons for the high variability are not entirely clear. However, it can be assumed that the length of the follicular phase and therefore the exposure time of oestrogen on the hypothalamus (see Chap. 6), the level of basal LH concentration, age, and other individual factors play a role. Because of this, it may be useful to perform a diagnostic cycle to determine the individual hormone profile and to estimate the individual E2 threshold for an LH surge before the first NC-IVF therapy is performed.

In summary,

estimation of the onset of the LH surge plays a relevant role in the timing of follicular aspiration in NC-IVF. However, the onset of the LH surge is quite variable and seems to vary individually.

10.6 Practical Conclusions

- In NC-IVF and minimal stimulation IVF, leading follicles should ideally be aspirated if ≥16 mm in size.
- Follicles with a size of 13–15 m can also be aspirated if E2 concentration is high.
- Follicles with a size of 21–22 mm can be aspirated. However, aspiration of even larger follicles should only be performed if the level of E2 concentration is high, indicating a functional follicle.

- The thickness of the endometrium does not play a relevant role in the timing of aspiration. Follicular aspiration can be delayed using GnRH antagonists (plus gonadotropins if antagonists are given >1 day), but whether this is associated with higher pregnancy rates is unclear.

References

1. Wirleitner B, Okhowat J, Vištejnová L, Králíčková M, Karlíková M, Vanderzwalmen P, Ectors F, Hradecký L, Schuff M, Murtinger M. Relationship between follicular volume and oocyte competence, blastocyst development and live-birth rate: optimal follicle size for oocyte retrieval. Ultrasound Obstet Gynecol. 2018;51:118–25.
2. Mohr-Sasson A, Orvieto R, Blumenfeld S, Axelrod M, Mor-Hadar D, Grin L, Aizer A, Haas J. The association between follicle size and oocyte development as a function of final follicular maturation triggering. Reprod Biomed Online. 2020;40:887–93.
3. Helmer A, Magaton I, Stalder O, Surbek D, Stute P, von Wolff M. Optimal timing of ovulation triggering to achieve highest success rates in natural cycles – an analysis based on follicle size and estradiol concentration in Natural cycle IVF. Front Endocrinol. in press. 2021;(Suppl 1):i414–5.
4. Palatnik A, Strawn E, Szabo A, Robb P. What is the optimal follicular size before triggering ovulation in intrauterine insemination cycles with clomiphene citrate or letrozole? An analysis of 988 cycles. Fertil Steril. 2012;97:1089–94.e1-3.
5. Shalom-Paz E, Marzal A, Wiser A, Hyman J, Tulandi T. Does optimal follicular size in IUI cycles vary between clomiphene citrate and gonadotrophins treatments? Gynecol Endocrinol. 2014;30:107–10.
6. Hancock KL, Pereira N, Christos PJ, Petrini AC, Hughes J, Chung PH, Rosenwaks Z. Optimal lead follicle size for human chorionic gonadotropin trigger in clomiphene citrate and intrauterine insemination cycles: an analysis of 1,676 treatment cycles. Fertil Steril. 2020:S0015-0282(20)32540-1.
7. Ectors FJ, Vanderzwalmen P, Van Hoeck J, Nijs M, Verhaegen G, Delvigne A, Schoysman R, Leroy F. Relationship of human follicular diameter with oocyte fertilization and development after in-vitro fertilization or intracytoplasmic sperm injection. Hum Reprod. 1997;12:2002–5.
8. Orvieto R, Mohr-Sasson A, Blumenfeld S, Nahum R, Aizer A, Haas J. Does a large (>24 mm) follicle yield a competent oocyte/embryo? Gynecol Obstet Invest. 2020;85:416–9.
9. Weiss NS, van Vliet MN, Limpens J, Hompes PGA, Lambalk CB, Mochtar MH, van der Veen F, Mol BWJ, van Wely M. Endometrial thickness in women undergoing IUI with ovarian stimulation. How thick is too thin? A systematic review and meta-analysis. Hum Reprod. 2017;32:1009–18.
10. Magaton I, Helmer A, Roumet M, Stute P, Von Wolff M. Clomiphene citrate stimulated cycles-additional gonadotrophin stimulation increases endometrium thickness without increasing implantation rate. Facts Views Vis. 2022;14:77–81.
11. Magnusson Å, Wennerholm UB, Källén K, Petzold M, Thurin-Kjellberg A, Bergh C. The association between the number of oocytes retrieved for IVF, perinatal outcome and obstetric complications. Hum Reprod. 2018;33:1939–47.
12. Kasius A, Smit JG, Torrance HL, Eijkemans MJ, Mol BW, Opmeer BC, Broekmans FJ. Endometrial thickness and pregnancy rates after IVF: a systematic review and meta-analysis. Hum Reprod Update. 2014;20:530–41.
13. von Wolff M, Fäh M, Roumet M, Mitter V, Stute P, Griesinger G, Kohl SA. Thin endometrium is also associated with lower clinical pregnancy rate in unstimulated menstrual cycles: a study based on natural cycle IVF. Front Endocrinol (Lausanne). 2018;9:776.

14. Magaton I, Helmer A, Roumet M, Stute P, Von Wolff M. High dose gonadotropin stimulation increases endometrial thickness but this gonadotropin induced thickening does not have an effect on implantation. Gynecol Obstet Hum Reprod. in press.
15. Gadalla MA, Huang S, Wang R, Norman RJ, Abdullah SA, El Saman AM, Ismail AM, van Wely M, Mol BWJ. Effect of clomiphene citrate on endometrial thickness, ovulation, pregnancy and live birth in anovulatory women: systematic review and meta-analysis. Ultrasound Obstet Gynecol. 2018;51:64–76.
16. von Wolff M, Nitzschke M, Stute P, Bitterlich N, Rohner S. Low-dosage clomiphene reduces premature ovulation rates and increases transfer rates in natural-cycle IVF. Reprod Biomed Online. 2014;29:209–15.

Chapter 11
Inhibition of Premature Ovulation in Natural Cycle and Minimal Stimulation IVF

Michael von Wolff

11.1 Background

Inhibition of premature ovulation is always performed in conventional IVF, often in minimal stimulation IVF and sometimes in natural cycle IVF (NC-IVF). In conventional IVF and minimal stimulation IVF, GnRH analogous are usually used. In NC-IVF, inhibition of ovulation is more complex. Ovulation can be inhibited by GnRH antagonists, clomiphene citrate and different non-steroidal anti-inflammatory drugs (NSAIDs), such as ibuprofen, indomethacin and diclofenac (Tables 11.1 and 11.2). Physicians and patients must find the right balance between the effectiveness of the medication and its side effects.

Other medications such as progestogens (progestin primed ovarian stimulation, PPOS), GnRH agonists or oral GnRH antagonists are usually not useful in NC-IVF and minimal stimulation IVF. PPOS does not allow a fresh transfer to be performed, GnRH agonists require too many injections, and the effect of oral GnRH antagonists lasts too long.

11.2 Inhibition with GnRH Antagonists

Inhibition of ovulation using GnRH antagonists is a standard procedure routinely performed in conventional IVF therapy. The aim is to inhibit the release of luteinizing hormone, LH, and thus inhibit the LH surge. Cetrorelix or ganirelix is usually

M. von Wolff (✉)
Division of Gynecological Endocrinology and Reproductive Medicine, University Women's Hospital, University of Bern, Bern, Switzerland
e-mail: Michael.vonwolff@insel.ch

Table 11.1 Frequently used medications to inhibit and thereby to postpone ovulation in NC-IVF and minimal stimulation IVF

Medication	Dose	Advantage	Disadvantage
GnRH antagonist (ganirelix, cetrorelix)	0.25 mg, 1 injection s.c.	Effective inhibitor for at least 24 h.	Expensive. Injection required.
Clomiphene citrate	25–50 mg per day orally [4]	Effective inhibitor. Additional stimulatory effect on folliculogenesis. Cheap.	Some side effects at doses >25 mg per day. Needs to be given for several days.
NSAID—Ibuprofen	3 × 400 mg per day orally [5]	Can still be started if LH surge has already been started. Almost no gastrointestinal side effects. Cheap.	Postpones ovulation for a few hours.
NSAID—Indomethacin	3 × 50 mg per day orally [16, 21]	Probably more effective than ibuprofen. Can still be started if LH surge has already been started. Cheap.	Postpones ovulation for several hours. Gastrointestinal side effects possible.
NSAID—diclofenac	25 mg 24 and 8 h before follicle aspiration or every 6–8 h orally or rectally [6]	Probably more effective than ibuprofen. Can still be started if LH surge has already been started. Cheap.	Postpones ovulation for several hours. Rectal application might be inconvenient. Oral application might cause gastrointestinal side effects.

used at a daily dose of 0.25 mg s.c. The following special features should be noted when using GnRH antagonists in NC-IVF and minimal stimulation IVF:

- Maximum blood concentrations of GnRH antagonists are reached approximately 1 h after injection. The half-life, depending on the dose and the preparation, is about 20–30 h [1, 2]. This means that the medication can be expected to suppress LH release a few hours longer than 24 h.
- The effectiveness of a single injection is less effective because multiple injections for several days, as administered in conventional IVF, have a cumulative effect [3]. Furthermore, the high E2 concentrations in conventional IVF have an additional LH-suppressing effect. Because of this, it is possible that a single injection of GnRH antagonists does not effectively inhibit LH surge.
- GnRII antagonists also inhibit the release of the follicle stimulating hormone, FSH [2, 3]. Because of this, if GnRH antagonists are administered for more than 1 day, gonadotropins such as HMG or FSH must be added in a dose of approx. 50–75 IU per day.

Table 11.2 Medications, indications and doses used for inhibition of ovulation in NC-IVF and minimal stimulation IVF in different centres, specialized in NC-IVF and/or minimal stimulation IVF (see also Chap. 15)

Centre	Medication[a]	Indication[a]	Dose, duration of treatment[a]
Bern, Switzerland [4, 5]	Clomiphene citrate	In women who have previously ovulated prematurely.	25 mg per day orally, starting around day 4 of the cycle until the day of ovulation triggering.
	Ibuprofen, diclofenac	If LH surge has already started.	Ibuprofen 3 × 400mg or diclofenac 3 × 25 mg per day, starting as soon as possible if increased LH is detected, until the morning of follicle aspiration 1–2 days later. (see Chap. 15).
	GnRH antagonist injections (ganirelix or cetrorelix)	To postpone aspiration for 1 day, i.e., if follicle is still too small.	1 injection, 0.25 mg, s.c. at 4 pm the day before HCG is given.
Tokyo, Japan, [6]	Diclofenac	If LH surge has already started.	25 mg rectally, 8 h and 14 h before oocyte retrieval 1–2 days later (see Chap. 15).
New York, U.S.	Clomiphene citrate	In all patients.	50 mg per day orally, starting around day 3 of the cycle until the day of ovulation triggering.
	Ibuprofen	In all patients.	3 × 400 mg orally, starting at the time of ovulation triggering.

[a] See also Chap. 15

In summary,

GnRH antagonists are very effective in delaying ovulation by about 1 day. If GnRH antagonists are used for longer than 1 day, gonadotropins must be added.

11.3 Inhibition with Clomiphene Citrate

Clomiphene citrate was already described as a stimulant in IVF therapy before the first IVF baby was born [7]. MacDougall et al. (1994) [8] showed 1994 that the addition of 100 mg of clomiphene citrate per day from day 2 to day 6 reduced the rate of premature ovulations.

In recent years, clomiphene has only been administered in a dose of 50 mg [9] or 25 mg [4], since even at a low dose, clomiphene stimulates slightly follicular growth but the side effects are much lower than in a daily dose of 100 mg [4].

The mechanism of action and the pharmacokinetics of clomiphene are still not fully understood. Clomiphene contains a mixture of two isomers, about 62% in the enclomifene (trans) and 38% in the zuclomifene (cis) form. It is assumed that the main stimulatory effects of clomiphene are due to enclomifene [10].

Enclomifene probably has oestrogen antagonistic effects and therefore inhibits positive feedback at the level of the hypothalamus [11] and suppresses the

LH surge. As enclomifene is eliminated rapidly within about 1 day [12, 13], clomiphene tablets are usually given once a day until the day of ovulation trigger.

In contrast, zuclomiphene, which probably has oestrogen agonist effects at the pituitary level [11], is eliminated within several days. Low concentrations are still detectable 21 days after 5-day treatment and are therefore still detectable in the luteal phase [12, 14]. This is probably the reason for cyst formations in consecutive stimulation cycles if higher doses of clomiphene citrate are used (see Chap. 5).

The effect of clomiphene citrate is different in obese and non-obese patients, which might explain some of the variation in the clinical response to the drug [14]. Absorption kinetics are not different, but maximum concentrations are lower in obese patients which might be due to differences in distribution and clearance. As women undergoing NC-IVF are usually non-obese, 25 mg/day of clomiphene citrate are usually sufficient to inhibit ovulation. Substantial stimulation of follicular growth, however, requires higher doses such as 50 mg per day, especially in women with polycystic ovary syndrome or in obese women.

The ovulation inhibitory effect of clomiphene citrate has already been demonstrated in a randomized controlled study with 30 participants by MacDougall et al. (1994) [8]. The addition of 100 mg of clomiphene citrate per cycle day from day 2 to day 6 in NC-IVF cycles led to more follicles >14 mm (2.4 ± 0.3 versus 0.9 ± 0.2) compared to cycles without clomiphene, and to reduced rate of premature ovulations (0% versus 71%).

Ingerslev et al. confirmed these results in 2001 [15]. 132 women were randomized to receive 100 mg clomiphene per day from cycle day 3–7 versus no clomiphene. The clomiphene group performed significantly better in terms of number of cycles with oocyte aspirations (86% versus 65%), collected oocytes per aspiration (1.8 versus 0.9), embryo transfers per started cycle (53% versus 25%) and pregnancy [15] rate per started cycle (18% versus 4%).

Von Wolff et al. (2014) [4], performed a study in which women received (non-randomized) either 25 mg clomiphene citrate per day from cycle day 7 until the day of ovulation triggering or no clomiphene. The clomiphene group also performed significantly better in terms of number of cycles with oocyte aspirations (93% versus 72%), collected oocytes per aspiration (0.8 versus 0.6) and embryo transfers per started cycle (54% versus 40%). Pregnancy rates per started cycle (14% versus 11%) were statistically not different.

These studies demonstrate that either high doses of clomiphene citrate can be given for around 5 days, or a lower dose can be given until the day of ovulation triggering.

However, the side effects are different: In women taking 100 mg clomiphene citrate per day, Ingerslev et al. (2001) [15] described hot flushes in 31.5% and nausea in 12.6% of the patients. In women taking only 25 mg clomiphene citrate per day, von Wolff et al. (2014) [4] described hot flushes in only 5% and nausea in 0% of cases and these side effects were described as being mild.

Therefore, 25 mg clomiphene citrate per day taken until the day of ovulation triggering to inhibit ovulation can be given. 50 mg per day can be a better option in obese women.

In summary,

clomiphene citrate is an effective drug to inhibit ovulation with few side effects at low doses.

11.4   Inhibition with NSAIDs

11.4.1   Effect of NSAIDs on Ovulation

Inhibition of ovulation using NSAIDs was already described as a case report by Nargund and Wei (1996) [16] using indomethacin.

The concept of NSAIDs is based on the knowledge that rupture of the follicle is due to an acute inflammatory reaction, in which ovarian prostaglandins play an important role (see Chap. 6). Inhibiting the synthesis of prostaglandins by NSAIDs, inhibitors of cyclooxygenase, COX, should thus delay or decrease the inflammatory reaction and thereby postpone ovulation.

The COX enzyme, which is the rate-limiting step in the prostaglandin synthesis, exists in two isoforms, COX-1 and COX-2. Whereas COX-1 is expressed in most human cells, and has an important role in maintaining cell homeostasis, cell signalling and platelet aggregation, COX-2 is upregulated during inflammation by cytokines, hormones and inflammatory mediators. Regarding ovulation, a study using COX-2 deficient mice showed that COX-2 deficiency led to defective ovulation and fertilization [17].

Since the ovulation-inhibiting effect is predominantly based on the inhibition of COX-2, NSAIDs with a higher COX-2 inhibiting effect are probably more effective in terms of ovulation inhibition. Figure 11.1 shows the ratio of COX-1 and COX-2 selectivity of different NSAIDs. Among the NSAIDs commonly used for ovulation inhibition, diclofenac has a strongest ovulation-inhibiting effect, followed by indomethacin and ibuprofen.

According to Fig. 11.1, selective COX-2 inhibitors such as celecoxib might have an even stronger ovulation-inhibiting effect. Studies have indeed shown that the inhibition of ovulation by selective COX-2 inhibitors such as rofecoxib, which was withdrawn from the market because of concerns about increased risk of heart attack and stroke, is so strong [18] that they had initially even been discussed as emergency contraceptives [19].

However, since it has been shown in animals that the administration of prostaglandin synthesis inhibitors can lead to disruption of embryo implantation and miscarriage, the very potent COX-2 inhibitors are contraindicated in pregnancy and should therefore not be used in NC-IVF therapy. There is also no data on whether very strong COX inhibition could lead to inhibition of the detachment of the

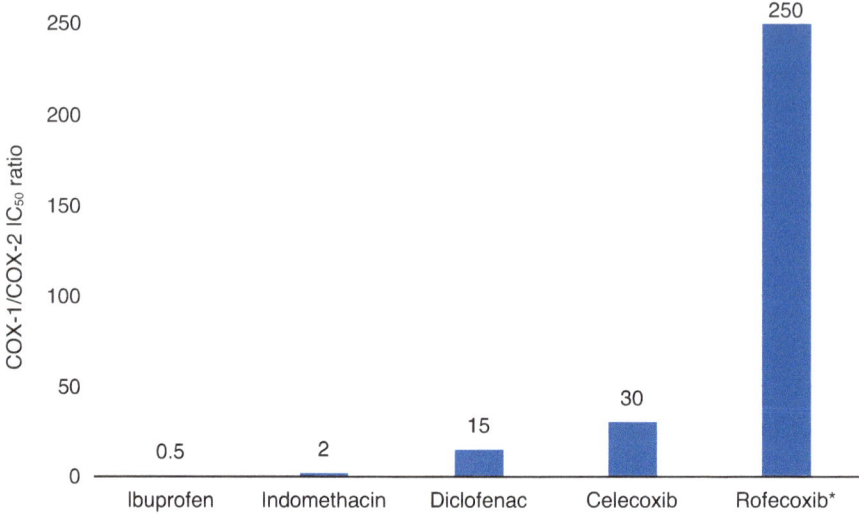

Fig. 11.1 Relative COX-1/COX-2 selectivity of different NSAIDs (IC_{50}: half-maximal inhibitory concentration) (according to [20]). (*withdrawn from the market). Higher values (>1) indicate greater selectivity for COX-2

cumulus oophorus complex from the follicular wall, which would reduce the number of retrieved oocytes.

11.4.2 Effect of NSAIDs on Ovulation in IVF Therapies

Diclofenac, indomethacin and ibuprofen are the most commonly used NSAIDs in NC-IVF. The effect of diclofenac was analysed by Kawachiva et al. (2012) [6]. They performed a retrospective analysis of NC-IVF treatment cycles with and without diclofenac. A spontaneous LH surge (LH 10–30 IU/mL) was detected in 1865 cycles. Of these, 962 women took 25 mg diclofenac rectally every 6 h, 903 women (control group) did not. Aspiration was scheduled for the following day in the afternoon or 2 days later in the morning. The premature ovulation rate in the diclofenac group was 3.6% versus 6.8% in the control group. Oocytes were collected in 75.3% versus 65.6% and fertilized oocytes were retrieved in 55.3% versus 44.5% of the cycles.

The effect of indomethacin was analysed by Nargund et al. (2001) [21]. They performed a retrospective analysis of NC-IVF cycles. In 42 cycles in which a beginning LH surge was detected on a Friday, women took 50 mg indomethacin three times a day to avoid aspiration on Sunday. Only one follicle ruptured before follicle aspiration on the following Monday (3 days after the start of indomethacin). Fertilized oocytes were retrieved in 71% of the cycles.

The effect of ibuprofen was analysed by Kohl Schwartz et al. (2020) [5]. A beginning LH surge (LH 10–30 IU/mL) was detected in 63 women. The women took 400 mg ibuprofen every 8 h until the morning of the follicle aspiration 2 days later. Even though the follicle aspiration was substantially delayed the premature ovulation rate was only 20.6%. Oocytes were collected in 65.1%, and fertilized oocytes were retrieved in 54% of cycles.

The effect of ibuprofen has also been analysed in a prospective, controlled study, performed in the infertility centre in Bern, Switzerland. The preliminary study results are the following ones:

5000 IE hCG was administered to 24 women undergoing NC-IVF treatment as soon as the follicle was mature but the LH concentration analysed in the morning was still <10 U/mL. Starting with the hCG injection in the afternoon, the women received 3 × 400 mg ibuprofen until follicular aspiration. The follicular aspiration was not performed after 36 h as usual, but 42 h after hCG administration. 18 women performing a diagnostic cycle served as the control group. The control group also received 5000 IE hCG, but no ibuprofen. 42 h after HCG administration, ultrasound was used to check whether ovulation had occurred. In the group of women with HCG and ibuprofen, ovulation had occurred in only 4/24 (16.7%) of cases, in the control group without ibuprofen in 14/18 (78%) of cases. The study (Clinical trials. gov: study number NCT02571543h) is expected to be published in 2023.

These four studies are the only ones that allow a statement on the effectiveness of NSAIDs in NC-IVF.

Kadoch et al. (2008) [22], Rijken-Zijlstra et al. (2013) [23] and others also conducted studies, but mostly with minimal stimulation IVF therapies. In the studies by Kadoch et al. and Rijken-Zijlstra et al. all patients took indomethacin, even though they were also treated with daily GnRH antagonist injections. Therefore, the concepts of these studies do not allow any definite conclusion to be made regarding the efficacy of NSAID to reduce the risk of premature ovulation.

Therefore, the data on the efficacy of NSAIDs in NC-IVF is very limited. Consistent with the efficacy of the various NSAIDs shown in Fig. 11.1, diclofenac and indomethacin appear to be slightly more effective than ibuprofen in inhibiting ovulation. However, a study directly comparing the different NSAIDs has never been performed.

The studies also show that even though NSAIDs apparently effectively inhibit the enzyme cyclooxygenase and thereby inhibit ovulation, this effect does not seem to affect the detachment of cumulus oophorus complexes from the follicular wall, which would otherwise lead to a reduction in the oocyte yield.

11.4.3 Side Effects of NSAIDs

When choosing NSAIDs as an ovulation inhibiting medication, their side effects must also be taken into account.

Table 11.3 Comparison of toxicity for gastrointestinal complications of NSAIDs with ibuprofen as reference (according to [24])

Comparator	Studies, n	Pooled relative risk	95% CI
Ibuprofen	–	1.0	–
Diclofenac	8	1.8	1.4–2.3
Indomethacin	11	2.4	1.9–3.1

The most important side effects of NSAIDs are gastrointestinal symptoms (Table 11.3). Since NSAIDs are used off label and since NC-IVF should be performed as gently as possible, drugs with as few side effects as possible should be preferred.

According to Henry et al. (1996) [24], ibuprofen has the least side effects. A meta-analysis examining over 1000 ibuprofen-treated subjects [25] showed that fewer adverse effects were reported in the ibuprofen group than in the placebo group (27.4% versus 31.7%). The frequency of digestive system adverse events was comparable for ibuprofen (12.1%) and placebo (11.0%); there was no significant difference for any specific digestive system.

Another meta-analysis also revealed that the number of severe side effects was not higher for ibuprofen than for placebo. Gastroendoscopy showed that ibuprofen produced little or no injury to the gastrointestinal system when taken at 1600 mg/day for 3 days and 2400 mg/day for 1 day [26].

In summary,

NSAIDs delay ovulation in the short term without adversely affecting detachment of the cumulus oophorus complex and oocyte quality. Indomethacin and diclofenac seem to be slightly more effective than ibuprofen, but have more gastrointestinal side effects.

11.5 Practical Conclusions

- Ovulation can be inhibited with GnRH antagonists, clomiphene citrate and NSAIDs. The medications have different functions and therefore different indications, advantages and disadvantages.
- If GnRH antagonists are given for more than 1 day, gonadotropins need to be added to compensate for the decrease of FSH concentration.
- GnRH antagonists can be used to postpone ovulation for around 1 day, clomiphene citrate to reduce the overall risk of premature ovulation, and NSAIDs can be used if the LH surge has already started.
- Clomiphene citrate given at a dosage of 25 and 50 mg per day not only inhibits ovulation but also slightly stimulates follicle growth.
- The NSAIDs with the apparently highest ovulation-inhibiting effect are diclofenac and indomethacin, the one with the lowest side effects is ibuprofen.

References

1. Rabinovici J, Rothman P, Monroe SE, Nerenberg C, Jaffe RB. Endocrine effects and pharmacokinetic characteristics of a potent new gonadotropin-releasing hormone antagonist (Ganirelix) with minimal histamine-releasing properties: studies in postmenopausal women. J Clin Endocrinol Metab. 1992;75:1220–5.
2. Behre HM, Klein B, Steinmeyer E, McGregor GP, Voigt K, Nieschlag E. Effective suppression of luteinizing hormone and testosterone by single doses of the new gonadotropin-releasing hormone antagonist cetrorelix (SB-75) in normal men. J Clin Endocrinol Metab. 1992;75:393–8.
3. Behre HM, Böckers A, Schlingheider A, Nieschlag E. Sustained suppression of serum LH, FSH and testosterone and increase of high-density lipoprotein cholesterol by daily injections of the GnRH antagonist cetrorelix over 8 days in normal men. Clin Endocrinol (Oxf). 1994;40:241–8.
4. von Wolff M, Nitzschke M, Stute P, Bitterlich N, Rohner S. Low-dosage clomiphene reduces premature ovulation rates and increases transfer rates in natural-cycle IVF. Reprod Biomed Online. 2014;29:209–15.
5. Kohl Schwartz AS, Burkard S, Mitter VR, Leichtle AB, Fink A, Von Wolff M. Short-term application of ibuprofen before ovulation. Facts Views Vis Obgyn. 2020;12:179–84.
6. Kawachiya S, Matsumoto T, Bodri D, Kato K, Takehara Y, Kato O. Short-term, low-dose, non-steroidal anti-inflammatory drug application diminishes premature ovulation in natural-cycle IVF. Reprod Biomed Online. 2012;24:308–13.
7. Lopata A, Brown JB, Leeton JF, Talbot JM, Wood C. In vitro fertilization of preovulatory oocytes and embryo transfer in infertile patients treated with clomiphene and human chorionic gonadotropin. Fertil Steril. 1978;30:27–35.
8. MacDougall MJ, Tan SL, Hall V, Balen A, Mason BA, Jacobs HS. Comparison of natural with clomiphene citrate - stimulated cycles in in vitro fertilisation: a prospective randomized trial. Fertil Steril. 1994;61:1052–7.
9. Teramoto S, Kato O. Minimal ovarian stimulation with clomiphene citrate: a large-scale retrospective study. Reprod Biomed Online. 2007;15:134–48.
10. Earl JA, Kim ED. Enclomiphene citrate: a treatment that maintains fertility in men with secondary hypogonadism. Expert Rev Endocrinol Metab. 2019;14:157–65.
11. Goldstein SR, Siddhanti S, Ciaccia AV, Plouffe L Jr. A pharmacological review of selective oestrogen receptor modulators. Hum Reprod Update. 2000;6:212–24.
12. Mikkelson TJ, Kroboth PD, Cameron WJ, Dittert LW, Chungi V, Manberg PJ. Single-dose pharmacokinetics of clomiphene citrate in normal volunteers. Fertil Steril. 1986;46:392–6.
13. Ghobadi C, Mirhosseini N, Shiran MR, Moghadamnia A, Lennard MS, Ledger WL, Rostami-Hodjegan A. Single-dose pharmacokinetic study of clomiphene citrate isomers in anovular patients with polycystic ovary disease. J Clin Pharmacol. 2009;49:147–54.
14. Ghobadi C, Amer S, Lashen H, Lennard MS, Ledger WL, Rostami-Hodjegan A. Evaluation of the relationship between plasma concentrations of en- and zuclomiphene and induction of ovulation in anovulatory women being treated with clomiphene citrate. Fertil Steril. 2009;91:1135–40.
15. Ingerslev HJ, Højgaard A, Hindkjaer J, Kesmodel U. A randomized study comparing IVF in the unstimulated cycle with IVF following clomiphene citrate. Hum Reprod. 2001;16:696–702.
16. Nargund G, Wei CC. Successful planned delay of ovulation for one week with indomethacin. J Assist Reprod Genet. 1996;13:683–4.
17. Lim H, Paria BC, Das SK, Dinchuk JE, Langenbach R, Trzaskos JM, Dey SK. Multiple female reproductive failures in cyclooxygenase 2-deficient mice. Cell. 1997;91:197–208.
18. Pall M, Fridén BE, Brännström M. Induction of delayed follicular rupture in the human by the selective COX-2 inhibitor rofecoxib: a randomized double-blind study. Hum Reprod. 2001;16:1323–8.

19. Weiss EA, Gandhi M. Preferential cyclooxygenase 2 inhibitors as a nonhormonal method of emergency contraception: a look at the evidence. J Pharm Pract. 2016;29:160–4.
20. Brune K, Patrignani P. New insights into the use of currently available non-steroidal anti-inflammatory drugs. J Pain Res. 2015;8:105–18.
21. Nargund G, Waterstone J, Bland J, Philips Z, Parsons J, Campbell S. Cumulative conception and live birth rates in natural (unstimulated) IVF cycles. Hum Reprod. 2001;16:259–62.
22. Kadoch IJ, Al-khaduri M, Phillips SJ, et al. Spontaneous ovulation rate before oocyte retrieval in modified natural cycle IVF with and without indomethacin. Reprod Biomed Online. 2008;16:245–9.
23. Rijken-zijlstra TM, Haadsma ML, Hammer C, et al. Effectiveness of indometacin to prevent ovulation in modified natural-cycle IVF: a randomized controlled trial. Reprod Biomed Online. 2013;27:297–304.
24. Henry D, Lim LL, Garcia Rodriguez LA, et al. Variability in risk of gastrointestinal complications with individual non-steroidal anti-inflammatory drugs: results of a collaborative meta-analysis. BMJ. 1996;312(7046):1563–6.
25. Kellstein DE, Waksman JA, Furey SA, Binstok G, Cooper SA. The safety profile of nonprescription ibuprofen in multiple-dose use: a meta-analysis. J Clin Pharmacol. 1999;39:520–32.
26. Lanza FL. Endoscopic studies of gastric and duodenal injury after the use of ibuprofen, aspirin, and other nonsteroidal anti-inflammatory agents. Am J Med. 1984;77:19–24.

Chapter 12
Ovulation Triggering in Natural Cycle and Minimal Stimulation IVF

Michael von Wolff

12.1 Background

Ovulation triggering is essential in natural cycle IVF (NC-IVF) and minimal stimulation IVF. Without triggering of ovulation, timing of follicle aspiration is imprecise leading to low success rates.

Different medications such as urinary human chorionic gonadotropin (hCG), recombinant hCG as well as GnRH agonist (GnRHa) injections and GnRH agonist nasal spray can be used to trigger ovulation. As the medications have different effects, advantages and disadvantages, they cannot simply be replaced by one other.

Table 12.1 describes frequently used medications to trigger ovulation and Table 12.2 shows medications, doses and the time interval between triggering and aspiration in three centres specialized in NC-IVF and/or minimal stimulation IVF.

12.2 Medications to Trigger Ovulation

12.2.1 Triggering with hCG

HCG is, like LH, a complex heterodimeric glycoprotein with a molecular weight of $\approx$40 kDa compared to recombinant LH of $\approx$30 kDa. Along with thyroid-stimulating hormone (TSH) and FSH, hCG and LH share a common 92-amino acid α subunit. The ß subunits are different, hCG has an extension at its carboxyl terminus.

M. von Wolff (✉)
Division of Gynecological Endocrinology and Reproductive Medicine, University Women's Hospital, University of Bern, Bern, Switzerland
e-mail: Michael.vonwolff@insel.ch

© The Author(s), under exclusive license to Springer Nature Switzerland AG 2022   115
M. von Wolff (ed.), *Natural Cycle and Minimal Stimulation IVF*,
https://doi.org/10.1007/978-3-030-97571-5_12

Table 12.1 Frequently used medications to trigger ovulation, typical doses and characteristics

Medication	Dose	Advantage	Disadvantage
uhCG, subcutaneous injections	5,000 IU; 10,000 IU	Low price.	Injection required. Adverse events (mainly Injection site-reaction): 33% [3]
Choriogonadotropin alfa, subcutaneous injections	6500 IU (250 µg)	Less injection site reactions than uhCG.	Injection required. Adverse events (mainly Injection site-reaction): 21% [3].
GnRH agonists, subcutaneous injections	Triptorelin, 0.2 mg	No OHSS in conventional IVF.	Injection required. Luteal phase negatively affected in conventional IVF.
GnRH agonists, intranasal spray	Buserelin, 300–600 µg; Nafarelin, 200 µg	No injection required. In NC-IVF luteal phase support is possibly not required[a]	Luteal phase negatively affected in conventional IVF.

[a] A RCT to test if luteal phase support can be avoided in NC-IVF will be finished in 2023 (see below)

Table 12.2 Medications used for ovulation triggering in centres specialized in NC-IVF and/or minimal stimulation IVF (see also Chap. 15)

Centre	IVF technique	Medication[a]	Time interval between triggering and aspiration[a]
Bern, Switzerland (von Wolff et al., 2014 [4]; Kohl-Schwartz et al., 2020 [5])	NC-IVF; Minimal stimulation IVF	Urinary HCG, 5000 IU s.c.	36 h
Tokyo, Japan, (Teramoto et al., 2007 [6]; Kato et al., 2012 [7])	NC-IVF; Minimal Stimulation IVF	3 × 1 intranasal hub of 0.15 mg buserelin = 0.45 mg in total.	34–35 h
New York, U.S.	NC-IVF; Minimal stimulation IVF	Choriogonadotropin alfa 500 µg s.c.; Triptorelin 0.05 mg s.c.	34–36 h

[a] See also Chap. 15

HCG is commonly used to trigger ovulation as it binds to and activates the same receptor as LH, the LH/choriogonadotropin receptor (LHCGR) (see Chap. 6). However, the pharmacokinetics of hCG and LH are not the same:

- The receptor exposure is different. Compared to the LH surge, hCG concentration increases faster after the injection and decreases much slower due to its slower clearance. Therefore, LHCGR receptor exposure is longer for hCG than for LH.

- The molecular structure is different. Therefore, hCG has a slower plasma metabolic clearance than LH, which consists of a rapid clearance of hCG in the first 5–9 h following injection and a slower clearance the following day. After 36 h, the calculated half-life of hCG is 2.3 days, as compared to LH with a half-life of around 1 h [1]. In women with tubal pregnancies who underwent salpingectomy, hCG half-life was approx. one day just after the operation and around two days between day 1 and 3 after the operation [2].
- The hCG peak is, in contrast to the LH surge, not accompanied by a simultaneous FSH surge. FSH presumably acts synergistically with LH to promote the optimal environment for final oocyte maturation and ovulation. FSH promotes formation of LH receptors in luteinizing granulosa cells and seems to promote oocyte nuclear maturation and cumulus expansion. FSH has a role in maintaining gap junctions between the oocyte and cumulus cells and, thus, may have an important role in signalling pathways (see Chap. 6).

However, even though the pharmacokinetics of hCG and LH are quite different, hCG induces ovulation very effectively. It is cheap and the medication and the injections can easily be handled by patients. Regarding its efficacy, it does not matter if urinary hCG or recombinant hCG is chosen [3].

The disadvantage of hCG, based on its long half-life and therefore its luteotropic activity, is the risk of ovarian stimulation syndrome (OHSS), especially in women with a high ovarian response in IVF treatments.

In summary,

even though the pharmacokinetics of hCG and LH are different, hCG is very effective in triggering ovulation.

12.2.2   Triggering with GnRH Agonists

GnRH agonists (GnRHa) are an alternative medication to trigger ovulation. GnRHa stimulate the endogenous release of LH from the pituitary gland resulting in a simultaneous LH and FSH surge, which is more natural than the hCG peak. However, the GnRHa-induced LH surge is not the same as the natural LH surge:

- The GnRHa-induced LH surge profile is different. The GnRHa-induced LH surge consists of two clearly defined phases, a fast increase of LH and a slow decrease. In contrast, the natural LH surge is variable in configuration, amplitude and duration. The surge can be single-peaked, plateauing, double-peaked and multiple peaked [8].
- The GnRHa-induced LH surge is shorter. The GnRHa-induced LH surge consists of a short ascending limb (4 h) and a long descending limb (20 h), lasting in total for 24–36 h, whereas the natural LH surge lasts for around 3–6 days [8]. Thus, the total amount of gonadotropins released during the surge is significantly reduced when GnRHa is used to trigger ovulation.

GnRHa can be applied as subcutaneous injections or as intranasal spray. Absorption is slightly faster by intranasal application [9]. The sensitivity of the pituitary gland for intranasally applied GnRHa varies throughout the cycle. The magnitude and the rate of gonadotropin release are greatest during the late follicular and luteal phase when LH is required for final follicle maturation, for ovulation and for luteal body support. LH peaks around 4 h after nasal application [10]. After subcutaneous application, LH peaks a little bit later [9].

The shorter duration of the endogenous LH surge induced by GnRHa triggering seems to play a key role for the reduced risk of OHSS when GnRHa is used instead of hCG to trigger ovulation.

hCG induces a higher risk of OHSS due to its longer half-life creating a long-lasting hCG effect. Luteal bodies are stimulated for around 1 week by hCG, which triggers the release of vasoactive substances such as vascular endothelial growth factor (VEGF). In contrast, the GnRHa-induced LH surge is much shorter than the hCG surge and even shorter than the natural LH surge. Therefore, the luteal bodies are less stimulated by LH and therefore dissolve a few days after ovulation. In line with this, the luteal phase is insufficient if GnRHa are used instead of hCG. Therefore, luteal phase support is required if fresh embryo transfer is performed. High doses of progesterone, additional hCG injections [11] or dual triggering with GnRHa and hCG (see Chap. 6) are needed to support the luteal phase.

GnRHa can also be administered as an intranasal spray. The nasal application of GnRHa is discussed in the following chapter.

12.3   Ovulation Triggering in NC-IVF and Minimal Stimulation IVF

12.3.1   NC-IVF Without Triggering of Ovulation

Many patients wish to perform NC-IVF without any medications and therefore also without triggering of ovulation. Indeed, it is possible to perform NC-IVF without triggering as shown below. However, it is challenging, and the success rate is limited.

Follicle aspiration needs to be performed in the short time window when the LH surge induced resumption of the meiosis has started and the cumulus oophorus complex has already detached from the follicular wall, but the follicle has not yet ovulated (see Chap. 6). This time window takes only few hours. By triggering of ovulation with hCG, etc., this time window is exactly defined and therefore follicle aspiration is performed around 33–36 h after the trigger (Table 12.2).

Without triggering, many consecutive blood tests are required to identify the beginning LH surge. And even if the beginning LH surge is identified, the timing of aspiration is imprecise as the time course of the increase of LH concentration leading to the LH surge and the LH surge itself varies individually and from cycle to cycle.

Therefore, NC-IVF without ovulation triggering requires a good understanding of the regulation of the LH surge. The commonest time for the LH surge (as detected in blood) is between 05:00 and 09:00 in the morning. Repeated serum testing showed that 45% of LH surges commence at this time. The GnRHa triggered increase in LH is probably initiated by the reduction of melatonin [12] as a result of light exposure in the morning. The increased GnRH release induced by reduced melatonin due to the increasing daylight in spring is also the driver of the increased sexual hormone production in some animals.

LH is secreted in pulses, on average one pulse every 90 min. As the half-life of LH is around 1 h, its serum levels fluctuate considerably. The duration of LH surge also varies as well as its configuration, amplitude and duration.

Therefore, it is very difficult to determine exactly the beginning of the LH surge. An accurate determination of the LH peak requires several blood tests, which is usually not feasible in clinical routine.

Elizabeth A. Lenton, a pioneer of NC-IVF [13], investigated the extent to which NC-IVF is possible without ovulation triggering [14]. Lenton set up an IVF-programme with a 7-day service and with working hours from 07:00 (7 AM) to 21:00 (9 PM). Follicle aspiration took place between 09:00 (9 AM) and 17:00 (5 PM) [14].

According to Lenton (2007) [14], 534 NC-IVF cycles without ovulation triggering were performed in 1991–1992. LH was measured at regular intervals between 08:00 and 20:00. An LH surge >10 IU/L was followed by further measurements to interpolate the start of the LH surge.

Table 12.3 Protocol for scheduling follicle aspiration, depending on the hour in the day when LH surge was expected to have started. LH was analysed between 08 AM and 08 PM 7 days per week and start of LH surge was calculated by interpolation of several measurements. Only the aspirations printed in bold were aspirated at the ideal time (adapted from Lenton (2007) [14])

Time of start of LH surge	Interval between LH surge and aspiration	Time of follicle aspiration	Interval between LH surge and aspiration	Time of follicle aspiration
8 PM	37 h	09 AM		
10 PM	**35 h**	**09 AM**		
12 AM	**35 h**	**11 AM**		
02 AM	**35 h**	**1 PM**		
04 AM	**35 h**	**3 PM**		
06 AM	**35 h**	**5 PM**		
08 AM	33 h	5 PM		
10 AM	31 h	5 PM	47 h	09 AM
12 noon	29 h	5 PM	45 h	09 AM
2 PM	27 h	5 PM	43 h	09 AM
4 PM	25 h	5 PM	41 h	09 AM
6 PM			39 h	09 AM

An aspiration could be scheduled in 495 cycles. As follicle aspirations could not be performed at night, most aspirations that should have been carried out before 08:00 (8 AM) were performed at around 09:00 (9 AM) with some delay in the morning (Table 12.3). To reduce the risk of premature ovulation, these women received indomethacin. Most aspirations that were scheduled after 20:00 (8 PM) were already performed at around 17:00 (5 PM) in the late afternoon and therefore earlier than required, some at 09:00 (9 PM) and therefore later than required. Table 12.3 demonstrates the scheme for scheduling the follicle aspirations.

Based on this, it can be assumed that a higher percentage of patients had already ovulated in the morning (due to an intervall between LH surge and aspiration >35 h), and that often no oocyte could be obtained in follicle aspirations in the afternoon (due to an intervall between LH surge and aspiration <35 h). This assumption was confirmed in the clinical data (Fig. 12.1).

The outcome of the IVF cycles, performed 1991–1992 was as follows:

534 cycles were started. The age range of the women was 23–47 years with 7.6% aged 40 years and above. 39 cycles (7.3%) were cancelled due to poor E2 profile, short follicular phases or small or ambiguous LH surges.

495 cycles were scheduled for egg collection. In 403/495 cycles (81%), an oocyte was retrieved. In 43 cycles (8.7%), an oocyte could not be collected due to premature ovulation. In 48 cycles (9.7%), no oocyte was aspirated.

An embryo transfer was achieved in 257/495 cycles (52%). 38 clinical pregnancies were counted, which corresponds with a pregnancy rate of 14.8% per embryo transfer, 9.4% per aspirated oocyte and 7.7% per cycle scheduled for oocyte collection. The clinical pregnancy rate per initiated cycle was 7.1%. Data on live birth rates was not provided.

Even though the interpretation of this data is difficult due to the limited information regarding the age of the women, the data presented indicates that NC-IVF is possible without ovulation triggering. However, the data also clearly indicates that the treatment effort is high and the success rate low.

In summary,

NC-IVF without ovulation triggering is difficult, requires many consultations throughout the day and high flexibility of the IVF centre. However, since it is possible in principle, it can be performed in individual cases at special request.

12.3.2 NC-IVF and Minimal Stimulation IVF with hCG to Trigger Ovulation

Since ovulation triggering is necessary to make the treatment as effective and simple as possible, hCG is usually administered to induce ovulation. The time interval between hCG administration and follicular aspiration is around 34–36 h. Table 12.2 shows the doses and time intervals between injection and follicular aspiration in three large centres/networks, specialized in NC-IVF and/or minimal stimulation IVF centres.

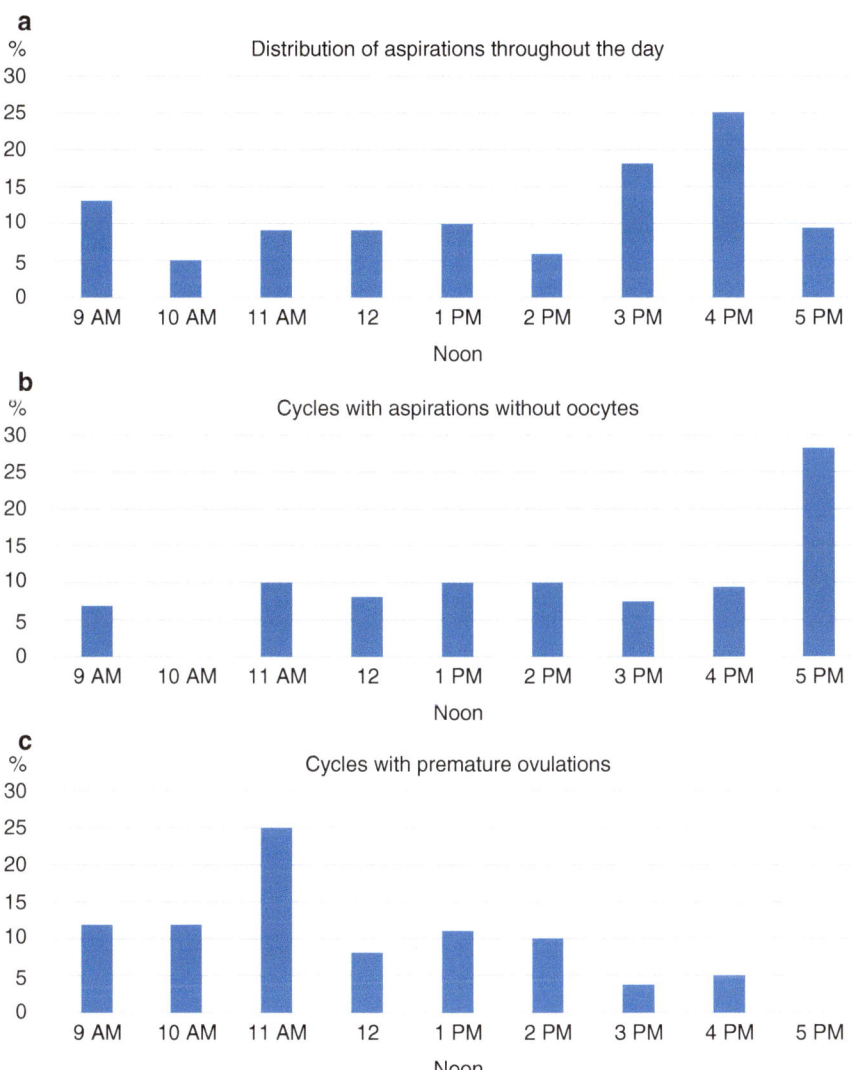

Fig. 12.1 (**a**) The distribution of 495 scheduled NC-IVF follicle aspirations throughout the day. An even distribution would result in approximately 11% of procedures in each interval. There were relatively more procedures than expected towards the end of the day. (**b**) The distribution of 48 cycles in which the follicle was aspirated but no oocyte was found despite vigorous flushing. (**c**) The equivalent distribution of 43 cycles in which ovulation occurred prior to or during aspiration (adapted from Lenton (2007) [14])

12.3.3 NC-IVF and Minimal Stimulation IVF with Nasal GnRH Agonists to Trigger Ovulation

Ovulation induction with subcutaneously injected GnRH analogues (GnRHa) does not make sense in NC-IVF and minimal stimulation IVF. The main intention of ovulation induction with GnRHa is to avoid OHSS which is very rare in NC-IVF and minimal stimulation IVF.

However, nasal administration of GnRHa is an option for some women who require NC-IVF without any injections.

In Japan, GnRHa is administered intranasally to avoid self-injections of the patients. Kato and Teramoto administered 300 μg buserelin 32–35 h [6] or 600 μg buserelin 30–34 h [7] before follicle aspiration in minimal stimulation IVF cycles. Luteal phase support was performed with 3 × 10 mg oral dydrogesterone per day [6].

Schmidt-Sarosi (1995) [15], administered two 400 μg intranasal doses of nafarelin 16 h apart before follicle aspiration in clomiphene citrate-stimulated intrauterine insemination cycles. Luteal phase support was performed with 400 μg nafarelin every 16 h between day 6 and day 10 after ovulation triggering.

A study is being prepared (see below; clinical.trials.gov: NCT04850261), based on the Kato Ladies Clinic in Tokyo (see Chap. 28) using GnRHa nasal spray for ovulation induction. The aim of the study is to use GnRHa nasal spray for ovulation induction and thereby not to apply any injections. This treatment would further simplify NC-IVF treatments and would possibly reduce treatment-related stress.

In summary,

intranasal application of GnRHa is a technique which is easy and avoids injections. However, the necessity to support the luteal phase after intranasal application of GnRHa still needs to be evaluated.

12.3.4 Future Perspectives of Ovulation Triggering in NC-IVF

One of the philosophies of NC-IVF is to use as few hormones as possible and to reduce the treatment-related stress as much as possible. Several studies have already shown that the follicular phase and the luteal phase [16] can be completely natural without any stimulation and luteal phase support. However, triggering of ovulation still requires an injection with an unnatural medication such as hCG.

It would be ideal to perform NC-IVF without any injections to reduce treatment-related stress even further [17]. Based on the studies by Teramoto et al. (2007) [6], Kato et al. (2012) [7] and Schmidt-Sarosi et al. (1995) [15] and on a pilot study performed in the infertility centre in Bern, Switzerland, a randomized controlled trial ("Injection free IVF"; study number: clinical.trials.gov: NCT04850261) is being prepared. It will be investigated whether ovulation induction with 200 μg nafarelin (1 hub) is possible in NC-IVF. In addition, the patient's therapy-related stress will be investigated.

Study protocol:

The patients will be randomized to be allocated to intervention A or B.

Intervention A:

As soon as the expected follicle size is >15 mm, ovulation will be induced by injecting 5000 IU hCG. Follicle aspiration, including flushing of the follicle will be performed 36 h later. The transfer of the embryo will be performed 2–5 days after the aspiration. To determine E2 and progesterone concentrations, blood will be taken 10 ± 1 days after hCG administration. Pregnancy will be confirmed or excluded by hCG testing in serum or urine 14–21 days after follicle aspiration. If hCG testing is positive, clinical pregnancy will be confirmed by vaginal ultrasound 1–4 weeks later.

Intervention B:

Intervention B will be performed identically to Intervention A with the following exception: Instead of injecting subcutaneous hCG, the patients will administer 1 hub of a GnRHa spray intranasally (200 µg nafarelin) to induce ovulation.

If there is no pregnancy achieved in the first treatment cycle, the patients switch to the respective other intervention (cross-over design).

The treatment-related stress will be evaluated using the Fertility Quality of Life (FertiQoL) [18] core questionnaire and a set of VAS questions concerning the level of discomfort encountered in the treatment.

12.4 Practical Conclusions

- NC-IVF is also possible without ovulation triggering, but many consultations are required, the IVF centre needs to be very flexible and the treatment is less effective.
- In NC-IVF and minimal stimulation IVF, ovulation triggering can be performed using hCG, GnRHa injections and GnRHa intranasal spray.
- In NC-IVF ovulation triggering with hCG does not require luteal phase support. Whether ovulation triggering with GnRHa nasal spray can also be performed without luteal phase support, which would further simplify NC-IVF treatment, is currently under investigation.

References

1. The European Recombinant LH Study Group. Human recombinant luteinizing hormone is as effective as, but safer than, urinary human chorionic gonadotropin in inducing final follicular maturation and ovulation in in vitro fertilization procedures: results of a multicenter double-blind study. J Clin Endocrinol Metab. 2001;86:2607–18.
2. Hajenius PJ, Mol BW, Ankum WM, van der Veen F, Bossuyt PM, Lammes FB. Clearance curves of serum human chorionic gonadotrophin for the diagnosis of persistent trophoblast. Hum Reprod. 1995;10:683–7.

3. Youssef MA, Abou-Setta AM, Lam WS. Recombinant versus urinary human chorionic gonadotrophin for final oocyte maturation triggering in IVF and ICSI cycles. Cochrane Database Syst Rev. 2016;4:CD003719.

4. von Wolff M, Nitzschke M, Stute P, Bitterlich N, Rohner S. Low-dosage clomiphene reduces premature ovulation rates and increases transfer rates in natural-cycle IVF. Reprod Biomed Online. 2014;29:209–15.

5. Kohl Schwartz AS, Calzaferri I, Roumet M, Limacher A, Fink A, Wueest A, Weidlinger S, Mitter VR, Leeners B, Von Wolff M. Follicular flushing leads to higher oocyte yield in monofollicular IVF: a randomized controlled trial. Hum Reprod. 2020;35:2253–61.

6. Teramoto S, Kato O. Minimal ovarian stimulation with clomiphene citrate: a large-scale retrospective study. Reprod Biomed Online. 2007;15:134–48.

7. Kato K, Takehara Y, Segawa T, Kawachiya S, Okuno T, Kobayashi T, Bodri D, Kato O. Minimal ovarian stimulation combined with elective single embryo transfer policy: age-specific results of a large, single-Centre, Japanese cohort. Reprod Biol Endocrinol. 2012;10:35.

8. Direito A, Bailly S, Mariani A, Ecochard R. Relationships between the luteinizing hormone surge and other characteristics of the menstrual cycle in normally ovulating women. Fertil Steril. 2013;99:279–285.e3.

9. Chrisp P, Goa KL. Nafarelin. a review of its pharmacodynamic and pharmacokinetic properties, and clinical potential in sex hormone-related conditions. Drugs. 1990;39:523–51.

10. Monroe SE, Blumenfeld Z, Andreyko JL, Schirock E, Henzl MR, Jaffe RB. Dose-dependent inhibition of pituitary-ovarian function during administration of a gonadotropin-releasing hormone agonistic analog (Nafarelin). J Clin Endocrinol Metab. 1986;63:1334–41.

11. Benadiva C, Engmann L. Intensive luteal phase support after GnRH agonist trigger: it does help. Reprod Biomed Online. 2012;25:329–30.

12. Zimmermann RC, Schröder S, Baars S, Schumacher M, Weise HC. Melatonin and the ovulatory luteinizing hormone surge. Fertil Steril. 1990;54:612–8.

13. Lenton EA, Woodward B. Natural-cycle versus stimulated-cycle IVF: is there a role for IVF in the natural cycle? J Assist Reprod Genet. 1993;10:406–8.

14. Lenton EA. Natural cycle IVF with and without terminal HCG: learning from failed cycles. Reprod Biomed Online. 2007;15:149–55.

15. Schmidt-Sarosi C, Kaplan DR, Sarosi P, Essig MN, Licciardi FL, Keltz M, Levitz M. Ovulation triggering in clomiphene citrate-stimulated cycles: human chorionic gonadotropin versus a gonadotropin releasing hormone agonist. J Assist Reprod Genet. 1995;12:167–74.

16. von Wolff M, Kohl Schwartz A, Stute P, Fäh M, Otti G, Schürch R, Rohner S. Follicular flushing in natural cycle IVF does not affect the luteal phase—a prospective controlled study. Reprod Biomed Online. 2017;35:37–41.

17. Haemmerli Keller K, Alder G, Loewer L, Faeh M, Rohner S, von Wolff M. Treatment-related psychological stress in different in vitro fertilization therapies with and without gonadotropin stimulation. Acta Obstet Gynecol Scand. 2018;97:269–76.

18. Boivin J, Takefman J, Braverman A. The fertility quality of life (FertiQoL) tool: development and general psychometric properties. Fertil Steril. 2011;96:409–415.e3.

Chapter 13
Follicle Aspiration in Natural Cycle and Minimal Stimulation IVF

Michael von Wolff

13.1 Background

In natural cycle IVF (NC-IVF) and minimal stimulation IVF, follicle aspiration with high oocyte retrieval rate and with low pain intensity is essential. The number of follicles is low, requiring aspiration with maximum efficacy. Monthly cycles and aspirations require aspirations with low risk and low pain intensity.

Aspirations in NC-IVF and minimal stimulation IVF with a low number of follicles and without analgesia are different from aspiration in conventional IVF with many follicles and analgesia or anaesthesia. It requires different needle sizes, different aspiration techniques and specific experience.

13.2 Size and Type of Aspiration Needle

In conventional IVF, large-lumen aspiration needles can be used to shorten the aspiration time because anaesthesia is usually administered. However, in case if only analgesia or sedation is administered, the size of the needle matters as the painfulness of the aspiration correlates with the size of the needle.

Aziz et al. (1993) [1] compared 16G and 18G aspiration needles. 35 women under sedation and intramuscular analgesia with pethidine underwent aspiration. Each ovary was randomized to be aspirated either first or second and by one of two different needles. Significantly greater pain was perceived by patients when the larger needle was being used. When aspirated with the 16G needle, 57% of the

M. von Wolff (✉)
Division of Gynecological Endocrinology and Reproductive Medicine, University Women's Hospital, University of Bern, Bern, Switzerland
e-mail: Michael.vonwolff@insel.ch

© The Author(s), under exclusive license to Springer Nature Switzerland AG 2022   125
M. von Wolff (ed.), *Natural Cycle and Minimal Stimulation IVF*,
https://doi.org/10.1007/978-3-030-97571-5_13

women reported a pain score of 3–4 (5: extremely painful), and when using an 18G needle, 23% of the women reported such a high pain score. The oocyte yield was not different.

Awonga et al. (1996) [2] compared 15G, 17G and 18G needles. 112 women under sedation and intravenous analgesia with pethidine underwent aspiration. They were randomized to be aspirated with one of the needles. When aspirated with the 15G needle, 44% of the women reported severe to intolerable pain, when aspirated with a 16G needle 22%, and when using an 18G needle, 16% of the women reported severe to intolerable pain. The duration of the aspiration and the oocyte yield were not different.

Wikland et al. (2011) [3] compared a 15G needle with a hybrid needle with a thin 21G needle tip. 257 women under oral analgesia and local anaesthesia (paracervical block) underwent aspiration. They were randomized to be aspirated with one of the needles. The aspiration pressure was between 90 and 120 mmHg. The overall pain was significantly lower in women with the 21G needle. Significantly more patients (40 of 126) had less than expected vaginal bleeding in the 21G group when compared with the 15G group (24 of 124; 32% versus 19%; 95% CI 1.7–23.0%). No differences were found between the two needles with regard to aspiration time, oocyte yield, fertilization, cleavage rate, number of good quality embryos, number of embryos for freezing and pregnancy rate.

These studies clearly prove that thin needles cause less pain. Furthermore, oocyte yield and the IVF outcome are apparently not different. However, in all studies, aspiration was performed in conventional IVF with many follicles and patients received analgesia, sedation or local anaesthesia. Therefore, the setting of these studies cannot be compared with the setting of NC-IVF and minimal stimulation IVF in which only one or few follicles are aspirated and in which aspiration is usually performed without anaesthesia or analgesia.

In NC-IVF and minimal stimulation IVF, very thin needles between 19G and 21G (Table 13.1) are usually used. It can be assumed that the aspiration time is longer, however, due to the low number of follicles, this does not play a relevant role. According to Kohl Schwartz et al., 2020 [4], the aspiration in NC-IVF with one follicle takes only 26 s (interquartile range 22–30 s).

When using very thin needles, the reduced pain must be weighed against the associated longer aspiration time and greater flexibility of the needle. The greater flexibility of the needle can be problematic when aspirating many follicles, in sonophobic conditions, and if the pelvic floor is quite firm possibly causing the aspiration needle to deviate from the aspiration line.

Thin needles allow trans-uterine aspirations without anaesthesia, e.g. if the ovaries are located and fixed behind the uterus as in some endometriosis patients. In the infertility centre in Bern, Switzerland, transfundal aspirations are performed in NC-IVF and minimal stimulation IVF with 19G needles and without touching the uterine cavity (Table 13.2). With this needle size, aspiration is still tolerable and the needle is stiff enough not to bend and to deviate. Transuterine follicle aspiration is only slightly more painful than normal follicular aspiration, as the peritoneum, but not the myometrium is the most pain sensitive.

Table 13.1 Aspiration needles used and aspiration techniques applied in centres specialized in NC-IVF and/or minimal stimulation IVF

Centre	IVF technique	Needle size	Needle type	Aspiration pressure	Aspiration technique	Analgesia
Bern, Switzerland (Kohl Schwartz et al., 2020) [4]	NC-IVF, Minimal stimulation IVF	19G	Monoluminal	220 mm Hg	Aspiration and follicle flushing	None
Tokyo, Japan, (Kato et al., 2012) [5]; Teramoto et al., 2019) [6]	NC-IVF, Minimal stimulation IVF	21G	Monoluminal	250 mm Hg[a]	Aspiration only	None
New York, U.S.	Minimal stimulation IVF	19–21G	Monoluminal	150 mm Hg	Aspiration and follicle flushing as needed	None, 10 mg diazepam if needed

[a] If several degenerated oocytes were retrieved in previous cycles, the aspiration pressures are reduced to approximately 200 mmHg

Table 13.2 Cases with transuterine and transfundal aspiration without anaesthesia, using 19G aspiration needles in women with endometriosis undergoing minimal stimulation IVF (Infertility centre Bern, Switzerland, performed in 2020)

Age.	Endometriosis	Aspirated oocytes, n	Transfer performed	Pregnancy	Live birth	Complications
36	rAFS IV	1	No (no fertilization)	–	–	No
36	rAFS IV	1	Yes	Yes	Yes	No
41	rAFS IV	1	Yes	No	No	No
39	rAFS I	2	Yes	Yes	Yes	No

In monofollicular NC-IVF, the use of a 21G needles is possible, whereas in minimal stimulation with many follicles, 19G needles might be more advantageous. 19G needles are a good compromise between painfulness, flexibility and aspiration time.

Very thin needles are always single-lumen needles. The disadvantage of single-lumen needles is that if flushing of the follicles is performed, the flushing medium needs to pass the full length of the tubing and the needle. However, as single-lumen needles have been successfully used for aspirations in combination with follicular flushing [4], they can also be recommended if flushing is needed.

To possibly improve the efficacy of follicular flushing, double-lumen needles have been designed. Double-lumen needles are usually thicker (total thickness minimum 17G), as they consist of an outer flushing lumen and an inner aspiration lumen. These needles allow effective flushing, but the disadvantage is the more painful aspiration due to its size.

Needles with a thick double-lumen shaft and a thin single-lumen needle tip have been designed to combine the advantages of a double-lumen needle with those of a thin single-lumen needle. These hybrid needles, such as the *Steiner-Tan needle* (https://www.ivffuture.com/steiner-tan-needle/) [7] or the *Sense™ Double Lumen* needle (Vitrolife - Oocyte retrieval needles) have a thick shaft of around 19G and a 5–7 cm long needle tip of minimum 21G (*Steiner-Tan needle)* or 20G (*Sense™ Double Lumen* needle).

If very thin needles are used, the negative aspiration pressure is usually increased to reduce aspiration time.

Table 13.2 shows the negative aspiration pressure used by large centres specialized in NC-IVF and/or minimal stimulation IVF. The IVF centre in Bern uses 19G needles and the pressure is 220 mm Hg, the centre in Tokyo uses 21G needles and the pressure is 250 mmHg and the centre in New York uses 19–21G needles and the aspiration pressure is 150 mmHg. These centres perform a very high number of cycles (see Chap. 25) without reporting adverse effects induced by high negative aspiration pressures. The centre in Tokyo reduces the pressure to approximately 200 mmg if several degenerated oocytes were retrieved in previous cycles.

In summary,

for NC-IVF and minimal stimulation IVF without anaesthesia and analgesia, aspiration needles of size 19–21G should be used, as they are significantly less painful. Centres can choose between different needle types such as mono-lumen, double-lumen and hybrid needles.

13.3   Analgesia

In conventional IVF, pain relief is required in most women undergoing follicle aspiration. A Cochrane analysis revealed that simultaneous use of sedation, combined with analgesia such as opiates and further enhanced by paracervical block or acupuncture, resulted in better pain relief than occurred with one modality alone [8]. However, all techniques reviewed were associated with a high degree of patient satisfaction.

With NC-IVF or minimal stimulation IVF, follicle aspiration is much less painful. As aspiration is usually performed on just one ovary, only one or few follicles are aspirated and aspiration takes much less time.

In a survey at the IVF centre Bern, Switzerland, 30 women undergoing NC-IVF were asked how painful they experienced the follicular aspiration compared to venous blood sampling. The aspiration was performed with a 19G needle and three follicular flushings. 85% of the women reported that the aspiration was equally or less painful than blood sampling. 15% described it as more painful (Fig. 13.1).

It should be noted, however, that aspiration without anaesthesia requires a different technique than aspiration with anaesthesia. The low pain intensities mentioned in Fig. 13.1 can only be achieved with sufficient expertise.

In most aspirations, the ovary is located close to the vaginal wall with the follicle very close to the ultrasound probe. In these cases, follicle aspiration is easy to perform.

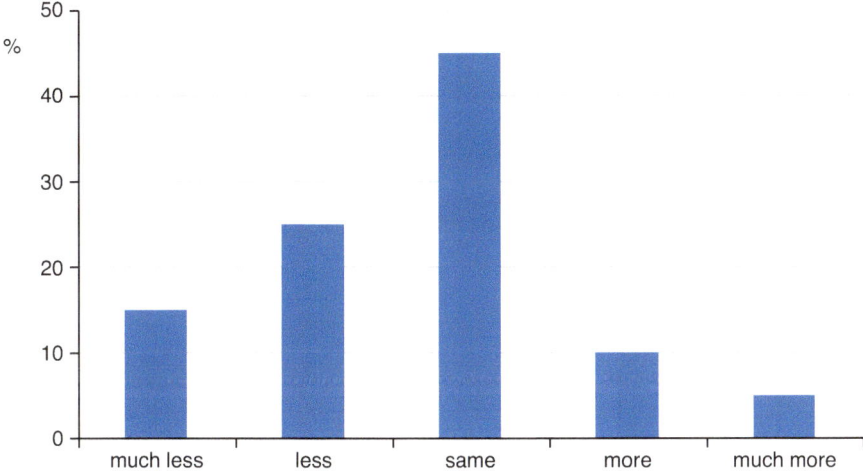

Fig. 13.1 Percentage of women with a given pain intensity compared to venous blood sampling during follicle aspiration with three follicular flushings without analgesia using a 19G single-lumen needle in NC-IVF (*n* = 30, data IVF centre Bern, Switzerland)

Aspiration is difficult, however, if

- the follicle is not located very closely to the ultrasound probe, so that the dense ovarian medulla must be penetrated to reach the follicle,
- the ovary is very mobile, i.e., in slim women,
- the ovary is located far cranially, which is common in obese women and in women with intra-abdominal adhesions, e.g., in endometriosis.

In these cases, it is recommended that

- the patient is not fasting to avoid hypoglycaemia,
- the patient is distracted, e.g., by engaging her in an interesting conversation. Some patients also benefit from being shown the aspiration procedure on the ultrasound monitor,
- the needle is additionally drilled during insertion so as not to push the ovary cranially, as this can lead to peritoneal stimulus with a drop in blood pressure and collapse,
- the aspiration is stopped immediately for a few minutes at the first signs of a drop in blood pressure, recognizable by increasing paleness or dizziness of the patient.

Taking these measures into account, aspirations can be easily performed without any analgesia.

If analgesia is desired, it is possible to give non-steroidal analgesics, e.g., ibuprofen 400 mg, 1–2 h before aspiration. Local infiltration of the vaginal wall with an anaesthetic or a paracervical block is also an option. However, the effectiveness of these measures is limited. Some centres offer sedation, i.e. with diazepam 10 mg 30 min before aspiration in very anxious patients.

In summary,

analgesia or even anaesthesia is not necessary for NC-IVF or minimal stimulation IVF. The key to successful follicle aspirations with low pain intensity is use of thin needles, distraction of the patient and clinical experience with aspirations without anaesthesia.

13.4   Follicle Flushing

Three different aspiration needles can be used for follicle flushing:

- A single-lumen needle with one tubing, where the aspiration and flushing medium are passed through the same needle channel and tubing, resulting in a dead volume of 1.2 mL (19G). The needles have a minimum thickness of 21G. The flushing medium is injected into the tubing via an adapter (e.g. 19G needle: Kohl Schwartz et al. (2020) [4]; 21G needle: Kato et al. (2018) [5]). These needles are easy to handle, can be very thin but create the largest dead volume.
- A single-lumen needle with two separate aspiration and flushing tubings and a thin needle tip (19G, 21G) and a thicker needle shaft (16G) resulting in a dead volume of 0.4 mL (19G) (e.g. 19G needle: Sense™ double lumen, Vitrolife; 21G needle: Wikland et al. (2011) [3]). These needles are easy to handle, have a very thin needle tip and create a lower dead volume. However, due to the two tubings in which the fluid exchange is reduced, fluid temperature inside the tubings can easily drop.
- A hybrid needle which is a double-lumen needle with two separate aspiration and flushing tubings with a thin single-lumen needle tip. The double-lumen part is rather thick but the size of the needle tip has a minimum size of 21G resulting in a minimal dead volume (Hybrid needle with needle tip 21G: Steiner-Tan Needle® [7]). These needles are less easy to handle, have a very thin needle tip and create a very low dead volume. However, due to the two separate tubings, fluid temperature inside the tubings can easily drop.
- A double-lumen needle with two separate aspiration and flushing tubings, in which the aspiration and flushing fluid is passed through different channels, resulting in no dead volume at all. The needles have a minimum thickness of 17G (e.g. 17G needle: Xiao et al. (2018) [9]). These needles are easy to handle, are rather thick but create no dead volume at all. However, due to the two tubings, fluid temperature inside the tubings can easily drop.

As the different needle types have not yet been evaluated in one clinical study, their practicability and effectiveness cannot be compared. However, it is certain that thin needles or needles with thin needle tips create least pain, tissue injury and lower risk for bleedings [3].

The single-lumen needle has the advantage of easy handling, but has the disadvantage that part of the aspirate remains in the needle and in the tubing system during the follicular flushing procedure. The flushing medium is flushed back into the follicle with each flushing. Therefore, the flushing procedure with a single-lumen needle is possibly less effective than with a single-lumen needle with two tubings, with a hybrid or with a double-lumen needle, requiring more flushing steps.

However, single-lumen needles have the advantage of lower risk of a temperature drop in the tubings as the tubings are constantly flushed. Temperature has been shown to be very critical for oocyte function as cooling results in dysfunction of the meiotic spindles [10].

As all needle types described above are used elsewhere and as single-lumen needles with one tubing, single-lumen needles with 2 tubings and double-lumen needles are also used within the network IVF-Naturelle® for aspiration and flushing, it is possibly less the needle system itself but it is rather the experience of the physicians that matters.

When evaluating the effectiveness of the flushing procedure, a distinction must be made between:

- polyfollicular IVF (conventional IVF with normal or high response),
- oligofollicular IVF (conventional IVF with poor or low response, minimal stimulation IVF),
- monofollicular IVF (natural cycle IVF; minimal stimulation IVF with one follicle).

For conventional, mainly polyfollicular IVF, a meta-analysis with 10 randomized controlled trials including 928 women was performed [11]. The study showed that follicular flushing revealed little or no difference in the live birth rate (OR 0.95, 95% CI: 0.58–1.56).

For poor responders, mainly oligofollicular IVF, a meta-analysis with 3 randomized controlled trials including 210 women was performed. This meta-analysis showed that in oligofollicular IVF, as also described in polyfollicular IVF, follicle flushing increases neither the oocyte retrieval rate (Table 13.3) nor the live birth rate (Table 13.4) [12].

Table 13.3 Comparison of the number of mature (metaphase II) oocytes retrieved in aspirations with flushing of the follicles versus aspiration only in poor responders (summary of a meta-analysis [12])

Included studies	Aspiration and flushing. Number of oocytes, mean ± SD	Aspiration only. Number of oocytes, mean ± SD	Mean difference (95% CI)	Heterogeneity, I^2
Haydardedeoglu 2017	2.1 ± 0.1	1.9 ± 0.1	0.2 (0.16–0.24)	
Mok-Lin 2013	2.5 ± 1.3	3.3 ± 1.9	−0.8 (−1.7 to 0.1)	
Von Horn 2017	2.1 ± 1.6	1.6 ± 1.2	0.5 (−0.12 to 1.12)	
Overall result			0.09 (−0.40 to 0.59)	64%[a]

[a] Indicates substantial heterogeneity of studies (www.handbook-5-1.cochrane.org)

Table 13.4 Comparison of the live birth rate after aspirations with flushing of the follicles versus aspiration only in poor responders (summary of a meta-analysis [12])

Included studies	Aspiration with flushing. Events/total	Aspiration only. Events/total	Mean difference (95% CI)	Heterogeneity, I^2
Overall result	13/105	16/105	0.81 (0.42–1.58)	36%[a]

[a] Indicates moderate heterogeneity of studies (www.handbook-5-1.cochrane.org)

Table 13.5 Effect of follicle aspiration plus 5 flushings versus aspiration only in NC-IVF, using a 19G single-lumen aspiration needle [4]

	Flushing group n, %	Aspiration only group n, %	Mantel-Haenszel risk difference % (95% CI)	p-value
Intention to treat analysis (cycles)	$n = 83$	$n = 81$		
Retrieved oocytes (retrieved oocytes/ cycle)	69 (83.1%)	51 (63.0%)	20.6% (7.1%,33.2%)	0.005
Metaphase II (MII) oocytes (MII oocytes/cycle)	64 (77.1%)	48 (59.3%)	18.2% (3.9%,31.7%)	0.02
Fertilized oocytes (fertilized oocytes/cycle)	53 (63.9%)	38 (46.9%)	16.9% (1.5%,31.5%)	0.05
Embryo transfers (transfer rate/cycle)	52 (62.7%)	38 (46.9%)	15.7% (0.3%,30.4%)	0.06
Implantations (implantation rate/cycle)	12 (14.5%)	10 (12.4%)	1.9% (−8.4%,12.1%)	0.89
Clinical pregnancies (pregnancy rate/cycle)	9 (10.8%)	9 (11.1%)	−0.5% (−9.9%,9.0%)	0.93
Live births (live birth rate/cycle)	7 (8.4%)	8 (9.9%)	−1.66% (−10.4%, 7.1%)	0.72

No meta-analysis has yet been published for monofollicular IVF. However, the data published so far suggest an increased success rate with follicle flushing.

In a retrospective study with 164 NC-IVF cycles, flushing increased the oocyte yield from 44.5% to 80.5% [13].

In a prospective study with 146 semi-NC-IVF aspirations with very little gonadotropin stimulation, the percentage of good embryos was 37.8% in the group with flushing and 28.8% in the group without flushing. The implantation rates were 44.1% and 24.1%, respectively [14].

A recent randomized controlled study analysed 164 women undergoing NC-IVF without and with 5 flushings (Table 13.5, Fig. 13.2). The study revealed higher oocyte yield and a non-significantly higher transfer rate in the flushing group. However, an increased live birth rate could not be shown.

In summary,

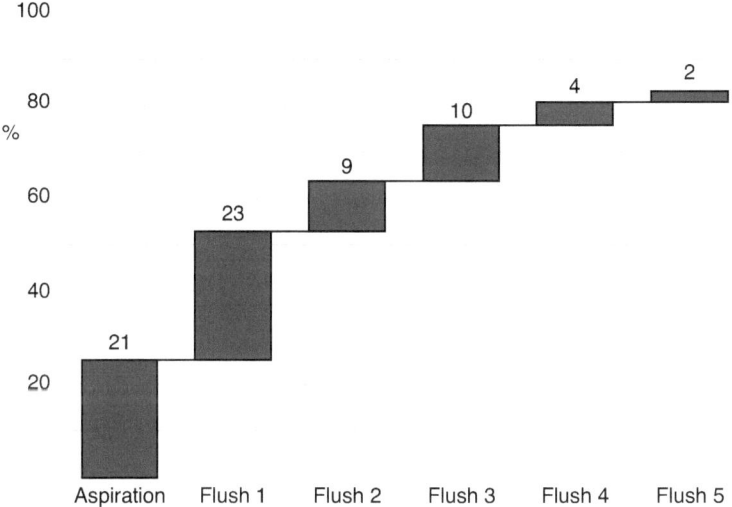

Fig. 13.2 Retrieval of oocytes per flushing step in NC-IVF using a 19G single-lumen aspiration needle (numbers above the boxes: collected oocytes per aspiration/flush, total number of aspirated oocytes: n = 69) (Reprinted with permission from [4])

follicular flushing seems to be beneficial in monofollicular IVF. Flushing of the follicles can be performed with different needle types and sizes and with different aspiration techniques. It is not yet known if flushing also increases live birth rate.

13.5   Practical Conclusions

- In NC-IVF and minimal stimulation IVF, follicle aspiration does usually not require anaesthesia or analgesia.
- Thin needles with a size of 19G to 21G should be preferred to reduce pain of aspiration.
- Single-lumen, double-lumen and hybrid needles are available. General recommendations which needle should be used cannot be given.
- Flushing should be considered in monofollicular IVF but not in oligofollicular and polyfollicular IVF.

References

1. Aziz N, Biljan MM, Taylor CT, Manasse PR, Kingsland CR. Effect of aspirating needle calibre on outcome of in-vitro fertilization. Hum Reprod. 1993;8:1098–00.
2. Awonuga A, Waterstone J, Oyesanya O, Curson R, Nargund G, Parsons J. A prospective randomized study comparing needles of different diameters for transvaginal ultrasound-directed follicle aspiration. Fertil Steril. 1996;65:109–13.

3. Wikland M, Blad S, Bungum L, Hillensjö T, Karlström PO, Nilsson S. A randomized controlled study comparing pain experience between a newly designed needle with a thin tip and a standard needle for oocyte aspiration. Hum Reprod. 2011;26:1377–83.
4. Kohl Schwartz AS, Calzaferri I, Roumet M, Limacher A, Fink A, Wueest A, Weidlinger S, Mitter VR, Leeners B, Von Wolff M. Follicular flushing leads to higher oocyte yield in monofollicular IVF: a randomized controlled trial. Hum Reprod. 2020;35(10):2253–61. https://doi.org/10.1093/humrep/deaa165.
5. Kato K, Ezoe K, Yabuuchi A, Fukuda J, Kuroda T, Ueno S, Fujita H, Kobayashi T. Comparison of pregnancy outcomes following fresh and electively frozen single blastocyst transfer in natural cycle and clomiphene-stimulated IVF cycles. Hum Reprod Open. 2018;2018:hoy006.
6. Teramoto S, Osada H, Sato Y, Shozu M. Pregnancy and neonatal outcomes of small follicle-derived blastocyst transfer in modified natural cycle in vitro fertilization. Fertil Steril. 2019;111:747–52.
7. von Horn K, Depenbusch M, Schultze-Mosgau A, Griesinger G. Randomized, open trial comparing a modified double-lumen needle follicular flushing system with a single-lumen aspiration needle in IVF patients with poor ovarian response. Hum Reprod. 2017;32:832–5.
8. Kwan I, Wang R, Pearce E, Bhattacharya S. Pain relief for women undergoing oocyte retrieval for assisted reproduction. Cochrane Database Syst Rev. 2018;5:CD004829. https://doi.org/10.1002/14651858.CD004829.pub4.
9. Xiao Y, Wang Y, Wang M, Liu K. Follicular flushing increases the number of oocytes retrieved in poor ovarian responders undergoing in vitro fertilization: a retrospective cohort study. BMC Womens Health. 2018;18:186.
10. Wang WH, Meng L, Hackett RJ, Odenbourg R, Keefe DL. Limited recovery of meiotic spindles in living human oocytes after cooling-rewarming observed using polarized light microscopy. Hum Reprod. 2001;16:2374–238.
11. Georgiou EX, Melo P, Brown J, Granne IE. Follicular flushing during oocyte retrieval in assisted reproductive techniques. Cochrane Database Syst Rev. 2018;4:CD004634.
12. Neumann K, Griesinger G. Follicular flushing in patients with poor ovarian response: a systematic review and meta-analysis. Reprod Biomed Online. 2018;36:408–15.
13. von Wolff M, Hua YZ, Santi A, Ocon E, Weiss B. Follicle flushing in monofollicular in vitro fertilization almost doubles the number of transferable embryos. Acta Obstet Gynecol Scand. 2013;92:346–8.
14. Méndez Lozano DH, Fanchin R, Chevalier N, Feyereisen E, Hesters L, Frydman N, Frydman R. The follicular flushing duplicate the pregnancy rate on semi natural cycle IVF. J Gynecol Obstet Biol Reprod (Paris). 2007;36:36–41.

Chapter 14
Luteal Phase Support in Natural Cycle and Minimal Stimulation IVF

Michael von Wolff

14.1 Background

In conventional IVF, luteal phase support is mandatory. The supraphysiological oestradiol (E2) blood concentration reduces the secretion of luteinizing hormone, LH, leading to premature luteolysis.

In natural cycle IVF (NC-IVF) and minimal stimulation IVF, treatment conditions are different to conventional IVF. E2 and progesterone concentrations are much lower or even normal, and gonadotropin suppressing medications such as GnRH analogues are not or are only given for a short period of time. On the other hand, follicles are usually flushed (see Chap. 13), which reduces the number of granulosa cells.

Therefore, to provide an individual and effective luteal phase support in NC-IVF and minimal stimulation IVF, a good understanding of the endocrinology and physiology of the luteal phase (see Chap. 8) and the effects of ovarian stimulations on the function of the luteal body is required.

14.2 Luteal Phase Support in Conventional IVF

In conventional IVF with high-dose gonadotropin stimulation and downregulation of endogenous gonadotropin secretion with GnRH antagonists or GnRH agonists, luteal phase support is mandatory.

M. von Wolff (✉)
Division of Gynecological Endocrinology and Reproductive Medicine, University Women's Hospital, University of Bern, Bern, Switzerland
e-mail: Michael.vonwolff@insel.ch

135

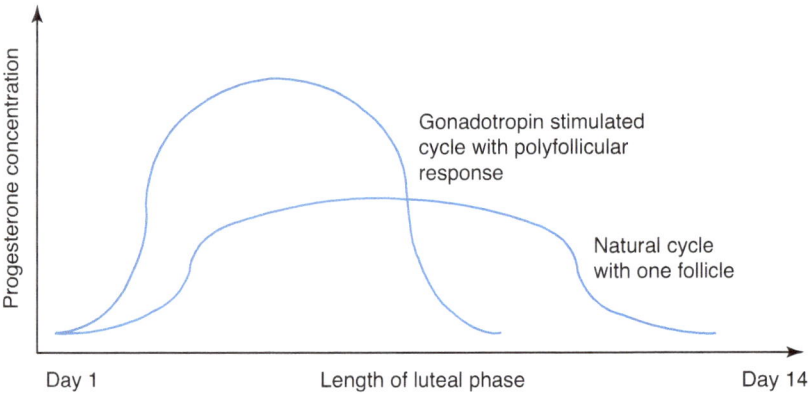

Fig. 14.1 Abnormal corpus luteum function following ovarian stimulation for in vitro fertilization. Abnormally raised progesterone levels during the early luteal phase coincide with premature luteolysis (according to [1])

The large number of mature follicles develop into luteal bodies leading to initially very high initial progesterone concentration in blood (Fig. 14.1). The high progesterone concentration drops prematurely, resulting in luteal phase insufficiency [1]. If luteal phase support with progesterone is administered during conventional IVF treatment, the IVF success rate is almost doubled. According to a meta-analysis including five randomized controlled studies with 642 patients, progesterone supplementation increases live birth or ongoing pregnancy rate almost two-fold (OR 1.77; 95% CI 1.09–2.86) [2].

14.2.1 Endocrinological Causes of Luteal Phase Insufficiency in Conventional IVF

The main cause for luteal phase insufficiency is thought to be supraphysiological E2 concentration, which suppresses the release of luteinizing hormone (LH) [1]. LH is required for the maintenance of the luteal body until, at the onset of pregnancy, the trophoblast produces human chorionic gonadotropin (hCG), which takes over the function of LH.

Ovulation triggering with GnRH agonists reduces pituitary LH release and thereby induces premature luteolysis.

It is possible that the initially high progesterone concentrations in the luteal phase also contribute to the LH-suppressing effect as progesterone modulates hypothalamic GnRH secretion by decreasing GnRH pulse frequency [3].

It was previously assumed that luteal phase insufficiency is less pronounced when GnRH antagonists are used, since the LH-suppressing effect of GnRH agonists last for longer than that of GnRH antagonists [4]. However, this does not seem to be the case since luteal progesterone serum concentrations are the same with GnRH agonist and GnRH antagonist protocols [5].

14.2.2   Dose, Mode of Application and Type of Progestogens

Luteal phase support can be performed with progestogens, with luteal hCG injections and with luteal GnRH agonist injections. All these techniques are largely equivalent in their effect in conventional IVF [2].

Micronized progesterone can be administered orally and vaginally. If administered orally, attention should be paid to the rapid decrease in concentration after ingestion [6]. Therefore, micronized progesterone should be administered several times a day when given orally.

With vaginal administration, the blood concentrations are largely stable for about 24 h [6]. The vaginal application of 200, 400, and 600 mg micronized progesterone leads largely the same blood concentrations on day 10 and 14 of the luteal phase in conventional IVF [7].

However, to definitely exclude fluctuations in concentration, micronized progesterone is usually administered 2–3 times daily and with a total dose of 400–600 mg per day when administered vaginally. The effect on the pregnancy rate is the same at low and high doses [2].

To increase the effect of vaginally administered micronized progesterone, bioadhesive substances were added in the medication Crinone® 8%. The bioadhesive vaginal gel contains micronized progesterone in an emulsion system. The progesterone carrier vehicle is an oil in water emulsion containing the water swellable, but insoluble polymer, polycarbophil. The progesterone is partially soluble in both the oil and water phase of the vehicle, with the majority of the progesterone existing as a suspension. These lead to a constantly slow and sustained release. Therefore, Crinone® 8% only needs to be applied once per day.

The recently published Lotus I [8] and Lotus II studies [9] have shown that vaginal micronized progesterone can be replaced by oral dydrogesterone as it has, like progesterone, only limited suppressive effects on the hypothalamus–pituitary axis. Both studies even revealed a non-significant increase in the live birth rate if dydrogesterone was used. However, dydrogesterone has so far only be studied in a dose of 10 mg orally three times a day and was administered in the Lotus studies until the 12th week of pregnancy.

14.2.3   Timing of Luteal Phase Support

Luteal phase support by luteal phase supplementation usually started in the evening on the day of follicular aspiration. However, as the progesterone concentration in blood is initially very high (Fig. 14.1), this is not absolutely necessary. Accordingly, luteal phase supplementation can also be started up to the fifth day after follicular aspiration [10].

Luteal phase supplementation can be discontinued on the day of a positive pregnancy test, as hCG then takes over the effect of LH and prevents luteolysis [10]. In clinical practice, however, luteal phase supplementation is administered for much longer. According to a survey conducted among reproductive physicians worldwide, luteal phase supplementation is administered until at least the eighth week of pregnancy in 72% of the 408 IVF centres surveyed in 82 countries [11].

In summary,

in conventional IVF, luteal phase support is always required due to luteal phase insufficiency induced by supraphysiological E2 concentration which suppress LH release. Vaginal micronized progesterone or oral dydrogesterone is most commonly used to supplement the luteal phase. Ovulation triggering with GnRH agonists reduces pituitary LH release and thereby induces premature luteolysis.

14.3 Luteal Phase Support in NC-IVF

In NC-IVF, luteal phase support is usually performed by luteal phase supplementation and is only required in cases of luteal phase insufficiency, defined by short luteal phase or premenstrual spotting (Table 14.1).

The length of the luteal phase in natural cycles is, according to the analysis of App recordings of more than 600,000 cycles, 12.4 ± 2.4 days (mean $\pm$ SD) [12].

Table 14.1 Different NC-IVF and minimal stimulation IVF treatments and suggested luteal phase supplementations, started anytime between aspiration and transfer, and stopped around 14 days after aspiration

Treatments	Luteal phase supplementation required	Remarks and treatment examples
Natural cycle IVF (including hCG trigger, 1× GnRH antagonist, NSAID)	Not required	If luteal phase <12 days or if premenstrual spotting: See minimal stimulation IVF with gonadotropin stimulation and low response
Natural cycle IVF with low-dose clomiphene citrate (including hCG trigger, 1× GnRH antagonist, NSAID)	Not required	If luteal phase <12 days or if premenstrual spotting: See minimal stimulation IVF with gonadotropin stimulation and low response
Minimal stimulation IVF with letrozole stimulation	Probably required	Low-dose supplementation recommended: See minimal stimulation IVF with gonadotropin stimulation and low response
Minimal stimulation IVF with gonadotropin stimulation and low response (2–3 follicles)	Low-dose supplementation required	• Micronized progesterone vaginally 200 mg once daily or • Crinone® 8% once daily or • Dydrogesterone orally 10 mg twice daily.
Minimal stimulation IVF with gonadotropin stimulation and normal/high response (>2–3 follicles)	Normal dose supplementation required	• Micronized progesterone vaginally 200 mg twice daily or • Crinone® 8% vaginally once daily or • Dydrogesterone orally 10 mg three times daily.

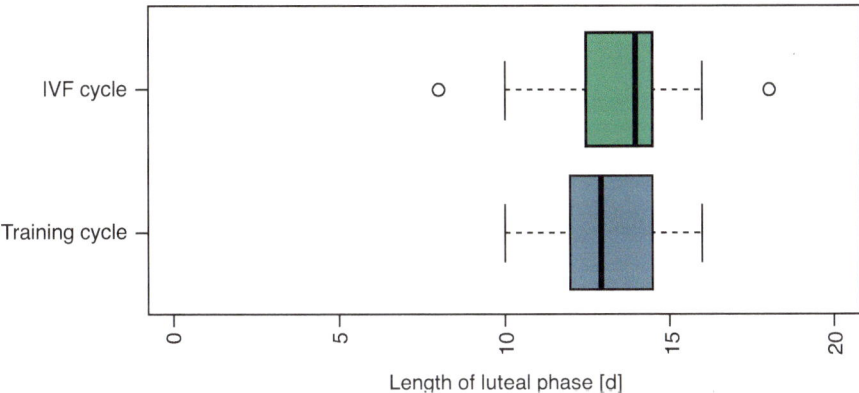

Fig. 14.2 Length of the luteal phases in natural IVF cycles (IVF cycle) compared to natural non-IVF cycles (Training cycle) of 23 women, both triggered with 5000 IU hCG. Follicles in IVF cycles were aspirated and also flushed 3 times (according to [13])

This is roughly in line with natural cycles triggered with 5000 IU hCG with a cycle length of 13 (12; 14.5) days (median and interquartile ranges) (Fig. 14.2) [13]. According to Bull et al. (2019) [12], the length of the luteal phase increases slightly with age, beginning at the age of 30 years. At the age of 25–30 years, the length of the luteal phase is 12.4 ± 2.2 days and at the age of 31–35 years, it is 12.9 ± 2.3 days (see Chap. 8).

According to these numbers, most women have a luteal phase lasting at least 12 days. Therefore, the length of the luteal phase is unphysiologically reduced only if it is shorter than 12 days.

Follicle flushing could theoretically have an impact on the function of the luteal body due to the reduction of granulosa cells. However, according to a controlled study in which the length of the luteal phase (Fig. 14.2) was analysed in 23 NC-IVF cycles with three follicular flushings, intraindividually compared with control cycles without aspiration, flushing did not have a relevant impact on the length of the luteal phase [13]. Follicle aspiration and flushing shortened the luteal phase in 7 women (30.4%), the length of the luteal phase was not affected in 4 women (17.4%) and in 12 women (52.2%) the length was increased. Statistically, aspiration and flushing did not shorten the luteal phase. Median duration of the luteal phase was 13 days (interquartile range 12d, 14.5d) in control cycles and 14 days (interquartile range 12.5d, 14.5d) in aspiration and flushing cycles.

Luteal serum concentrations of progesterone were also analysed and compared in 23 cycles and were also not different (Fig. 14.3).

Accordingly, luteal phase supplementation is only required in NC-IVF cycles if the luteal phase is shorter than 12 days, or if premenstrual spotting indicates luteal phase insufficiency.

If however, progesterone should be supplemented, vaginal micronized progesterone 200 mg per day is sufficient according to the studies performed in conventional IVF.

Fig. 14.3 Progesterone concentration in natural IVF cycles (IVF cycle) compared to natural non-IVF cycles (Training cycle) of 23 women, both triggered 5000 IU hCG. Follicles in IVF cycles were aspirated and flushed 3 times (according to [13]). Early luteal phase: day 2–3, mid-luteal phase day 6–7, and late luteal phase day 10–11 after ovulation/aspiration. Presentation of median with interquartile ranges and whiskers with maximum length of 1.5 interquartile ranges (according to [13])

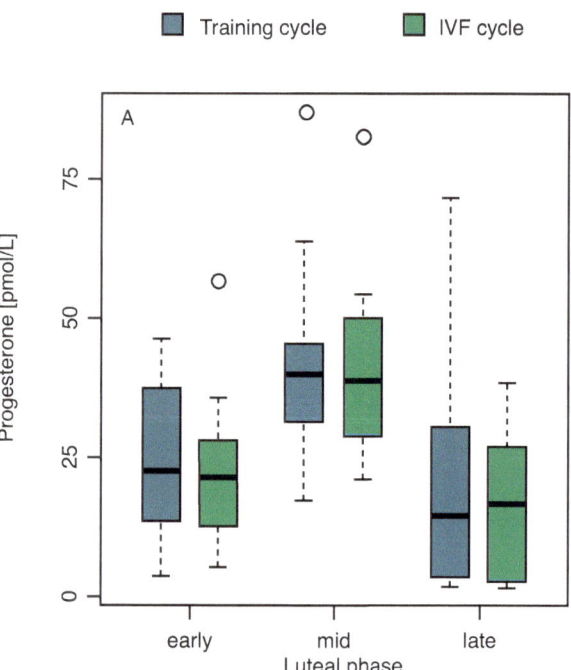

Supplementation should be started any time between follicle aspiration and embryo transfer and should be given until the day of the pregnancy test around 14 days after aspiration. For practical reasons and to improve adsorption, vaginal supplementation is usually performed in the evening before sleep.

Some centres induce ovulation with GnRH agonists (GnRHa) as intranasal spray in NC-IVF and minimal stimulation IVF (see Chap. 12). Triggering ovulation with GnRHa in conventional IVF dysregulates the luteal phase. Whether the luteal phase is also dysregulated in NC-IVF is still unknown and is currently being evaluated in a prospective controlled study (see Chap. 12). Therefore, ovulation triggering with GnRH agonist intranasal spray is still combined with luteal phase support.

Table 14.2 describes the luteal phase supports given in the large centres specialized in NC-IVF and/or minimal stimulation IVF.

In NC-IVF, possible luteal phase supplements are as follows:

- No luteal phase supplementation if luteal phase ≥12 days and no premenstrual spotting.
- If luteal phase <12 days and premenstrual spotting: Micronized progesterone once daily, administered vaginally in the evening, starting between aspiration and embryo transfer until pregnancy test, i.e., approx. 14th day after follicular aspiration. Alternatively, dydrogesterone can be administered orally twice daily.

Table 14.2 Luteal phase supplementation in centres specialized in NC-IVF and/or minimal stimulation IVF (see also Chap. 15)

Centre	IVF technique	Luteal phase support[a]
Bern, Switzerland (von Wolff et al. (2017) [13])	NC-IVF	Only if luteal phase <12 days or premenstrual spotting: 200 mg micronized progesterone intravaginally in the evening.
	Minimal stimulation IVF	Depending on the number of follicles, 200 mg micronized progesterone intravaginally once or twice daily.
Tokyo, Japan, (Kato et al. (2012) [20], Onogi et al. (2020) [21])	NC-IVF, minimal stimulation IVF	Cleavage stage embryo transfer (day 2): Dydrogesterone 3 × 10 mg/d orally, starting on the day of transfer for 10 days. Blastocyst transfer: Progesterone additionally administered intravaginally (800 mg/d) along with oral dydrogesterone for 7 days if luteal function is insufficient (progesterone concentration on the day of ovulation triggering 8–11 ng/mL). Blastocyst transfer is cancelled if progesterone concentration is <8 ng/mL.
New York, U.S.	NC-IVF, minimal stimulation IVF	Not required if freezing of blastocysts. In case of fresh transfer: Progesterone vaginally.

[a] See also Chap. 15

14.4 Luteal Phase Support in Minimal Stimulation IVF

Minimal stimulation IVF is a heterogeneous group of different stimulations (see Chaps. 2 and 15). Accordingly, luteal phase support must be adjusted for each stimulation protocol, taking into account the patient's ovarian response (Table 14.1). Roughly speaking, a distinction should be made between the following stimulations with regard to luteal phase supplementation:

14.4.1 Minimal Stimulation IVF with Clomiphene Citrate

When stimulating with clomiphene citrate, the same rules apply as with NC-IVF, i.e., no luteal phase support is required if the luteal phase is of normal length. The reason is the increased LH baseline concentrations due to clomiphene citrate. Due to the half-life of the clomiphene isomer zuclomifene [14, 15] (see Chap. 11), which lasts several days, this effect also persists in the luteal phase and thus seems to prevent premature luteolysis. A meta-analysis of three randomized controlled trials including 606 patients who had undergone stimulation with clomiphene citrate followed by intrauterine insemination demonstrated this (Table 14.3). According to

Table 14.3 Clinical pregnancy rates in women undergoing clomiphene citrate stimulation and intrauterine insemination with and without luteal phase support. (Summary of a meta-analysis [16])

Included studies	Sample size, n	Risk ratio (95% CI)	Heterogeneity, I^2
6 studies, overall result	606	0.85 (0.52-1.41)	0%*

*indicates very low heterogeneity of studies (www.handbook-5-1.cochrane.org)

this meta-analysis, the pregnancy rate is not higher with luteal phase support (RR 0.85, 95% CI: 0.52–1.41).

In minimal stimulation IVF with clomiphene citrate, possible luteal phase supplementations are as follows:

- No luteal phase supplementation if luteal phase ≥12 days and no premenstrual spotting.
- If luteal phase <12 days and premenstrual spotting: Micronized progesterone once daily, administered vaginally in the evening, starting between aspiration and embryo transfer until pregnancy test, i.e., approx. 14th day after follicular aspiration. Alternatively, dydrogesterone can be administered orally twice daily.

14.4.2 Minimal Stimulation IVF with Letrozole Stimulation

Letrozole stimulation leads to an inhibition of the aromatization of intrafollicular androgens and therefore to a reduction in E2 production. As a result, serum E2 concentrations decrease, which increases pituitary secretion of FSH.

Furthermore, the intrafollicular androgen/E2 ratio is shifted towards higher relative androgen concentrations. Such a dysbalance has also been described in women with high AMH serum concentrations, affecting the endocrine milieu in follicular fluid [17].

In some cases letrozole is administered up to the day of hCG administration. Since letrozole has a half-life of 2–4 days [18], the inhibition of aromatization of androgens to E2 (see Chap. 8) continues into the luteal phase and affects the function of the luteal body. It can be assumed that letrozole also affects the function of luteal phase antral follicles by inhibiting aromatization of androgens to E2 and thereby to reduce E2 blood concentrations.

All these effects are in line with a study by Mai et al. (2017) [19]. The 5-day administration of 2.5 mg letrozole, starting on the day of hCG administration, leads to a significant reduction in the risk of ovarian hyperstimulation syndrome (OHSS) in women with conventional IVF. This supports the concept of letrozole to affect the function of the luteal bodies.

For this reasons, luteal phase supplementation is recommended for minimal stimulation IVF.

In minimal stimulation IVF with letrozole stimulation, possible luteal phase supplements are as follows:

- Micronized progesterone 200 mg daily, vaginally, starting between aspiration and embryo transfer until pregnancy test, i.e., approx. 14th day after follicular aspiration.
- Crinone® 8% once daily vaginally. Duration of therapy as for micronized progesterone.
- Dydrogesterone 10 mg twice daily orally. Duration of therapy as for micronized progesterone.

14.4.3 Minimal Stimulation IVF with Low-Dose Gonadotropins in Cycles with a Low Ovarian Response

This group includes cycles with a daily gonadotropin dose of up to 100 IU with a monofollicular or oligofollicular response.

In case of a monofollicular response, strictly speaking, the above procedure applies as with NC-IVF—in spite of the stimulation with gonadotropins. In case of an oligofollicular response, the increased E2 and progesterone concentrations may lead to suppression of LH, and luteal phase support is required.

These explanations show that based on the number of growing follicles, luteal phase support could be individualized. In practice, however, for the sake of simplicity, individualization is dispensed within favour of a uniform procedure.

In minimal stimulation IVF with low-dose gonadotropins in cycles with a low ovarian response, possible luteal phase supplements are as follows:

- Micronized progesterone 200 mg once daily, vaginally, starting between aspiration and embryo transfer until pregnancy test, i.e., approx. 14th day after follicular aspiration.
- Crinone® 8% once daily vaginally. Duration of therapy as for micronized progesterone.
- Dydrogesterone 10 mg twice daily orally. Duration of therapy as for micronized progesterone.

14.4.4 Minimal Stimulation IVF with Low-Dose Gonadotropins in Cycles with a High Ovarian Response

This group includes cycles with a daily gonadotropin dose of up to 100 IU but with a polyfollicular response.

From an endocrinological point of view, luteal phase support needs to follow the same principles as described for conventional IVF. However, the luteal phase

Table 14.4 Clinical pregnancy rates in women undergoing clomiphene citrate stimulation and intrauterine insemination with and without luteal phase support. (Summary of a meta-analysis [16])

Included studies	Sample size, n	Risk ratio (95% CI)	Heterogeneity, I^2
6 studies, overall result	927	1.56 (1.21-2.02)	0%*

*indicates very low heterogeneity of studies (www.handbook-5-1.cochrane.org)

supplementation doses can be reduced if the number of follicles and thus the E2 concentration in blood is rather low.

The necessity of luteal phase support in minimal stimulation IVF is confirmed by a meta-analysis with five randomized controlled studies including 927 patients who were stimulated with low-dose gonadotropins followed by intrauterine insemination [16] (Table 14.4). According to this meta-analysis, the pregnancy rate is higher with luteal phase support (RR 1.56, 95% CI: 1.21–2.02).

In minimal stimulation IVF with low-dose gonadotropins in cycles with a high ovarian response, possible luteal phase supplements are as follows:

- Micronized progesterone 200 mg twice daily, vaginally, starting between aspiration and embryo transfer until pregnancy test, i.e., approx. 14th day after follicular aspiration.
- Crinone® 8% once daily vaginally. Duration of therapy as for micronized progesterone.
- Dydrogesterone 10 mg three times daily orally. Duration of therapy as for micronized progesterone.

14.5   Practical Conclusions

- Luteal phase supplementation is not required in NC-IVF and in NC-IVF with clomiphene citrate stimulation in patients with a normal luteal phase length. However, if luteal phase is shorter than 12 days, luteal phase support is required.
- Luteal phase support is required in women undergoing minimal stimulation IVF treated with letrozole or with gonadotropins. The dose required for luteal phase support depends on the ovarian response.
- Injection free NC-IVF cycles are possible by using GnRH agonist intranasal spray. It is still unknown if luteal phase support is required in NC-IVF if ovulation is triggered with GnRH agonists.
- IVF centres use different luteal phase supplementations. Table 14.2 shows the supplementations used by three large centres /networks specialized in NC-IVF and/or minimal stimulation IVF.

References

1. Fauser BC, Devroey P. Reproductive biology and IVF: ovarian stimulation and luteal phase consequences. Trends Endocrinol Metab. 2003;14:236–42.
2. van der Linden M, Buckingham K, Farquhar C, Kremer JA, Metwally M. Luteal phase support for assisted reproduction cycles. Cochrane Database Syst Rev. 2015;2015:CD009154.
3. Skinner DC, Evans NP, Delaleu B, Goodman RL, Bouchard P, Caraty A. The negative feedback actions of progesterone on gonadotropin-releasing hormone secretion are transduced by the classical progesterone receptor. Proc Natl Acad Sci U S A. 1998;95:10978–83.
4. Frydman R, Cornel C, de Ziegler D, Taieb J, Spitz IM, Bouchard P. Prevention of premature luteinizing hormone and progesterone rise with a gonadotropin-releasing hormone antagonist, Nal-Glu, in controlled ovarian hyperstimulation. Fertil Steril. 1991;56:923–7.
5. Friedler S, Gilboa S, Schachter M, Raziel A, Strassburger D, Ron ER. Luteal phase characteristics following GnRH antagonist or agonist treatment—a comparative study. Reprod Biomed Online. 2006;12:27–32.
6. Norman TR, Morse CA, Dennerstein L. Comparative bioavailability of orally and vaginally administered progesterone. Fertil Steril. 1991;56:1034–9.
7. Tay PY, Lenton EA. The impact of luteal supplement on pregnancy outcome following stimulated IVF cycles. Med J Malaysia. 2005;60:151–7.
8. Tournaye H, Sukhikh GT, Kahler E, Griesinger G. A phase III randomized controlled trial comparing the efficacy, safety and tolerability of oral dydrogesterone versus micronized vaginal progesterone for luteal support in in vitro fertilization. Hum Reprod. 2017;32:1019–27.
9. Griesinger G, Blockeel C, Sukhikh GT, Patki A, Dhorepatil B, Yang DZ, Chen ZJ, Kahler E, Pexman-Fieth C, Tournaye H. Oral dydrogesterone versus intravaginal micronized progesterone gel for luteal phase support in IVF: a randomized clinical trial. Hum Reprod. 2018;33:2212–21.
10. Child T, Leonard SA, Evans JS, Lass A. Systematic review of the clinical efficacy of vaginal progesterone for luteal phase support in assisted reproductive technology cycles. Reprod Biomed Online. 2018;36:630–45.
11. Vaisbuch E, de Ziegler D, Leong M, Weissman A, Shoham Z. Luteal-phase support in assisted reproduction treatment: real-life practices reported worldwide by an updated website-based survey. Reprod Biomed Online. 2014;28:330–5.
12. Bull JR, Rowland SP, Scherwitzl EB, Scherwitzl R, Danielsson KG, Harper J. Real-world menstrual cycle characteristics of more than 600,000 menstrual cycles. NPJ Digit Med. 2019;2:83.
13. von Wolff M, Kohl Schwartz A, Stute P, Fäh M, Otti G, Schürch R, Rohner S. Follicular flushing in natural cycle IVF does not affect the luteal phase—a prospective controlled study. Reprod Biomed Online. 2017;35:37–41.
14. Ghobadi C, Amer S, Lashen H, Lennard MS, Ledger WL, Rostami-Hodjegan A. Evaluation of the relationship between plasma concentrations of en- and zuclomiphene and induction of ovulation in anovulatory women being treated with clomiphene citrate. Fertil Steril. 2009b;91:1135–40.
15. Ghobadi C, Mirhosseini N, Shiran MR, Moghadamnia A, Lennard MS, Ledger WL, Rostami-Hodjegan A. Single-dose pharmacokinetic study of clomiphene citrate isomers in anovular patients with polycystic ovary disease. J Clin Pharmacol. 2009a;49:147–54.
16. Green KA, Zolton JR, Schermerhorn SM, Lewis TD, Healy MW, Terry N, DeCherney AH, Hill MJ. Progesterone luteal support after ovulation induction and intrauterine insemination: an updated systematic review and meta-analysis. Fertil Steril. 2017;107:924–933.e5.
17. von Wolff M, Mitter VR, Jamir N, Stute P, Eisenhut M, Bersinger N. The endocrine milieu in naturally matured follicles is different in women with high serum anti-müllerian concentrations. Reprod Biomed Online. 2021;43:329–37.

18. Buzdar AU, Robertson JF, Eiermann W, Nabholtz JM. An overview of the pharmacology and pharmacokinetics of the newer generation aromatase inhibitors anastrozole, letrozole, and exemestane. Cancer. 2002;95:2006–16.
19. Mai Q, Hu X, Yang G, Luo Y, Huang K, Yuan Y, Zhou C. Effect of letrozole on moderate and severe early-onset ovarian hyperstimulation syndrome in high-risk women: a prospective randomized trial. Am J Obstet Gynecol. 2017;216:42.e1–42.e10.
20. Kato K, Takehara Y, Segawa T, Kawachiya S, Okuno T, Kobayashi T, Bodri D, Kato O. Minimal ovarian stimulation combined with elective single embryo transfer policy: age-specific results of a large, single-Centre, Japanese cohort. Reprod Biol Endocrinol. 2012;10:35.
21. Onogi S, Ezoe K, Nishihara S, Fukuda J, Kobayashi T, Kato K. Endometrial thickness on the day of LH surge: an effective predictor of pregnancy outcomes after modified natural cycle-frozen blastocyst transfer. Hum Reprod Open. 2020;17:hoaa060.

Chapter 15
Treatment Protocols for Natural Cycle and Minimal Stimulation IVF

Michael von Wolff, Keiichi Kato, and John Zhang

15.1 Background

There are a number of different treatment protocols for natural cycle IVF (NC-IVF) and minimal stimulation IVF. Even with NC-IVF, where it should be assumed that the treatments are carried out quite similarly, there are relevant differences between the centers.

Treatment protocols differ in the timing and frequency of follicle monitoring, measures to prevent premature ovulation (see Chap. 11), timing of follicle aspiration (see Chap. 10), triggering of ovulation (see Chap. 12), follicle aspiration (see Chap. 13), and luteal phase support (see Chap. 14).

In the case of minimal stimulation IVF, the protocols also differ in terms of the various medications used for follicle stimulation, their dose, the start of therapy and the duration of therapy.

This shows that treatment protocols can vary greatly between centers based on their experience and treatment principles. It also shows that NC-IVF and minimal stimulation IVF therapies are often highly individualized and tailored to the physiological requirements of the woman, the wishes of the couple, and even cultural circumstances.

M. von Wolff (✉)
Division of Gynecological Endocrinology and Reproductive Medicine, University Women's Hospital, University of Bern, Bern, Switzerland
e-mail: Michael.vonwolff@insel.ch

K. Kato
Kato Ladies Clinic, Tokyo, Japan
e-mail: k-kato@towako.net

J. Zhang
New Hope Fertility Center, New York, USA

For this reason, this chapter presents therapy protocols from three centers and networks. The presentation is descriptive and graphical and is supplemented by relevant information such as indications and special features. The protocols can be further modified in practice.

Costs, risks, and success rates of the therapy protocols are discussed in the Chaps. 18, 17, and 19.

15.2 Treatment Protocols by IVF-Naturelle® Centers

15.2.1 Natural Cycle IVF

15.2.1.1 References

This protocol has been published elsewhere regarding indications [1], psychological treatment stress [2], and success rates [1, 3–6] (Fig. 15.1).

15.2.1.2 Indications

This protocol can be performed in any women with regular cycles. Ideally in women <35 years, women with blocked tubes or couples with severe andrological factors [1], or in women who prefer IVF treatment cycles with the lowest possible hormone stimulation.

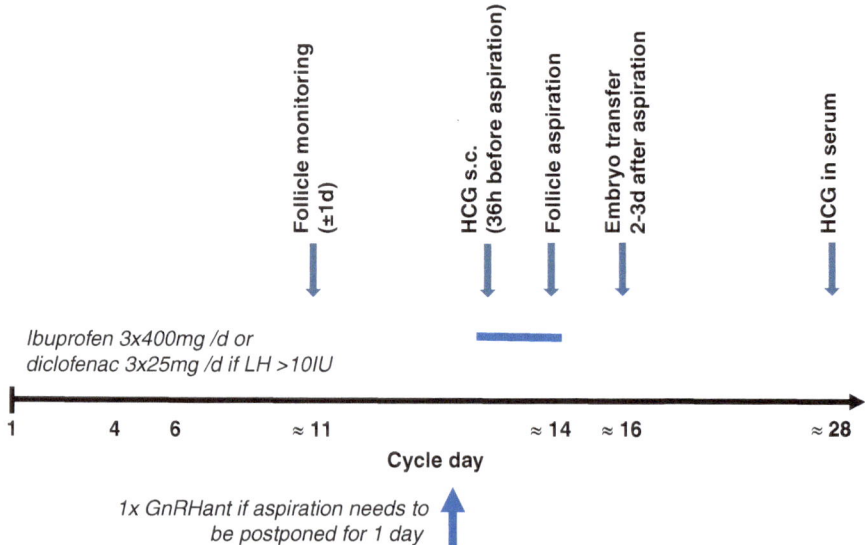

Fig. 15.1 Natural cycle IVF as performed in IVF-Naturelle® centers

This protocol is not suitable for women with a risk of premature ovulation. In this case, NC-IVF with low-dose clomiphene citrate should be considered.

15.2.1.3 Protocol

- 1st consultation on cycle day 11 ±1 at 8 am to 12 am (for 28 day cycles; for 27 day cycles on day 10 ±1, etc.).
- Monitoring of follicular growth: Evaluation of size of the follicle, thickness of the endometrium, concentration of E2 and luteinizing hormone (LH) in serum.
- Scheduling of day and time of the aspiration (8 am to 12 am). If scheduling of aspiration is not yet possible: scheduling of a 2nd consultation for monitoring of follicular growth.
- Triggering of ovulation with 5000 IE hCG s.c. if expected size of the follicle is 16–20 mm, if E2 concentration is >700–800 pmol/L (>190–220 ng/mL), and if LH concentration is <10 IU/L.
- Follicle aspiration 36 h after hCG triggering. Use of 19G aspiration needles and five follicle flushings.
- No luteal phase support required.
- hCG blood test 14 days after aspiration.

15.2.1.4 Special Situations

- If aspiration needs to be postponed for one day (due to the patient's agenda, if follicle is still too small or if endometrium is too thin): 1 injection of GnRH antagonist (GnRHant) (ganirelix or cetrorelix) 0.25 mg s.c. one day before hCG triggering at 4 pm.
- If LH concentration is 10–20 IU on the day of follicle monitoring (=beginning of LH surge, see Fig. 15.10): hCG 5000 IU s.c. to trigger ovulation in the evening of the same day, 36 h before follicle aspiration. Start ibuprofen 3 × 400mg or diclofenac 3 × 25mg orally immediately until the morning of follicle aspiration, which is scheduled 2 days later in the morning as early as possible.
- If LH concentration is >20 IU and E2 concentration is >800 pmol/L (>220 ng/mL) on the day of follicle monitoring (=halfway of LH surge, see Fig. 15.10): hCG 5000 IU s.c. to trigger ovulation as soon as possible. Start ibuprofen 3 × 400 mg or diclofenac 3 × 25 mg orally immediately until the morning of follicle aspiration which is scheduled for the following day around 12 pm.
- If LH concentration is >20 IU and E2 is <800 pmol/L (<220 ng/mL) on the day of follicle monitoring (=end of LH surge, see Fig. 15.10): hCG 5000 IU s.c. to trigger ovulation as soon as possible. Start ibuprofen 3 × 400 mg or diclofenac 3 × 25 mg orally immediately until the morning of follicle aspiration which is scheduled for the following day in the morning as early as possible.

- If luteal phase <12 days: Luteal phase support with micronized progesterone 1 × 200 mg vaginally or dydrogesterone 2 × 10 mg orally for 13 days, starting in the evening on the day of follicle aspiration.

15.2.2   Natural Cycle IVF with Low-Dose Clomiphene Citrate

15.2.2.1   References

This protocol has been published elsewhere regarding indications [1], psychological treatment stress [2], and success rates (Fig. 15.2) [1–6].

15.2.2.2   Indications

This protocol can be performed in any women with regular cycles. Ideally in women <35 y, women with blocked tubes, or couples with severe andrological factors [1].

As clomiphene citrate reduces the risk of premature ovulation [4], it is an alternative for women requiring NC-IVF who have experienced premature ovulation.

Not suitable for women with endometrial thickness <8 mm. In this case, minimal stimulation IVF with low-dose gonadotropins should be considered.

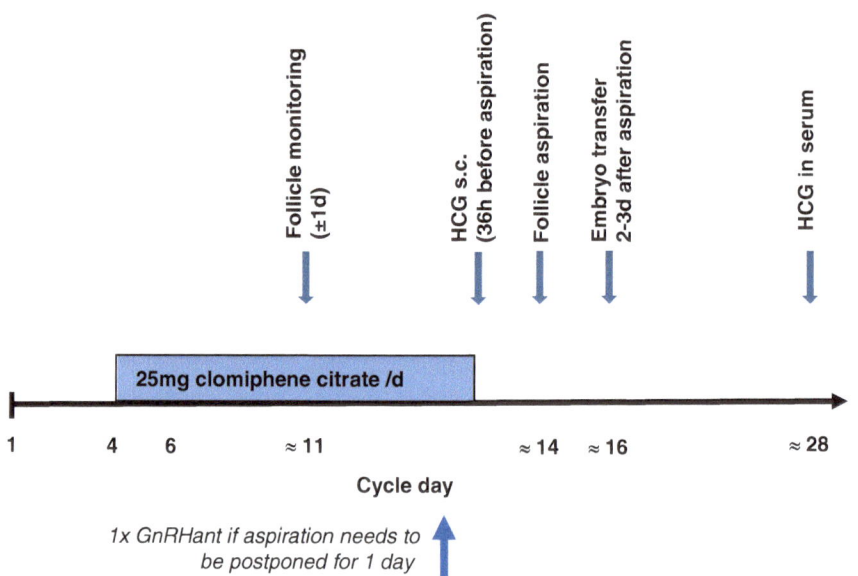

Fig. 15.2 Natural cycle IVF with low-dose clomiphene citrate as performed in IVF-Naturelle® centers

15.2.2.3   Protocol

- Clomiphene citrate 25 mg once daily is started in the morning around day 4 of the cycle until the morning of ovulation triggering.
- 1st consultation on cycle day 11 ±1 at 8 am to 12 am (for 28 day cycles; for 27 day cycles on day 10 ±1 etc.).
- Monitoring of follicular growth: Evaluation of size of the follicle, thickness of the endometrium, concentration of E2 and LH in serum.
- Scheduling of day and time of the aspiration (8 am to 12 am). If scheduling of aspiration is not yet possible: scheduling of a 2nd consultation for monitoring of follicular growth.
- Triggering of ovulation with 5000 IE hCG s.c. if expected size of the follicle is 16–20 mm and E2 is >1500 pmol/L (>400 ng/mL).
- Follicle aspiration 36 h after hCG. Use of 19G aspiration needles and five follicle flushings.
- No luteal phase support required.
- hCG blood test 14 days after aspiration.

15.2.2.4   Special Situations

- If endometrium thickness is <8 mm on the day of ovulation triggering or if endo-metrial thickness is reduced by treatment with clomiphene citrate by >1 mm, the protocol should not be continued. In this case, minimal stimulation IVF with low-dose gonadotropins should be considered (see Fig. 15.3).
- If the follicular phase is very short, clomiphene citrate should be started 1–2 days earlier.

15.2.3   Minimal Stimulation IVF with Low-Dose Gonadotropins

15.2.3.1   References

This protocol has not yet been published (Fig. 15.3).

15.2.3.2   Indications

This protocol can be performed in any women with regular or irregular cycles. It is especially suitable for women with irregular cycles and with premature ovulation in NC-IVF. Premature ovulation can be avoided with GnRHant started as soon as E2 concentration is >600–700 pmol/L (>160–190 ng/mL). If oocyte yield should be increased (as in women with increased age), minimal stimulation with gonadotropins and clomiphene citrate should be considered.

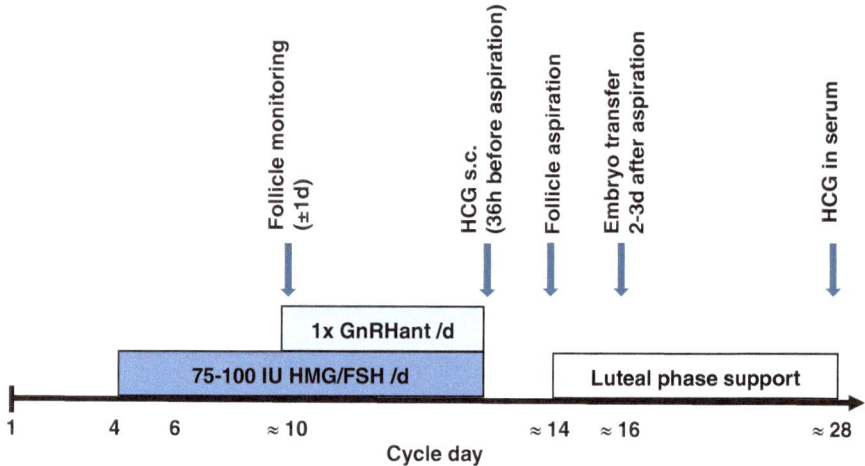

Fig. 15.3 Minimal stimulation IVF with low-dose gonadotropins as performed in IVF-Naturelle® centers

15.2.3.3 Protocol

- FSH or HMG 75–100 IU is started in the evening around day 4 of the cycle until the morning of ovulation triggering.
- 1st consultation on cycle day 10 ±1 at 8 am to 12 am (for 28 day cycle; for 27 day cycles on day 9 ±1, etc.).
- Monitoring of follicular growth: Evaluation of size of the follicle, thickness of the endometrium, concentration of E2 and LH in serum.
- Scheduling of day and time of the aspiration (8 am to 12 am). If scheduling of aspiration is not yet possible: scheduling of a 2nd consultation for monitoring of follicular growth. Start of GnRHant as soon as E2 >600-700pmol/L (>160-190ng/ml).
- Triggering of ovulation with 5000 IE hCG s.c. if expected size of the follicle is 16–20 mm and E2 is >800 pmol/L (>220 ng/mL).
- Follicle aspiration 36 h after hCG. Use of 19G aspiration needles and five follicle flushings.
- Luteal phase support with micronized progesterone 1 × 200 mg vaginally or dydrogesterone 2 × 10 mg orally for 13 days, starting in the evening on the day of follicle aspiration.
- hCG blood test 14 days after aspiration.

15.2.3.4 Special Situations

- If oocyte yield should be increased (as in women with increased age), minimal stimulation IVF with gonadotropins and clomiphene citrate should be considered (Fig. 15.4).

15.2.4   Minimal Stimulation IVF with Low-Dose Gonadotropins and Clomiphene Citrate

15.2.4.1   References

This protocol has not yet been published (Fig. 15.4).

15.2.4.2   Indications

This protocol can be performed in any women with regular or irregular cycles. It is especially suitable for women in whom an increased oocyte yield is required.

15.2.4.3   Protocol

- Clomiphene citrate 25 mg is started in the morning around day 4 of the cycle until the morning of ovulation triggering.
- FSH or HMG 75–100 IU/d is started in the evening around day 4 of the cycle until the day before ovulation triggering.
- 1st consultation on cycle day 11 ±1 at 8 am to 12 am (for 28 day cycles; for 27 day cycles on day 10 ±1, etc.).
- Monitoring of follicular growth: Evaluation of size of the follicle, thickness of the endometrium, concentration of E2 and LH in serum.

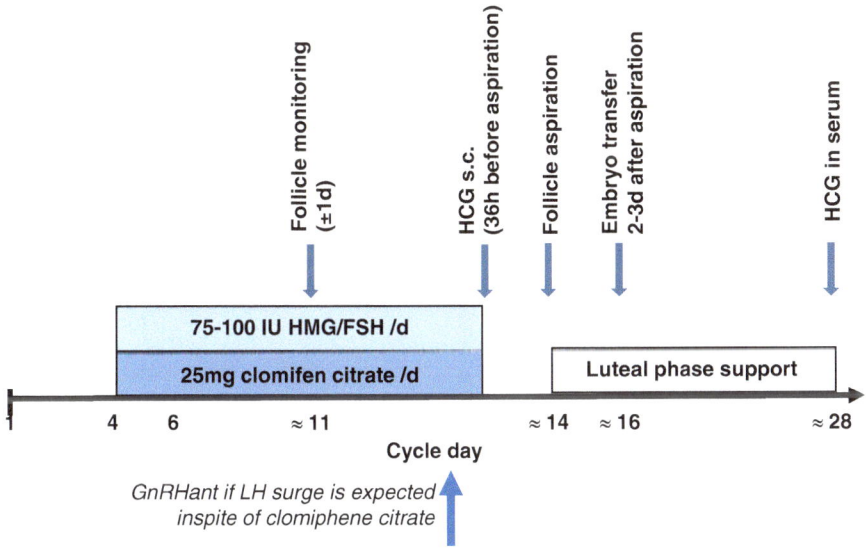

Fig. 15.4 Minimal stimulation IVF with low-dose gonadotropins and clomiphene citrate as performed in IVF-Naturelle® centers

- Scheduling of day and time of the aspiration (8 am to 12 am). If scheduling of aspiration is not yet possible: scheduling of a 2nd consultation for monitoring of follicular growth.
- Triggering of ovulation with 5000 IE hCG s.c. if expected size of the follicle is 16–20 mm and E2 is >1500 pmol/L (>400 ng/mL).
- Follicle aspiration 36 h after hCG. Use of 19G aspiration needles and five follicle flushings.
- Luteal phase support with micronized progesterone 1 × 200 mg vaginally or dydrogesterone 2 × 10 mg orally for 13 days, starting in the evening on the day of follicle aspiration. In case of high response, micronized progesterone 2 x 200mg vaginally or dydrogesterone 3 x 10mg orally.
- hCG blood test 14 days after aspiration.

15.2.4.4   Special Situations

- If aspiration needs to be postponed for 1 day (due to the patient's agenda, if follicles are still too small or endometrium too thin): 1 injection of GnRH antagonist (GnRHant) (ganirelix or cetrorelix) 0.25 mg s.c. one day before hCG triggering at 4 pm.
- If oocyte yield should be further increased (as in women with increased age) and if AMH concentration is sufficiently high, conventional IVF with high dose gonadotropin stimulation should be considered.

15.2.5   Minimal Stimulation IVF with Letrozole

15.2.5.1   References

This protocol has not yet been published (Fig. 15.5).

15.2.5.2   Indications

This protocol can be performed in any women, especially with those with polycystic ovarian syndrome (PCOS).

Not suitable for women with endometrial thickness <8mm. In this case, minimal stimulation with low-dose gonadotropins and letrozole (see Fig. 15.6) or minimal stimulation IVF with low-dose gonadotropins (see Fig. 15.3) should be considered.

15.2.5.3   Protocol

- Letrozole 5 mg (1 × 5 mg or 2 × 2.5 mg) is started in the morning around day 4 of the cycle and given for 5 days.

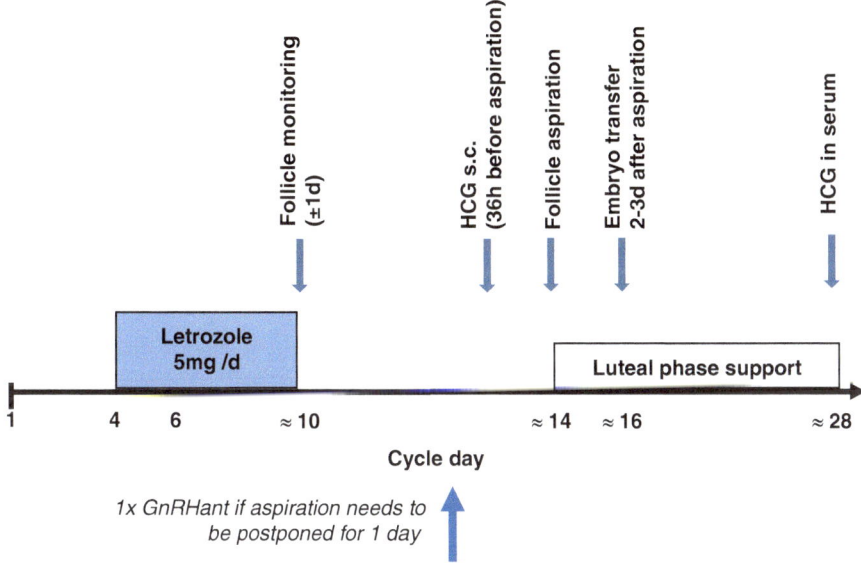

Fig. 15.5 Minimal stimulation IVF with letrozole as performed in IVF-Naturelle® centers

- 1st consultation on cycle day 10 ±1 at 8 am to 12 am (for 28 day cycles; for 27 day cycles on day 9 ±1, etc.).
- Monitoring of follicular growth: Evaluation of size of the follicle, thickness of the endometrium, concentration of E2 and LH in serum.
- Scheduling of day and time of the aspiration (8 am to 12 am). If scheduling of aspiration is not yet possible: scheduling of a 2nd consultation for monitoring of follicular growth.
- Triggering of ovulation with 5000 IE hCG s.c. if expected size of the follicle is 16–20 mm. Please note: E2 concentration is lower as usual due to letrozole.
- Follicle aspiration 36 h after hCG. Use of 19G aspiration needles and five follicle flushing.
- Luteal phase support with micronized progesterone 1 × 200 mg vaginally or dydrogesterone 2 × 10 mg orally for 13 days, starting in the evening on the day of follicle aspiration.
- hCG blood test 14 days after aspiration.

15.2.5.4 Special Situations

- If aspiration needs to be postponed for 1 day (due to the patient's agenda, if follicles are still too small or endometrium too thin): 1 injection of GnRH antagonist (GnRHant) (ganirelix or cetrorelix) 0.25 mg s.c. one day before hCG triggering at 4 pm.

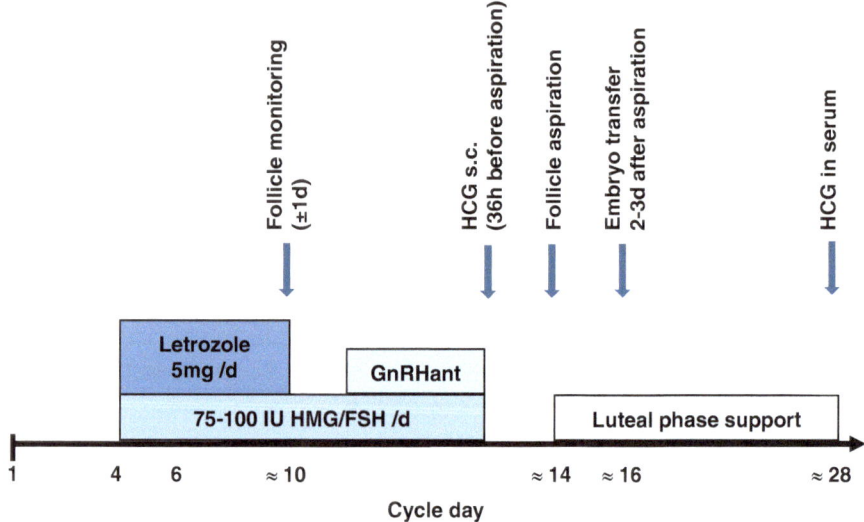

Fig. 15.6 Minimal stimulation IVF with low-dose gonadotropins and letrozole as performed in IVF-Naturelle® centers

- If oocyte yield should be further increased (as in women with increased age) and if AMH concentration is sufficiently high, minimal stimulation IVF with low-dose gonadotropins and letrozole should be considered (see Fig. 15.6).

15.2.6 Minimal Stimulation IVF with Low-Dose Gonadotropins and Letrozole

15.2.6.1 References

This protocol has not yet been published (Fig. 15.6).

15.2.6.2 Indications

This protocol can be performed in any women, especially with those with polycystic ovarian syndrome (PCOS). It is especially suitable for women in whom an increased oocyte yield is required.

15.2.6.3 Protocol

- Letrozole 5mg (1 × 5 mg or 2 × 2.5 mg) is started in the morning around day 4 of the cycle and is given for 5 days.

- FSH or HMG 75–100 IU 1×/d is started in the evening around day 4 of the cycle until the day before ovulation triggering.
- 1st consultation on cycle day 10 ±1 at 8 am to 12 am (for 28 day cycles; for 27 day cycles on day 9 ±1, etc.).
- Monitoring of follicular growth: Evaluation of size of the follicle, thickness of the endometrium, concentration of E2 and LH in serum.
- Scheduling of day and time of the aspiration (8 am to 12 am). If scheduling of aspiration is not yet possible: scheduling of a 2nd consultation for monitoring of follicular growth.
- Triggering of ovulation with 5000 IE hCG s.c. if expected size of the follicle is 16–20 mm. Please note: E2 concentration is lower as usual due to letrozole.
- Follicle aspiration 36 h after hCG. Use of 19G aspiration needles and five follicle flushings.
- Luteal phase support with micronized progesterone 1 × 200 mg vaginally or dydrogesterone 2 × 10 mg orally for 13 days, starting in the evening on the day of follicle aspiration. In case of high response micronized progesterone 2 x 200mg vaginally or dydrogesterone 3 x 10mg orally.
- hCG blood test 14 days after aspiration.

15.2.6.4 Special Situations

- If aspiration needs to be postponed for 1 day (due to the patient's agenda, if follicles are still too small or endometrium too thin): 1 injection of GnRH antagonist (GnRHant) (ganirelix or cetrorelix) 0.25 mg s.c. one day before hCG triggering at 4 pm.

15.3 Treatment Protocols by Kato Ladies Clinic, Japan

15.3.1 Natural Cycle IVF

15.3.1.1 References

This protocol has been published elsewhere (Fig. 15.7) [7, 8].

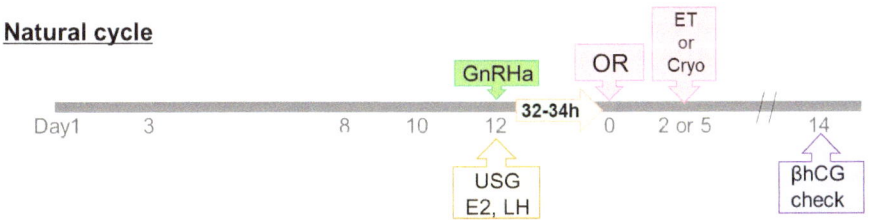

Fig. 15.7 Natural cycle IVF as performed in Kato Ladies clinic (*OR* Oocyte retrieval, *ET* Embryo transfer)

15.3.1.2 Indications

Natural cycle IVF is indicated in patients with a regular menstrual cycle and spontaneous ovulation regardless of the patient's age.

15.3.1.3 Protocol

- The only pharmaceutical intervention is final oocyte maturation with intranasal application of 3 hubs of the GnRHa buserelin (Suprecur® nasal solution, 3 hubs of each 0.15 mg = 0.45 mg in total) (Fig. 15.7).
- The medical examination on day 3 after menstruation is not mandatory and the first visit date can take place on day 10 depending on the patients' menstruation cycle.
- When the leading follicle reaches 18 mm in diameter with a concomitant serum E2 level of 250 pg/mL (900 pmol/L), oocyte maturation is triggered. Oocyte retrieval is performed 34–35 h later.
- Follicle aspiration is performed with 21G monoluminal needles without follicle flushing.
- Embryos are usually frozen either 2 (cleavage stage) or 5–7 days (blastocyst stage) after follicle aspiration and transferred later. The first line regimen of endometrial preparation for vitrified and warmed embryo transfer is natural ovulatory cycle except for patients with PCOS, luteal phase insufficiency, and pituitary dysfunction.
- If embryos are transferred fresh, embryo transfer is performed on day 2. Luteal phase support is provided with administration of dydrogesterone (3×10 mg/d) for 10 days, starting on the day of embryo transfer.

15.3.2 Minimal Stimulation IVF (Fig. 15.6)

15.3.2.1 References

This protocol has been published elsewhere (Fig. 15.8) [6, 7, 9].

15.3.2.2 Indications

Minimal stimulation cycle with clomiphene citrate (CC) IVF ± gonadotropins is indicated in group II ovulation disorders according to World Health Organization categorization. Thus, this approach is suitable for a large number of patients of various age groups.

15.3.2.3 Protocol

- The first patient consultation is scheduled on day 3 of the cycle (Fig. 15.8).

Minimal stimulation cycle

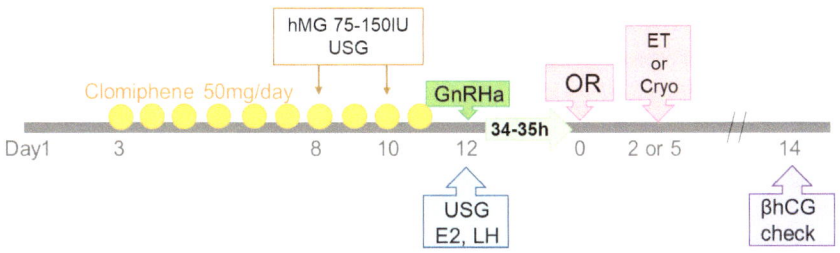

Fig. 15.8 Minimal stimulation IVF as performed in Kato Ladies clinic (*USG* Ultrasonography, *OR* Oocyte retrieval, *ET* Embryo transfer)

Administration of CC (50 mg/day) is started on day 3 and continued until right before triggering ovulation. Because CC is started on day 3, ovarian stimulation using CC starts before follicle recruitment. CC is administered for two purposes: for its main effect to promote follicular maturation and to inhibit LH surge, which is achieved through its anti-estrogenic effect.

- For patients with insufficient levels of follicle-stimulating hormone (FSH) because of negative feedback from follicle growth or delayed follicular growth, an appropriate dose of gonadotropins (75–150 IU per day) is administered. Considering the half-life of gonadotropins, alternate-day administration (rather than daily administration) is sufficient.
- Since the pituitary gland is not inhibited, oocyte maturation can be induced prior to retrieval by triggering an endogenous LH surge with intranasal application of 3×1 hub of each 0.15 mg buserelin = 0.45 mg in total.
- The criteria for confirming follicular maturation are a dominant follicle diameter of ≥ 18 mm and sufficient E2 levels relative to the number of growing follicles. Oocyte retrieval is performed 34–35 h later.
- Follicle aspiration is performed with 21G monoluminal needles without follicle flushing.
- Day 2 cleavage stage embryos are considered to be transferred directly without freezing. The criteria for fresh transfer in clomiphene citrate-based minimal stimulation cycle IVF are an endometrial thickness of ≥ 8 mm on the day of ovulation triggering [10]. Otherwise, embryos are vitrified either on day 2 or day 5–7 and transferred later in a thawing cycle. The first line regimen of endometrial preparation for thawing cycles is a natural ovulatory cycle except for patients with polycystic ovarian syndrome, luteal phase insufficiency, and pituitary dysfunction.
- Luteal phase support is performed in case of transfer of day 2 cleaved stage embryos with dydrogesterone (3×10 mg/d, orally) starting on the day of embryo transfer for 10 days. In case of blastocyst transfer, progesterone is additionally administered intravaginally (800 mg/d) along with oral dydrogesterone for 7 days if luteal function is insufficient (progesterone concentration on the day of ovulation triggering 8–11 ng/mL). Blastocyst transfer is cancelled if progesterone concentration is <8 ng/mL.

15.3.3   Attempts to Prevent Ovulation

It is necessary to determine how to adapt to the contradiction of securing time until oocyte maturation while ensuring oocyte retrieval before ovulation. Determining whether the LH surge has begun is the most important factor in oocyte retrieval during natural and minimal stimulation cycles. Figure 15.9 shows the physiological hormone dynamics and timing of ovulation. The timing of GnRHa administration and oocyte retrieval according to LH levels is shown in Fig. 15.10. If the LH surge

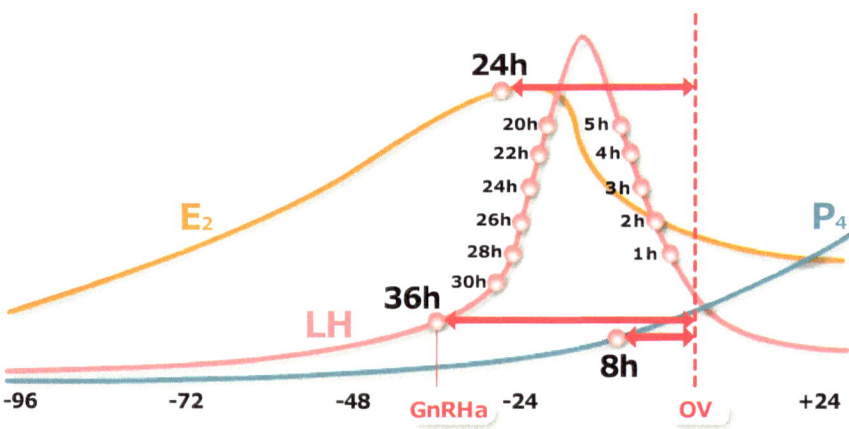

Fig. 15.9 Diagram of LH surge and expected time of ovulation (OV)

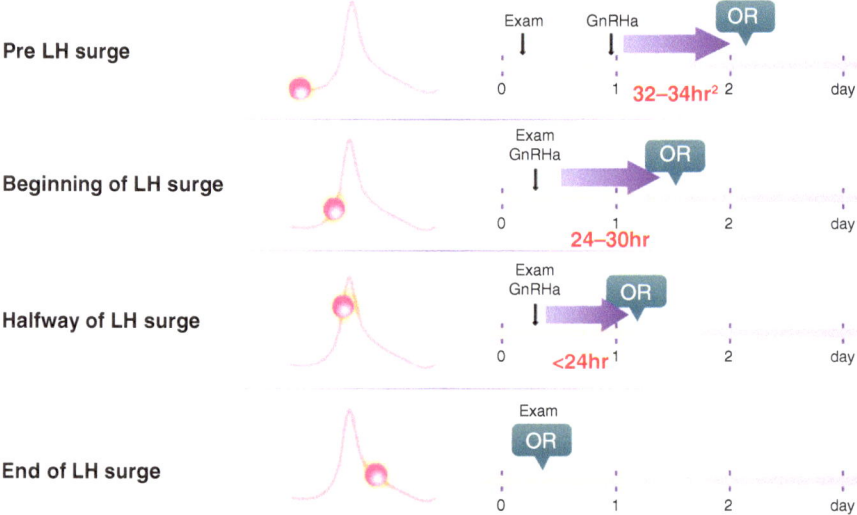

Fig. 15.10 LH surge and appropriate timing of oocyte retrieval (OR)

has already begun on the day of examination, GnRHa is administered immediately, and oocyte retrieval is performed at an appropriate time according to the LH levels. If the LH surge has already ended by the time of examination, ovulation is predicted to occur on the same day. Thus, oocyte retrieval is performed on the day of the examination.

The cyclooxygenase (COX) enzyme, COX-2, is induced by the LH surge in granulosa cells prior to ovulation. Non-steroidal anti-inflammatory drugs (NSAIDs) inhibit COX. Therefore, administration of NSAIDs is likely to reduce the rate of premature ovulation. At 8 and 14 h before the scheduled oocyte retrieval time, 25 mg of diclofenac is administered as a suppository. We confirmed that diclofenac administration reduced the rate of natural ovulation and increased the likelihood of obtaining mature oocytes [11].

15.4   Treatment Protocols by New Hope Fertility Center, New York, U.S.

15.4.1   Natural Cycle IVF

15.4.1.1   References

This protocol has not been published (Fig. 15.11).

15.4.1.2   Indications

NC-IVF is indicated in patients with a regular menstrual cycle, regardless of the age of the patient and the state of the ovarian reserve. It is also considered in patients with a history of suboptimal response and failure in conventional stimulation IVF cycles.

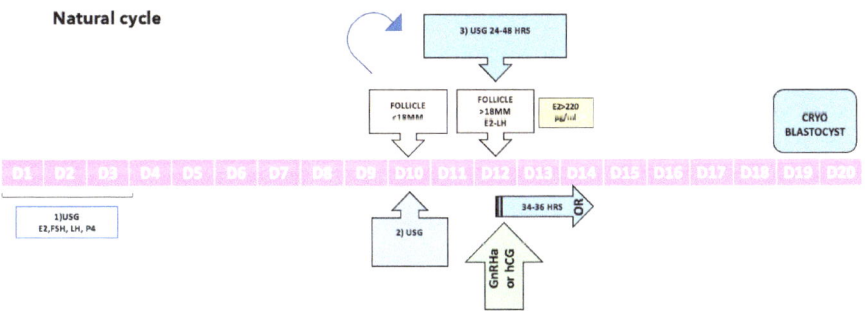

Fig. 15.11 Natural cycle IVF as performed in New Hope Fertility Center (*USG* ultrasound, *OR* Oocyte retrieval)

15.4.1.3 Protocol

- First consultation between day 1 and 3 of the cycle, ultrasonographic monitoring to record antral follicle count and endometrial thickness as well as serum hormone concentration: E2, FSH, LH, and progesterone (P4) (Fig. 15.11). In some patients, a first monitoring is considered on day 8–10 of the cycle, mainly in those who have had previous NC-IVF.
- Second assessment on day 10 of the cycle, ultrasound monitoring of follicular growth to evaluate follicle size, thickness, and endometrial pattern. If on this day, the measurement of the dominant follicle is <18 mm, a 3rd monitoring is programmed 24–48 h later.
- When the lead follicle has reached ≥18 mm, serum hormonal monitoring of E2 and LH is performed. With a serum E2 level >220 pg/mL (800 pmol/L), oocyte maturation is triggered by GnRHa triptorelin 0.05 mg s.c. or 250 µg HCG s.c.. Ibuprofen 400 mg every 8 h is started for ovulation prevention until oocyte retrieval.
- Oocyte retrieval is performed 34–36 h later, without anesthesia. In some patients, 10 mg diazepam is preceded 30 min before follicular aspiration. Use of 21G aspiration needles and follicular flushing is performed as needed.
- Generally, the embryo is frozen in the blastocyst stage to be transferred in a later cycle. In the case of fresh embryo transfer on day 5, luteal phase support is administered with progesterone 8% vaginal gel 2 times a day (Crinone® 8%).
- HCG blood test is performed 7 days after embryo transfer.

15.4.2 Minimal Stimulation IVF

15.4.2.1 References

The protocols have been published elsewhere (Fig. 15.12) [12–14].

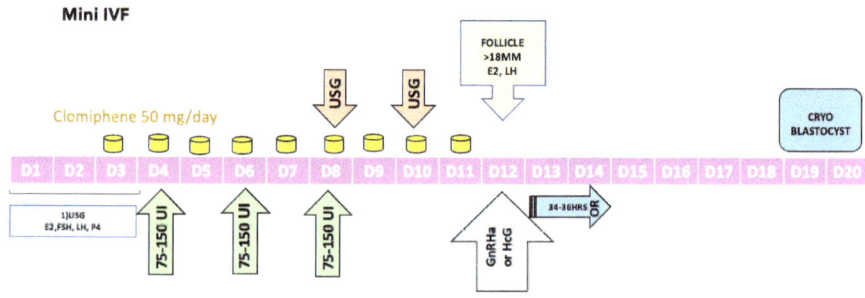

Fig. 15.12 Minimal stimulation IVF (Mini IVF®) as performed in New Hope Fertility Center (*USG* Ultrasonography, *OR* Oocyte retrieval)

15.4.2.2 Indications

The protocol indicated for women with regular or irregular cycles, patients at risk of ovarian hyperstimulation, and in cases where a higher oocyte yield is required.

15.4.2.3 Protocol

- First consultation between day 1 and 3 of the cycle, ultrasonographic monitoring to record antral follicle count and endometrial thickness as well as serum hormone concentration: E2, FSH, LH, and progesterone (P4) (Fig. 15.12).
- Clomiphene citrate (50 mg/day) is started on day 3 and subcutaneous administration of HMG (150 IU every 48 h) is started between day 4 and 5 depending on the FSH concentration on day 3 (FSH > 7.5 U = 75 IU HMG; FSH < 7.5 U = 150 IU HMG). Both medications are continued until the follicles have developed sufficiently for ovulation triggering.
- Ultrasound monitoring of follicular growth to evaluate follicles size and endometrial thickness is performed on day 8 of the cycle.
- Subsequent monitoring is carried out every 24 or 48 h depending on follicular development.
- The criteria to trigger final maturation are the size of the dominant follicle with a diameter of >18 mm and sufficient E2 level. Oocyte maturation is triggered by GnRHa triptorelin 0.05 mg s.c. or 250 µg HCG s.c.. Ibuprofen 400 mg every 8 h is started for ovulation prevention until oocyte retrieval. Hormonal control 24 h after trigger to adjust aspiration time if necessary.
- Oocyte retrieval is performed 34-36 hours later without anesthesia and in some patients 10 mg diazepam is preceded 30 min before follicular aspiration. Use of 21G aspiration needles and follicular flushing is performed as needed.
- Generally, the embryo is frozen in the blastocyst stage to be transferred in a later cycle. In the case of fresh embryo transfer on day 5, luteal phase support is administered with progesterone 8% vaginal gel 2 times a day (Crinone® 8%).
- Single embryos, selected by Embryo Ranking Intelligent Classification Algorithm, ERICA [15] are transferred.
- HCG blood test is performed 7 days after embryo transfer.

References

1. von Wolff M, Schwartz AK, Bitterlich N, Stute P, Fäh M. Only women's age and the duration of infertility are the prognostic factors for the success rate of natural cycle IVF. Arch Gynecol Obstet. 2019;299:883–9.
2. Haemmerli Keller K, Alder G, Loewer L, Faeh M, Rohner S, von Wolff M. Treatment-related psychological stress in different in vitro fertilization therapies with and without gonadotropin stimulation. Acta Obstet Gynecol Scand. 2018;97:269–76.
3. von Wolff M, Hua YZ, Santi A, Ocon E, Weiss B. Follicle flushing in monofollicular in vitro fertilization almost doubles the number of transferable embryos. Acta Obstet Gynecol Scand. 2013;92:346–8.

4. von Wolff M, Nitzschke M, Stute P, Bitterlich N, Rohner S. Low-dosage clomiphene reduces premature ovulation rates and increases transfer rates in natural-cycle IVF. Reprod Biomed Online. 2014;29:209–15.
5. Kohl Schwartz AS, Calzaferri I, Roumet M, Limacher A, Fink A, Wueest A, Weidlinger S, Mitter VR, Leeners B, Von Wolff M. Follicular flushing leads to higher oocyte yield in mono-follicular IVF: a randomized controlled trial. Human Reprod. 2020;35:2253–61.
6. Magaton IM, Helmer A, Roumet M, Stute P, von Wolff M. High dose gonadotropin stimulation increases endometrial thickness but this gonadotropin induced thickening does not have an effect on implantation. J Gynecol Obstet Hum Reprod. in press
7. Kato K, Takehara Y, Segawa T, Kawachiya S, Okuno T, Kobayashi T, Bodri D, Kato O. Minimal ovarian stimulation combined with elective single embryo transfer policy: age-specific results of a large, single-center Japanese cohort. Reprod Biol Endocrinol. 2012;10:35.
8. Silber SJ, Kato K, Aoyama N, Yabuuchi A, Skaletsky H, Fan Y, Shinohara K, Yatabe N, Kobayashi T. Intrinsic fertility of human oocytes. Fertil Steril. 2017;107:1232–7.
9. Abe T, Yabuuchi A, Ezoe K, Skaletsky H, Fukuda J, Ueno S, Fan Y, Goldsmith S, Kobayashi T, Silber S, Keiichi K. Success rates in minimal stimulation cycle IVF with clomiphene citrate only. J Assist Reprod Genet. 2020;37:297–304.
10. Nishihara S, Fukuda J, Ezoe K, Endo M, Nakagawa Y, Yamadera R, Kobayashi T, Kato K. Does the endometrial thickness on the day of the trigger affect the pregnancy outcomes after fresh cleaved embryo transfer in the clomiphene citrate-based minimal stimulation cycle? Reprod Med Biol. 2020;19:151–7.
11. Kawachiya S, Matsumoto T, Bodri D, Kato K, Takehara Y, Kato O. Short-term, low-dose, non-steroidal anti-inflammatory drug application diminishes premature ovulation in natural-cycle IVF. Reprod Biomed Online. 2012;24:308–13.
12. Zhang J, Chang L, Sone Y, Silber S. Minimal ovarian stimulation (mini-IVF) for IVF utilizing vitrification and cryopreserved embryo transfer. Reprod Biomed Online. 2010;21:485–95.
13. Zhang JJ, Merhi Z, Yang M, Bodri D, Chavez-Badiola A, Repping S, van Wely M. Minimal stimulation IVF vs conventional IVF: a randomized controlled trial. Am J Obstet Gynecol. 2016;214(96):e1–8.
14. Zhang J. Resurgence of minimal stimulation in vitro fertilization with a protocol consisting of gonadotropin releasing hormone-agonist trigger and vitrified-thawed embryo transfer. Int J Fertil Steril. 2016;10:148–53.
15. Chavez-Badiola A, Flores-Saiffe-Farías A, Mendizabal-Ruiz G, Drakeley AJ, Cohen J. Embryo Ranking Intelligent Classification Algorithm (ERICA): artificial intelligence clinical assistant predicting embryo ploidy and implantation. Reprod Biomed Online. 2020;41:585–93.
16. Teramoto S, Kato O. Minimal ovarian stimulation with clomiphene citrate a large-scale retrospective study. Reprod Biomed Online. 2007;15:134–48.

Chapter 16
Laboratory Aspects of Natural Cycle and Minimal Stimulation IVF

Markus Montag

16.1 Background

In contrast to stimulated cycles, natural cycle IVF (NC-IVF) and minimal stimulation IVF will usually yield few oocytes and mostly only one. The overall workflow is identical between NC-IVF and stimulated IVF cycles, and the same applies to related aspects like laboratory setting and equipment, training and experience of the embryologists, and the various aspects related to quality management as outlined in the guidelines for good practice in IVF laboratories by the European Society for Human Reproduction and Embryology (ESHRE) [1].

However, some details of the various procedures that are performed in the laboratory are different and/or can be adapted for optimization.

16.2 Preparation of Dishes

According to the low number of oocytes that are retrieved in NC-IVF and minimal stimulation IVF, the various dishes that are required for culture until insemination, for insemination by IVF or ICSI, and for subsequent culture until fertilization check and embryo transfer can be adapted accordingly. Firstly, for each type of dish that is routinely used in stimulated IVF cycles, only one may be needed. For NC-IVF cycles with insemination by IVF, a new dish is required from fertilization check until embryo transfer on day 2 or 3 due to the time needed for denudation. If insemination is done by ICSI, the dish used for culture after ICSI can be used for

M. Montag (✉)
ilabcomm GmbH, Sankt Augustin, Germany
e-mail: mmontag@ilabcomm.com

fertilization check and until embryo transfer on day 2 or 3 as checking only one oocyte can be done in less than 2 min, provided that the temperature is maintained by using properly heated workplaces and microscope stages.

Dishes that are set up with culture medium where the pH is only achieved by the sodium-bicarbonate buffer system must be prepared the day before. In general, dishes must be prepared in advance with sufficient time to adapt to the pH/CO_2 conditions as well as to the required temperature.

16.3 Isolation of the Cumulus–Oocyte Complex (COC)

The area for ovum pick-up (OPU) and subsequent isolation of the COC should preferably be located next to each other and allow for a direct communication between the clinician who performs OPU and the embryologist or technician who searches and isolates the COC. In case that no COC is found in the aspirate, OPU can be continued, and additional flushing may eventually allow to recover the COC in one of the subsequent aspirates.

16.4 Insemination by Conventional IVF

The process of insemination is identical to that used in conventional IVF. However, depending on the type and design of the culture dish used, it is advisable to have two additional droplets or wells, one for denudation and washing after insemination and one for fertilization check.

16.5 Processing of Oocytes and Insemination by ICSI

The quality of the oocyte is an important aspect in IVF in general. In stimulated cycles with multiple oocytes available, few immatures may be found among all oocytes. If only one oocyte is available, as in most NC-IVF cycles, maturity is important. Before denudation of the COC prior to ICSI, it may be advisable to check the presence of a first polar body under stereo-microscopic control, which is facilitated by careful and slow pipetting of the COC with a wide-diameter pipette ($>250 \, \mu m$). If no polar body is present, it is advisable to incubate the oocyte enclosed by the cumulus cells (CC) for another 2–4 h prior proceeding with denudation. Maturation after denudation will also occur, but maturation in the presence of CC and preferably within an intact COC is closer to natural conditions.

Denudation is performed as for standard ICSI and according to the time management of the laboratory. To streamline the process, it is advisable to perform denudation just prior ICSI and to continue with embryo culture under suitable incubation conditions.

16.6   Fertilization Check

Based on recent data, it is advisable to perform fertilization check as early as 16–16.5 h post-insemination to not miss the presence of pronuclei and to be able to assure the patient on proper (or failed) fertilization.

For conventional IVF, the inseminated oocyte must be carefully isolated from the COC by using suitable pipettes which are not too narrow to avoid any damage to the oocyte. For ICSI, fertilization can be immediately checked in the culture dish. Fertilization check is best performed using an inverted microscope equipped with interference contrast optics at 20× and 40× magnification.

16.7   Culture Conditions

Further culture after fertilization check should be performed in a standard culture medium under optimal conditions, which is a concentration of CO_2 that gives the proper pH according to the recommendation of the media manufacturer. Further, based on current knowledge, it is advisable to perform culture in a reduced oxygen atmosphere at 5% oxygen, independent of the anticipated time of culture before embryo transfer.

In principle, all aspects of quality control are applicable to stimulated IVF cycles, and the related equipment and consumables equally applied to natural or low stimulation cycle IVF.

16.8   Embryo Transfer

As the hormonal preparation for a NC-IVF cycle is fundamentally different to stimulated IVF, a potential negative effect of the stimulation and the trigger for ovulation induction on endometrial receptivity remain to be discussed. Regarding economics, a fresh transfer is advisable and is usually in the interest of the patient. Embryo transfer is performed as in stimulated IVF cycles and preferably using ultrasound guidance (Table 16.1).

Table 16.1 Differences in the laboratory procedures in NC-IVF, minimal stimulation IVF, and conventionally stimulated IVF

	NC-IVF	Minimal stimulation IVF	Conventionally stimulated IVF
Number of expected oocytes (see also Chap. 2)	1 (Monofollicular IVF)	1–3 (Oligofollicular IVF)	≥3 (Polyfollicular IVF)
Preparation of follicle aspiration	Preparation for 1–2 oocytes required. Possibly no oocytes, requiring discarding of all prepared material.	Preparation for few oocytes required.	Preparation for many oocytes required.
Follicle aspiration (see also Chap. 13)	Flushing medium possibly required.	No flushing medium.	No flushing medium.
Fertilization technique	IVF or ICSI	IVF or ICSI	IVF or ICSI
Embryo selection	Usually not performed.	Possibly performed.	Mostly performed.
Time lapse	Can be considered.	Can be considered.	Can be considered.
Assisted hatching/zona thinning	Usually not required.	Can be considered in subsequent frozen embryo transfer cycles.	Can be considered in subsequent frozen embryo transfer cycles.
Embryo transfer	Usually transfer of 1–2 fresh embryos on day 2–3.	Mostly transfer of 1 fresh or thawed embryo on day 2–3 or on day 5–6.	Mostly transfer of 1 fresh or thawed embryo on day 5–6.
PGT-A (see also Chap. 7)	Usually not performed.	Can possibly be performed.	Can be performed.

16.9 Special Add-on Laboratory Procedures

16.9.1 Follicle Flushing

Follicle flushing may be useful in monofollicular NC-IVF [2], which will require the preparation of approximately 15 mL of a suitable flushing medium for one follicle. Technical details and the procedure of follicle flushing are described in detail in the Chap. 13.

16.9.2 Embryo Selection

In general, procedures aimed to identify from the cohort of a patient's embryos the one with the highest implantation potential are not routinely applied in NC-IVF. In case that a patient presents with more than one embryo in a NC-IVF or minimal stimulation IVF cycle, it is up to the policy of the center on when to perform an embryo transfer. One option is to transfer the best embryo on day 2/3 and culture any remaining embryo(s) to the blastocyst stage, followed by vitrification. Alternatively, all embryos can be subjected to extended culture, followed by a fresh embryo transfer on day 5 or day 6 and vitrification of any remaining embryo(s) that reach the blastocyst stage by day 5 or day 6.

16.9.3   Time-Lapse Culture

Using a time-lapse incubation system for undisturbed culture and additional embryo selection parameters was initially suggested for stimulated IVF cycles only. Improved embryo development and clinical outcome following culture of inseminated oocytes in an undisturbed time-lapse system has recently been reported for NC-IVF and for minimal stimulation IVF cycles by the center with the largest number of NC-IVF and minimal stimulation IVF treatment cycles [3], which awaits confirmation by further studies. The same group also showed the potential use of time-lapse based algorithms for predicting pregnancy [4].

16.9.4   Assisted Hatching/Zona Thinning

30 years after the initial reports on assisted hatching (AH), the effect of this procedure on live birth rates in stimulated IVF cycles is still considered to be uncertain [5]. So far, no large clinical studies using AH in NC-IVF and minimal stimulation IVF have been presented and thus AH is not considered to be applied as a routine in NC-IVF and minimal stimulation IVF.

16.9.5   Preimplantation Genetic Testing for Aneuploidy (PGT-A)

Detection of chromosomal aberrations in human embryos by PGT-A is usually applied to identify one or more chromosomally normal or euploid embryos for embryo transfer and to increase the chance of achieving a pregnancy. One aspect is embryo selection according to PGT-A results to shorten the time to pregnancy. Another aspect is the psychological burden associated with failed implantation or even a miscarriage of an aneuploid embryo. Although there are no large studies on this subject in NC-IVF and minimal stimulation IVF, one study reported chromosomal aneuploidies in embryos from unstimulated cycles, which suggests that aneuploidy can be an issue in NC-IVF and minimal stimulation IVF as well [6].

Naturally the aspect of selection is not given in NC-IVF and for most minimal stimulation IVF cycles, whereas the psychological aspect may be of importance to some patients, especially after a previous treatment cycle that ended in a miscarriage. In the latter case, it may be an option to discuss the use of PGT-A with a patient if this technique is offered in a particular clinic.

16.10   Summary

The overall workflow is identical between NC-IVF, minimal stimulation IVF, and conventional IVF cycles, and the same applies to related aspects like laboratory setting and equipment, training and experience of the embryologists, and the various aspects related to quality management. However, some details of the various procedures that are performed in the laboratory are different and/or can be adapted for optimization.

References

1. De los Santos MJ, Apter S, Coticchio G, Debrock S, Lundin K, Plancha CE, et al. Revised guidelines for good practice in IVF laboratories. Hum Reprod. 2016;31:685–6.
2. Kohl Schwartz AS, Caluzaferri I, Roumet M, Limacher A, Fink A, Wuuest A, et al. Follicular flushing leads to higher oocyte yield in monofollicular IVF: a randomized controlled trial. Hum Reprod. 2020;35:2253–61.
3. Ueno S, Ito M, Uchiyama K, Okimura T, Yabuuchi A, Kobayashi T, Kato K. Closed embryo culture system improved embryological and clinical outcome for single vitrified-warmed blastocyst transfer: a single-center large cohort study. Reprod Biol. 2019;19:139–44.
4. Kato K, Ueno S, Berntsen J, Ito M, Shimazaki K, Uchiyama K, Okimura T. Comparing prediction of ongoing pregnancy and live birth outcome in patients with advanced and younger maternal age patients using KIDScore™ day 5: a large-cohort retrospective study with single vitrified-warmed blastocyst transfer. Reprod Biol Endocrinol. 2021;19:98.
5. Lacey L, Hassan S, Frank S, Seif MW, Ahsan AM. Assisted hatching on assisted conception (in vitro fertilisation (IVF) and intracytoplasmic sperm injection (ICSI)). Cochrane Database Syst Rev. 2021;3:CD001894.
6. Verpoest W, Fauser BC, Papanikolaou E, Staessen C, Van Landuyt L, Donoso P, Tournaye H, Liebaers I, Devroey P. Chromosomal aneuploidy in embryos conceived with unstimulated cycle IVF. Hum Reprod. 2008;23:2369–71.

Part IV
Costs, Risks and Success Rates

Chapter 17
Risks of Natural Cycle and Minimal Stimulation IVF

Michael von Wolff

17.1 Background

In addition to the success of IVF therapy, its risks also play a significant role. Couples are most concerned about the possible effects of hormone stimulation on the woman's health and psyche. From a reproductive medicine point of view, the risks of overstimulation syndrome with all the associated complications as well as the risks of follicle aspiration play the largest role.

When deciding on the various IVF therapies, it is important to bear in mind that the risk of overstimulation is greatest with conventional IVF, while the risk of follicular aspiration is probably more relevant with natural cycle IVF (NC-IVF) and minimal stimulation IVF, as more oocyte pick-ups are required on average.

The risks of IVF therapy for the health of children are also relevant. The effect on children's health is dealt with in Part V of this book, "Children's health."

17.2 Health Risks for Children

The IVF-related risks for children are dealt with in Part V of this book "Children's health." In Chap. 20, the malformation, obstetric and epigenetic risks are described and discussed, regardless of the type of IVF therapy. Chapter 21 describes specifically the child health risks associated with NC-IVF. Part V is concluded by Chap. 22 in which the risks of asthma and, in connection with this, the frequency of breast feeding in the different IVF therapies are presented.

M. von Wolff (✉)
Division of Gynecological Endocrinology and Reproductive Medicine, University Women's Hospital, University of Bern, Bern, Switzerland
e-mail: Michael.vonwolff@insel.ch

© The Author(s), under exclusive license to Springer Nature Switzerland AG 2022   173
M. von Wolff (ed.), *Natural Cycle and Minimal Stimulation IVF*,
https://doi.org/10.1007/978-3-030-97571-5_17

17.3   Risks of Ovarian Hyperstimulation Syndrome (OHSS)

OHSS was a feared complication, especially during the early years of IVF therapy. The goal at that time was to obtain as many oocytes as possible. Later it was found out that the cumulative success rate did not increase further with a very large number of oocytes which led to a reduction in the gonadotropin doses used and thus also to a reduction in OHSS rates. Another important step was the introduction of GnRH antagonist protocols, which were associated with a lower risk of OHSS compared to long-acting GnRH agonist protocols. According to a meta-analysis by Yang et al. (2021) [1] (Table 17.1), that included studies from 2015 to 2018, the risk of OHSS is increased with long-acting GnRH agonist protocols, with a relative risk of 1.63 (95% CI: 1.15–2.32). In the included studies, OHSS rate varied in the long-acting GnRH agonist group from 3.1% to 46.2%, whereas in the antagonist group, the rate varied from 2.0% to 21.1%.

A further decrease in risk results from the "freeze all" strategy and the use of GnRH agonists to trigger ovulation, which are used in cycles with an increased risk of OHSS [2].

With NC-IVF and minimal stimulation IVF therapies, the risk of OHSS is practically non-existent due to a low number of follicles.

17.4   Risks of Oocyte Pick-Up

The risk of a pelvic infection as a result of the follicle aspiration is very low and is less than 1% (Table 17.2).

The risk of relevant vaginal bleeding, which requires longer compression or tamponade, is also very low and is <1% (Table 17.2). More clinically relevant are the risks of bleeding into the abdomen leading to hemoperitoneum. In the study by Levi-Setti et al. (2018) [3], the risk of hemoperitoneum per oocyte pick-up was 0.23%, and 35% of these cases subsequently required laparoscopy or laparotomy.

Bleeding leading to a hemoperitoneum or peritoneal hematoma is probably often the cause of severe pain, requiring hospitalization, which occurs in <1% of follicle aspirations (Table 17.2).

Table 17.1 Risk for OHSS in women treated with long-acting GnRH agonists versus GnRH antagonists (Summary of a meta-analysis [1])

Included studies	GnRH agonist cycles: Events/total, n	GnRH antagonist cycles: Events/total, n	Risk ratio (95% CI)	Heterogeneity, I^2
7 studies, overall result	99/1769	62/1434	1.63 (1.15–2.32)	0%[a]

[a] Indicates very low heterogeneity of studies (www.handbook-5-1.cochrane.org)

Table 17.2 Complications observed due to follicle aspiration in patients undergoing IVF treatments

	Levi-Setti et al. (2018) [3]	Özaltin et al. (2018) [4]	Ludwig et al. (2006) [5]
Number of oocyte pick-ups	23.827	1.031	1.058
Pelvic infections	10 (0.04%)	8 (0.77%)	0
Major vaginal bleeding	2 (0.01%)	7 (0.7%)	1 (0.1%)
Hemoperitoneum	54 (0.23%)	No data	No data
Severe pain, requiring hospitalization	14 (0.6%)	1 (0.09%)	7 (0.7%)

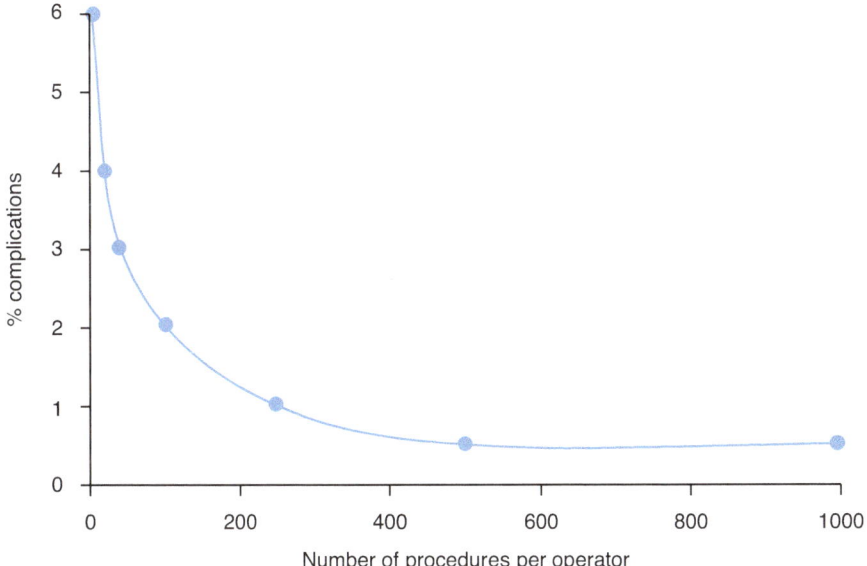

Fig. 17.1 Rate of surgical complications for single operator (% complications) versus number of procedures (follicle aspirations). Adjusted according to [3]

It should be noted that data about the risk of follicle aspirations are derived exclusively from conventional IVF therapies. Conventional IVF therapies are usually accompanied by a polyfollicular response, so that a large number of follicles are aspirated. Serum estradiol (E2) concentrations are also very high, which dilates the veins of the vaginal wall and pelvis, increasing the risk of bleeding. Finally, it is important to note that the studies used large-volume aspiration needles such as 16G [4, 5] or 17G [3], which are associated with greater tissue trauma and therefore a higher risk of bleeding.

Levi-Setti et al. (2018) [3] also evaluated whether the surgeon's experience played a role in the incidence of complications (Fig. 17.1). They found that the incidence was significantly higher for physicians who had performed <250 retrievals compared with those who had completed >250 retrievals (OR 0.63, 95% CI: 0.40–0.99).

17.5   Risk and Need Assessment in Different IVF Treatments

There is practically no risk of OHSS with NC-IVF or minimal stimulation IVF treatment. On the other hand, more treatment cycles are carried out on average until pregnancy occurs, and therefore more aspirations are performed (see Chap. 19). The more oocyte retrievals are performed, the higher the risk of infection or bleeding.

However, it should be noted that the risks from follicle aspirations in NC-IVF or minimal stimulation IVF treatment may be lower than in conventional IVF treatment.

In NC-IVF and minimal stimulation IVF, only one to very few follicles are aspirated. The E2 concentrations are also much lower, and the aspiration needles are much thinner. The aspiration needles used in the IVF centre in Bern, Switzerland have a volume of 19G, needles in the Kato Ladies Clinic in Tokyo and New Hope infertility Centre in New York have a volume of 21G (see Chap. 13).

It can therefore be assumed that the risk of complications is much lower in aspirations performed in NC-IVF and minimal stimulation IVF treatments. Even though data regarding the risks has not yet been published for different IVF treatments, personal experiences confirm this assumption. In the IVF centre in Bern, Switzerland, only one hemoperitoneum was reported in a series of 5000 aspirations using 19G aspiration needles performed between 2009 and 2020. The reported hemoperitoneum required a laparoscopy and revealed bleeding from the punctured ovary but no other injury.

A systematic analysis of the risks of follicle aspiration in NC-IVF and minimal stimulation IVF compared to conventional IVF is currently performed in the IVF-Naturelle® network (see Chap. 24). Results are expected in 2023.

Each IVF technique is associated with therapy-specific risks. Since the overall risks are very low, these risks are usually not a criterion for or against performing one of the different IVF techniques.

However, awareness of complications should be present, and efforts should be made to minimize the risk of infection and bleeding. A worldwide web-based survey of 155 IVF centres in 55 countries, performing 97,200 IVF cycles annually, revealed that centres use different strategies to minimize risk. However, the types of strategies used are inconsistent [6].

The examples in this chapter show that a thin aspiration needle, paired with much experience with follicle aspirations, is likely to be a major key to risk reduction. An ESHRE working group provides good practice recommendations covering technical aspects of ultrasound guided transvaginal oocyte retrieval [7].

17.6   Practical Conclusions

- Each IVF therapy has therapy-specific risks.
- However, the risks (OHSS due to ovarian stimulation and infection or bleeding due to follicle aspiration) are very low.

- The risks are usually not a decision criterion when choosing the IVF technique.
- Nevertheless, efforts should be made to minimize the risks, whether by avoiding excessively high stimulation doses, using the antagonist protocol or thin aspiration needles.

References

1. Yang R, Guan Y, Perrot V, Ma J, Li R. Comparison of the long-acting GnRH agonist follicular protocol with the GnRH antagonist protocol in women undergoing in vitro fertilization: a systematic review and meta-analysis. Adv Ther. 2021;38:2027–37.
2. Nelson SM. Prevention and management of ovarian hyperstimulation syndrome. Thromb Res. 2017;151(Suppl 1):S61–4.
3. Levi-Setti PE, Cirillo F, Scolaro V, Morenghi E, Heilbron F, Girardello D, Zannoni E, Patrizio P. Appraisal of clinical complications after 23,827 oocyte retrievals in a large assisted reproductive technology program. Fertil Steril. 2018;109:1038–1043.e1.
4. Özaltın S, Kumbasar S, Savan K. Evaluation of complications developing during and after transvaginal ultrasound—guided oocyte retrieval. Ginekol Pol. 2018;89:1–6.
5. Ludwig AK, Glawatz M, Griesinger G, Diedrich K, Ludwig M. Perioperative and postoperative complications of transvaginal ultrasound-guided oocyte retrieval: prospective study of >1000 oocyte retrievals. Hum Reprod. 2006;21:3235–40.
6. Bhandari H, Agrawal R, Weissman A, Shoham G, Leong M, Shoham Z. Minimizing the risk of infection and bleeding at trans-vaginal ultrasound-guided ovum pick-up: results of a prospective web-based world-wide survey. J Obstet Gynaecol India. 2015;65:389–95.
7. ESHRE Working Group on Ultrasound in ART, D'Angelo A, Panayotidis C, Amso N, Marci R, Matorras R, Onofriescu M, Turp AB, Vandekerckhove F, Veleva Z, Vermeulen N, Vlaisavljevic V. Recommendations for good practice in ultrasound: oocyte pick up. Hum Reprod Open. 2019;2019:hoz025.

Chapter 18
Costs for Natural Cycle and Minimal Stimulation IVF

Michael von Wolff

18.1 Background

When a couple first presents at a fertility centre, the conversation often comes to the question: "How much does the IVF treatment cost?" This question is absolutely understandable, but often not easy to answer.

In some countries, the answer might be as simple as: "IVF treatment is paid for by the health insurance system and therefore you do not need to pay anything".

In other countries, the answer might also be simple at first glance but is more complex: "IVF treatments are not paid for by the health insurance system and therefore everything need to be paid by yourself. However, the costs are difficult to calculate and depend on several factors such as the oocyte yield and transfer rate, how many cycles are required and whether expensive drugs are needed".

In in a third group of countries, the answer might be the following one: "A few IVF cycles are covered by the health insurance system, but no distinction is made between natural cycle IVF (NC-IVF), minimal stimulation IVF or conventional IVF therapy. Therefore and even though you might prefer NC-IVF treatments it is better to start the treatment with conventional IVF therapy to reduce costs per live birth because more oocytes are produced per cycle in case of normal ovarian reserve".

These examples show that "costs" have very different meanings and dimensions depending on the country's cost reimbursement system. They also show that "costs" are not easy to quantify, as the couple does not want to know how expensive an IVF cycle is, they are interested in how much they have to pay to get a child.

M. von Wolff (✉)
Division of Gynecological Endocrinology and Reproductive Medicine, University Women's Hospital, University of Bern, Bern, Switzerland
e-mail: Michael.vonwolff@insel.ch

© The Author(s), under exclusive license to Springer Nature Switzerland AG 2022   179
M. von Wolff (ed.), *Natural Cycle and Minimal Stimulation IVF*,
https://doi.org/10.1007/978-3-030-97571-5_18

However, this question cannot really be answered because the total number of IVF treatment cycles required can hardly be predicted. Therefore, the possibly best and only relevant answer might be the following one:

> For an average 50% probability of birth in your individual situation, an average of 1/2/3…
> cycles of NC-IVF/Minimal stimulation IVF/conventional IVF are required, which in total
> cost you 1/2/3… thousand euros, dollars, francs, yen.

Accordingly, this book chapter tries to compare the costs of different IVF treatment cycles. It also tries to compare the costs per live birth. The costs determined are the sums incurred by the fertility centre, the IVF laboratory and the medication. However, this does not mean that exactly these costs will be charged to the couple or reimbursed by the health insurance company. Furthermore, it should also be noted that the costs can vary due to differences in material, medication and personnel costs.

18.2   Treatment Costs in Mild vs. Conventional IVF Treatments

Van Tilborg et al. [1] performed an RCT and a cost analysis on poor responders, Heijnen et al. [2] on normal responders and Oudshoorn et al. [3] on hyper-responders. Patients either underwent mild IVF, defined as treatment dosage of 100–150 IE gonadotropins/day (see Chap. 2), or IVF with higher gonadotropin dosages.

In poor and normal responders, the cumulative treatment costs per achieved live birth was found to be lower in mild IVF, whereas in hyper-responders, no difference was found. Therefore, in poor and normal responders, mild IVF seems to be the economically better option (Table 18.1).

Table 18.1 Studies comparing the costs of different IVF therapies and the conclusions stated in the abstracts

Study	Comparison	Conclusions
Van Tilborg et al. [1]	Poor responders: Costs per live birth rates in mild vs. conventional IVF	"As an increased dose strategy was more expensive (delta costs/woman: €1099,– (95% CI, 562,– 1591,–)), standard FSH dosing was the dominant strategy in our economic analysis".
Heijnen et al. [2]	Normal responders: Costs per live birth rates in mild vs. conventional IVF	"However, a mild IVF treatment protocol can substantially reduce multiple pregnancy rates and overall costs".
Oudshoorn et al. [3]	Hyper-responders: Costs per live birth rates in mild vs. conventional IVF	"As dose reduction was not less expensive (€4.622,– vs. €4.714,–, delta costs/woman €92,– (95% CI: 479,– 325,–)), there was no dominant strategy in the economic analysis".

18.3   Treatment Costs in Natural Cycle and Minimal Stimulation vs. Conventional IVF Treatments

Data on these treatments is much poorer compared to mild IVF. Two studies calculated the costs of natural cycle IVF (NC-IVF) [4, 5], and two studies calculated the costs of minimal stimulation IVF [4, 6]. Ragni et al. [6] included only poor responder patients.

Minimal stimulation vs. conventional IVF was defined either [6] as 150 mg clomiphene citrate/day on cycle day 3–7 vs. 450 IE gonadotropins/day or [4] 150 IE gonadotropins/day plus GnRH antagonists started at follicle size of 14 mm vs. conventional IVF with 150–225 IE gonadotropins/day.

18.3.1   Treatment Costs per IVF Treatment Cycle

Table 18.2 shows the costs per IVF treatment cycle. The costs calculated by von Wolff et al. [5] for NC-IVF are approx. 50% lower than in the other studies. Von Wolff et al. calculated the costs based on the assumption that only in 50% of cycles an embryo transfer can be performed. Therefore, the laboratory and transfer costs were not incurred in cycles without a retrieved oocyte or without an embryo transfer. Furthermore, as apparently only von Wolff has taken into account the lower costs due to the lack of anaesthesia the cost comparison has to interpreted with care.

Table 18.2 Costs calculated by different studies for different IVF treatments

	NC-IVF vs. cIVF [4]	NC-IVF vs. cIVF [5]	Minimal stimulation IVF vs. cIVF [6]	Minimal stimulation IVF vs. cIVF [4]
Category of patients	Normal responders	All kinds of responders	Poor responders	Normal responders
Medications	No gonadotropins vs. 150–225 IE gonadotropins/day	No gonadotropins vs. ≈225 IE gonadotropins/day	Clomiphene citrate 150 mg/day day 3–7 vs. 450 IE gonadotropins/day	150 IE gonadotropins/day plus GnRH antagonist, started at follicle size of 14 mm vs. 150–225 IE gonadotropins/day
Mean number of oocytes retrieved per cycle	NC-IVF: 1	NC-IVF: 0.5*	Minimal stimulation IVF: 1.4	Minimal stimulation IVF: 1
Costs per cycle	€960,–vs.€2194,–	€431,–vs.€2188,–	€406,– vs. €791,–	€1156,– vs. €2194,–

*A transfer rate of 54% is included in the calculation

The comparison of the studies nevertheless allows the estimation that the costs of a conventional IVF stimulation cycle are approx. 2–3× higher than of NC-IVF and minimal stimulation IVF cycles.

18.3.2   Treatment Costs per Achieved Pregnancy or Live Birth

To calculate the costs per live birth, the costs per cycle need to be multiplied by the number of cycles required to achieve the same overall chance of a live birth. Such a calculation has roughly been performed in Fig. 19.1 in Chap. 19.

Furthermore, the costs for singleton and multiple pregnancies and the associated complications should ideally also be included in the calculation. However, such a complex calculation is hardly possible.

18.4   Practical Conclusions

- The therapy costs for NC-IVF treatment cycles are the lowest, followed by minimal stimulation IVF and conventional IVF.
- If the patient becomes pregnant during one of the first treatment cycles, the costs are lowest for NC-IVF.
- The average cost of treatment per pregnancy or live birth achieved depends also on the medical circumstances.
- In very poor responders NC-IVF, in poor responders minimal stimulation IVF, in normal responders mild IVF and in normal or hyper-responders conventional IVF treatment may be the most cost-effective treatments.
- National and regional reimbursement systems have an impact on treatment costs and can lead to a preference for certain IVF therapies.
- Internationally, costs can vary considerably, especially due to differences in personnel costs.
- Counselling on treatment costs per IVF treatment cycle as well as per average success rate should be part of the first IVF consultation.

References

1. van Tilborg TC, Torrance HL, Oudshoorn SC, Eijkemans MJC, Koks CAM, Verhoeve HR, Nap AW, Scheffer GJ, Manger AP, Schoot BC, Sluijmer AV, Verhoeff A, Groen H, Laven JSE, Mol BWJ, Broekmans FJM. OPTIMIST study group. Individualized versus standard FSH dosing in women starting IVF/ICSI: an RCT. Part 1: the predicted poor responder. Hum Reprod. 2017;32:2496–505.

2. Heijnen EM, Eijkemans MJ, De Klerk C, Polinder S, Beckers NG, Klinkert ER, Broekmans FJ, Passchier J, Te Velde ER, Macklon NS, Fauser BC. A mild treatment strategy for in-vitro fertilisation: a randomised non-inferiority trial. Lancet. 2007;369:743–9.

3. Oudshoorn SC, van Tilborg TC, Eijkemans MJC, Oosterhuis GJE, Friederich J, van Hooff MHA, van Santbrink EJP, Brinkhuis EA, Smeenk JMJ, Kwee J, de Koning CH, Groen H, Lambalk CB, Mol BWJ, Broekmans FJM, Torrance HL. OPTIMIST study group. Individualized versus standard FSH dosing in women starting IVF/ICSI: an RCT. Part 2: the predicted hyper responder. Hum Reprod. 2017;32:2506–14.

4. Groen H, Tonch N, Simons AH, van der Veen F, Hoek A, Land JA. Modified natural cycle versus controlled ovarian hyperstimulation IVF: a cost-effectiveness evaluation of three simulated treatment scenarios. Hum Reprod. 2013;28:3236–46.

5. von Wolff M, Rohner S, Santi A, Stute P, Popovici R, Weiss B. Modified natural cycle in vitro fertilization an alternative in vitro fertilization treatment with lower costs per achieved pregnancy but longer treatment time. J Reprod Med. 2014;59:553–9.

6. Ragni G, Levi-Setti PE, Fadini R, Brigante C, Scarduelli C, Alagna F, Arfuso V, Mignini-Renzini M, Candiani M, Paffoni A, Somigliana E. Clomiphene citrate versus high doses of gonadotropins for in vitro fertilisation in women with compromised ovarian reserve: a randomised controlled non-inferiority trial. Reprod Biol Endocrinol. 2012;10:114.

Chapter 19
Success Rates of Natural Cycle and Minimal Stimulation IVF

Michael von Wolff and Isotta Magaton

19.1 Background

The live birth rate is the most important parameter of success in IVF therapy. However, there is controversy about what it should be related to. In conventional IVF, the live birth rate is most often related to embryo transfer, however, other possible reference variables, such as the duration of IVF therapy, the number of consultations, the risks for mother and child and the total costs per pregnancy achieved, might be alternative variables. For natural cycle IVF (NC-IVF) or minimal stimulation IVF, such alternative variables are more useful as the number of retrieved oocytes is low and embryo selection is not performed.

Since success rates can be based on different reference variables and since they depend on factors that have different significance for the individual therapies, the following chapter will present the success rate from different perspectives. This should enable optimal counselling of the couple so that the best individual IVF treatment can be selected.

19.2 Definition of "Success"

"Success" in IVF therapy means getting pregnant and deliver a baby with the lowest possible risks and costs. The criteria "risks" and "costs" have already been dealt with in the previous chapters (see Chaps. 17 and 18). This chapter focuses on the chance of a live birth, i.e. the "live birth rate" as the "success rate".

M. von Wolff (✉) · I. Magaton
Division of Gynecological Endocrinology and Reproductive Medicine, University Women's Hospital, University of Bern, Bern, Switzerland
e-mail: Michael.vonwolff@insel.ch

The live birth rate is generally related to the transfer of embryos. The live birth rate per transfer is easy to calculate and allows a comparison of many IVF therapies and IVF centres. It is also easy to communicate to patients, as it seems to be a good measure of the success of IVF therapy.

But is it really a good measure? Comparing IVF therapies only based on success rate per transfer has some limitations due to a variety of factors that have a significant effect on the live birth rate per transfer, but not equally on the live birth rate per IVF therapy.

For example, Reig et al. [1], showed that the live birth rate per transfer is similar after PGT-A in women >42 years of age with 52.9% compared to 62.8% in women aged <35 years with 62.8%. However, as the transfer rate per cycle is significantly lower in women >42 years due to the high rate of aneuploid embryos [2], the live birth rate per initiated treatment cycle is much lower.

Thus, the success rate per transfer can be misleading and is usually of little help to the couple. The couple is primarily interested in the success rate of the overall IVF therapy and therefore in the success rate

- per total IVF treatment time,
- per number of consultations and thus absences from the workplace,
- per therapy-induced stress (see Chap. 23),
- per risk for mother and child (see Chap. 17),
- per treatment costs (see Chap. 18).

In other words, the couple wants to know when they will get a child, with what effort, what risk and at what cost.

This is the main difference between conventional IVF and NC-IVF or minimal stimulation IVF. In conventional IVF, a stimulation cycle including timing with contraceptive pills and a recovery cycle requires a period of up to 3 months. During this time, however, three NC-IVF and minimal stimulation IVF cycles can be carried out.

Accordingly, a comparison of the success rates of conventional IVF with NC-IVF and minimal stimulation IVF requires a complex calculation of various factors.

Such a calculation was carried out based on data from the IVF centre in Bern, Switzerland. The different treatment protocols were compared with regard to various parameters [3]. A comparison of the therapies was possible because embryo selection was not allowed in Switzerland until July 2017 and embryos were always transferred on day 2–3.

The pregnancy rate per treatment time was derived from this data (Fig. 19.1), and the number of necessary consultations and the relative costs (according to von Wolff et al. [4]) were calculated. Interestingly, the total success rates of these therapies per treatment time did not differ very much.

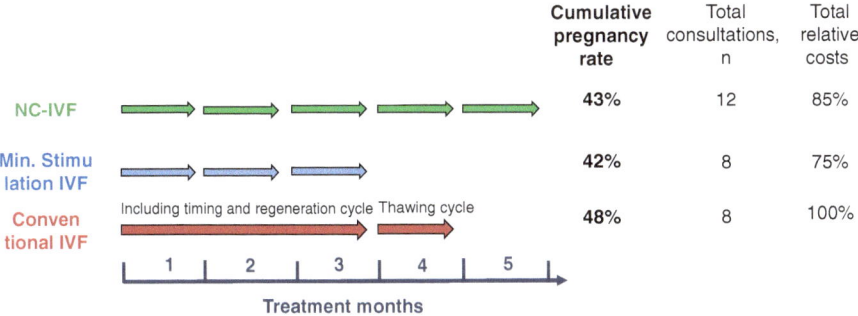

Fig. 19.1 Cumulative pregnancy rate, number of consultations and relative costs of different IVF treatments per treatment time (adapted from [3])

19.3   Prognostic Factors for Success

The previous chapter shows that the overall success rates of NC-IVF, minimal stimulation IVF and conventional therapies differ less than is commonly assumed. However, a high success rate of the individual therapy is only possible if the following therapy-specific prognostic factors are taken into account:

- effect of stimulation on the potential of oocytes and embryos to generate a pregnancy,
- effect of female age on the potential of embryos to generate a pregnancy,
- effect of duration and cause of infertility on the potential of embryos to generate a pregnancy,
- effect of endometrial thickness on the potential of embryos to generate a pregnancy.

19.3.1   Effect of Stimulation on the Potential of Oocytes and Embryos to Generate a Pregnancy

Stimulation can have an effect on oocyte quality and embryo quality as well as on endometrial function (see below). Both effects influence the implantation potential of the embryos.

The effect of gonadotropin stimulation can ideally be studied by comparing the implantation rates of NC-IVF and conventional IVF. Since this comparison is only possible if no embryo selection and no PGT-A are performed, this effect has only been investigated in a few studies.

Mitter et al. [5] retrospectively compared implantation, miscarriage and live birth rates for NC-IVF and conventional IVF cycles per transferred embryo in Switzerland. The comparison was possible because conventional IVF only included cycles performed before August 2017, i.e. before the introduction of embryo selection in Switzerland. The transfer took place 2–3 days after aspiration. Couples were

Table 19.1 Normal and poor responders: comparison of outcome parameters of day 2–3 transferred embryos [5]

	Conventional IVF	NC-IVF	Adjusted OR (95% CI)	P value
Cycles, *n*	524	453		
Age in years ± SD	35.1 ± 4.1	35.9 ± 3.8		0.023
Transferred embryos, *n*	985	462		
Amniotic sacs, *n* (%) (Implantation rate)	128/985 (13.0%)	83/462 (18.0%)	1.42 (1.10–1.84)	0.008
Miscarried amniotic sacs, *n* (%)	30/128 (23.4%)	19/83 (23.1%)	0.90 (0.52–1.54)	0.698
Live births, *n* (%)	99/1014 (9.8%)	60/468 (12.8%)	1.38 (1.01–1.88)	0.044

Table 19.2 Poor responders: comparison of outcome parameters of day 3 transferred embryos [6]

	Conventional cIVF	NC-IVF	P value
Women, *n*	355	230	
Age, mean (range)	41 (40–42)	41 (40–42)	n.s.
AMH (ng/mL), mean	1.46	0.58	0.02
Transferred embryos, *n*	845	277	
Implanted embryos, *n* (%)	70/845 (8.3%)	36/277 (13.0%)	0.047
Miscarried embryos, *n* (%)	27/70 (38.6%)	10/36 (27.8%)	n.s.
Live births, *n* (%)	51/845 (6.0%)	22/277 (7.9%)	n.s.

offered both treatment options regardless of ovarian reserve. The success rates were adjusted for the age of the woman and the cause of infertility. According to Table 19.1, the implantation and live birth rate per transferred embryo was higher with NC-IVF. The miscarriage rates, however, were the same.

De Marco et al. [6] (Table 19.2) also retrospectively compared both IVF therapies, but only in poor responders. In this group, a comparison of the therapies was also possible, as embryo selection was not performed due to the poor response. The embryos were transferred 3 days after aspiration.

This study also showed a higher implantation rate with NC-IVF. The miscarriage rate and the live birth rate were not significantly different.

Thus, the developmental potential of embryos seems to be higher with NC-IVF than with conventional IVF. However, it is still unclear whether the difference is due to an effect of stimulation on the embryos or on endometrial function.

The miscarriage rate does not seem to be different. This is in line with studies showing that gonadotropin stimulation does not lead to a higher aneuploidy rate (see Chap. 7).

19.3.2   Effect of Female Age on the Potential of Embryos to Generate a Pregnancy

The age of women plays an essential role in the success of IVF therapies. The decline in fertility with increasing female age is essentially due to disturbances in meiosis due to a functional defect of the spindle apparatus, which leads to aneuploidy of the embryos [2].

Silber et al. [7] impressively examined the live birth rate per oocyte analysing 14,159 oocytes leading to 1913 live births (Fig. 19.2). Since the oocytes were retrieved in NC-IVF therapies, it was possible to calculate the natural, age-dependent potential of oocytes to lead to a live birth and thus the intrinsic fertility. According to this study, this potential per oocyte leading to a live birth is approx. 25% at the age of 35 years, approx. 18% at the age of 37.5 years and approx. 10% at the age of 40 years.

von Wolff et al. [8] not only analysed the live birth rate per transferred embryo but also the clinical pregnancy rate (Fig. 19.3). They found that the pregnancy rate is still quite high in women around the age of 40 years but the increasingly higher miscarriage rate leads to a marked decline in live birth rates.

The age of the woman is therefore the most important limiting factor for the success of IVF therapy. Since only one or a few oocytes can be retrieved in NC-IVF and minimal stimulation IVF therapy, the success limiting effect of age is particularly great in these therapies. This means that if the woman is approaching the age of

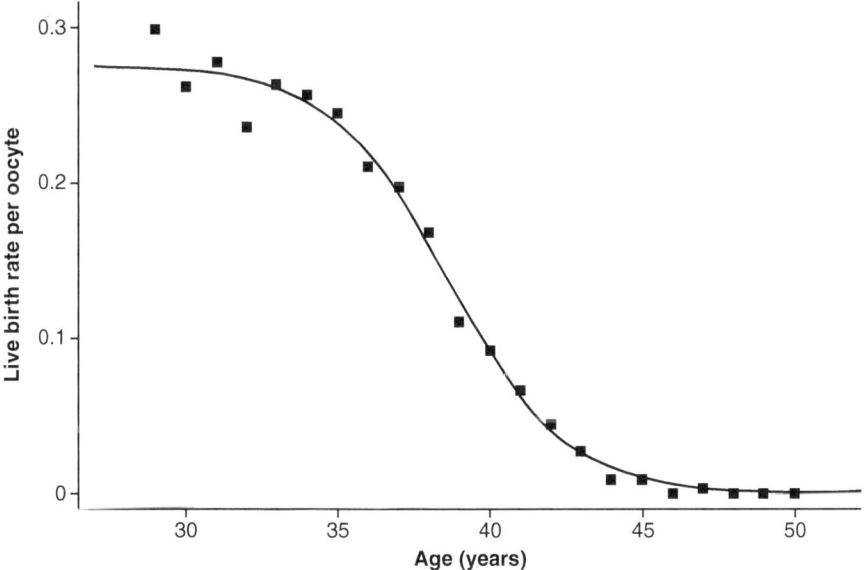

Fig. 19.2 Live birth rate per human oocyte in relation to female age, based on 14,185 oocytes and 1913 live births from single embryo transfers, generated by NC-IVF (adapted from [7])

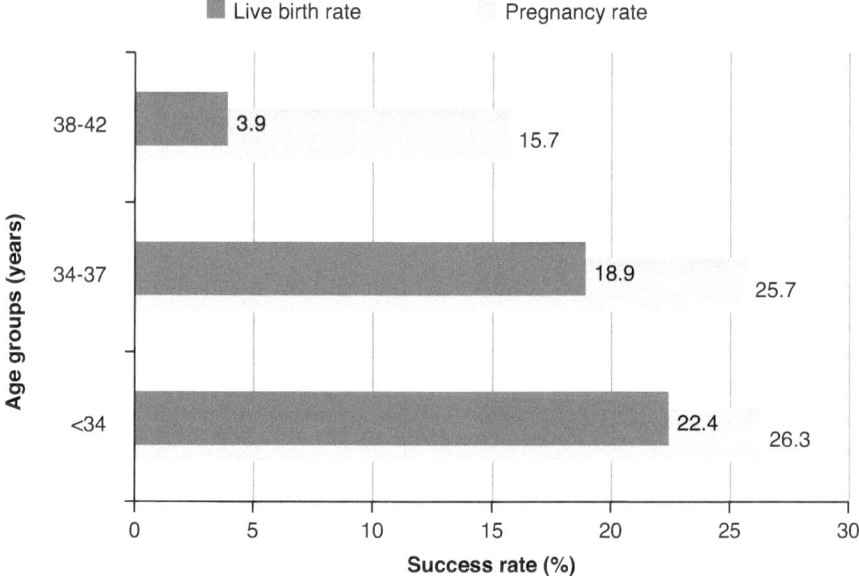

Fig. 19.3 Clinical pregnancy and live birth rates per day 2–3 embryo transfer in women in relation to women's age (adapted from [8])

40 years, those IVF therapies should be chosen which allow a higher oocyte yield. Therefore, if women approach the age of 40 years and if they still have a high ovarian reserve, minimal stimulation IVF or even conventional IVF should be the treatment of choice.

19.3.3 Effect of Duration and Cause of Infertility on the Potential of Embryos to Generate a Pregnancy

In conventional IVF therapy, the factors "low female age", "short duration of subfertility" and "low basal FSH" have been identified as positive prognostic factors [9, 10].

In NC-IVF, von Wolff et al. [8] identified "short duration of infertility" as a positive prognostic factor (Fig. 19.4) in addition to "low female age". In contrast, the "cause of infertility" could not be identified as a significant prognostic factor. However, the study by Wolff et al. suggests that a "severe andrological factor" is also a positive prognostic factor, whereas "idiopathic infertility" seems to be a negative prognostic factor. In the case of a severe andrological factor, IVF therapy is initiated with a shorter time delay than with idiopathic infertility. Accordingly, von Wolff et al. [8] demonstrated in NC-IVF a very high pregnancy rate of 36.7% per transferred embryo in young women (<34 years) with a short duration of infertility

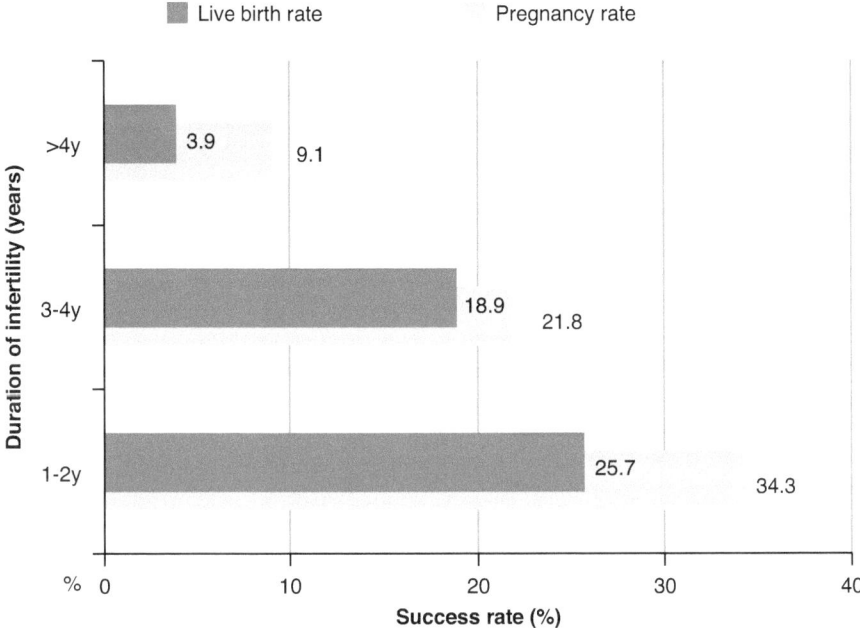

Fig. 19.4 Clinical pregnancy and live birth rates per day 2–3 transfer in women in relation to the duration of infertility in years (adapted from [8])

of only 1–2 years in combination with a severe andrological factor. In young women (<34 years) with idiopathic infertility, however, the pregnancy rate per transferred embryo was only 23.8%.

Thus, in addition to the female age as described above, other factors also limit the success of IVF therapy. This means that in the case of poor prognostic factors such as high female age and long duration or idiopathic infertility, IVF therapies with a high oocyte yield should be preferred.

19.3.4 Effect of Endometrial Thickness on the Potential of Embryos to Generate a Pregnancy

A thin endometrium is associated with a lower IVF success rate, not only in conventional IVF [11] but also in NC-IVF [12].

Theoretically, additional gonadotropin stimulation in women with a physiologically thin endometrium could be considered in order to achieve a thicker endometrium and thus a higher pregnancy rate through the higher serum oestradiol (E2) concentrations.

Magaton et al. [13], were able to show that the endometrium is significantly thicker by approx. 1.5 mm in conventional IVF therapy than in NC-IVF treatment on the day of ovulation triggering ($p < 0.001$). Magaton et al. were also able to show that the endometrium is significantly thicker by approx. 0.8 mm in women treated with 25 mg clomiphene + 75 IE human menopausal gonadotropins (HMG)/day than with clomiphene only on the day of follicle aspiration ($p < 0.001$) [14]. However, pregnancy rates were not increased in women with additional gonadotropin stimulation and thereby higher E2 concentrations.

Therefore, although endometrial thickness is positively associated with pregnancy rate in IVF treatments, additional gonadotropin stimulation to increase endometrial thickness is not beneficial.

19.4 Cumulative Live Birth Rate After Several IVF Treatment Cycles

If several consecutive IVF treatment cycles are performed, the pregnancy rate and live birth rates per cycle decrease over the course of therapy and finally reach a plateau.

This effect was impressively demonstrated in conventional IVF by Garrido et al. [15] (Fig. 19.5). With conventional IVF, the live birth rate decreased progressively with each transfer and reached a plateau after the transfer of approx. 10–15 embryos.

In NC-IVF or minimal stimulation IVF, this effect has hardly been studied.

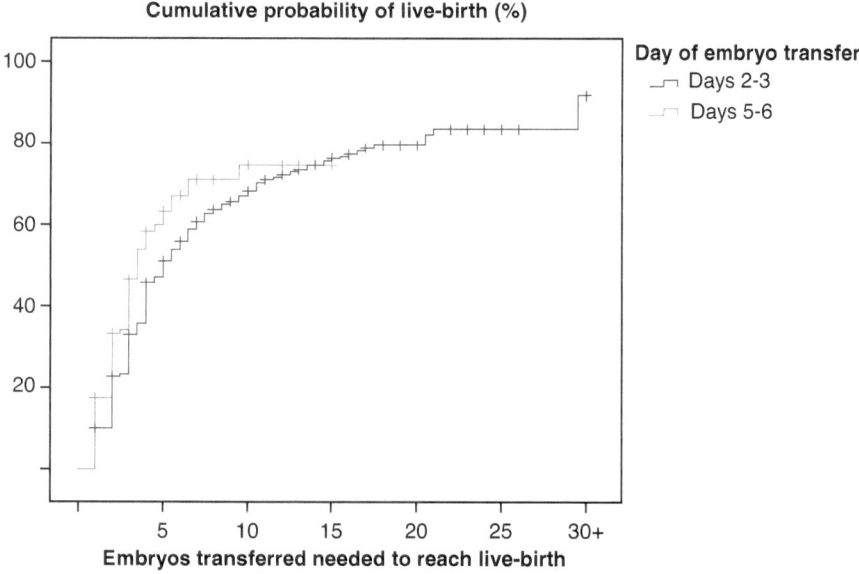

Fig. 19.5 Cumulative live birth rates in 11,429 women, undergoing 51,012 embryo transfers of day 2–3 and day 5–6 embryos (modified according to [15])

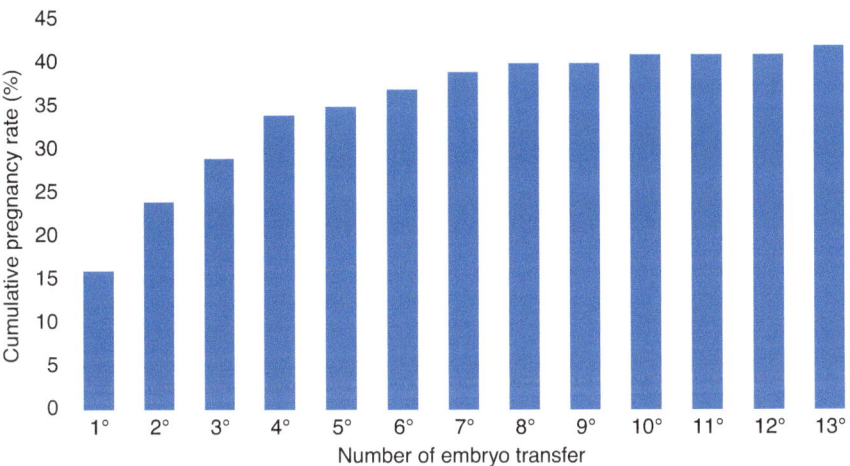

Fig. 19.6 Cumulative pregnancy rate in 210 women (36 ± 3.7 years (range 23–44 years)) undergoing 137 day 2–3 single embryo transfers (Infertility Centre, Bern, Switzerland)

Nargund et al. [16] published a small study on NC-IVF with 52 rather young women (mean 34 years, range 24–40 years) who underwent 182 NC-IVF treatment cycles. However, due to the small number of IVF cycles, there was considerable overall variability. Therefore, it was difficult to assess after which cycle the success rate flattened. After 10 cycles, the cumulative live birth rate was around 80%.

The IVF centre in Bern, Switzerland also evaluated the data of NC-IVF cycles. 210 women underwent 127 embryo transfers after NC-IVF cycles. Female age was 36 ± 3.7 years (range 23–44 years). Figure 19.6 shows the cumulative clinical pregnancy rates in relation to the number of treatment cycles with single embryos transferred on day 2–3. This evaluation showed that the success rate decreases after about 5 embryo transfers and reaches a plateau after about 10 transfers. Since the transfer rate in NC-IVF is approx. 50% per cycle [17], the plateau is reached after around 20 NC-IVF treatment cycles.

For minimal stimulation IVF, Abe et al. [18] published a large study with 839 women who completed 2541 cycles. The women received stimulation with 50–100 mg clomiphene citrate/day from day 3 until the day before ovulation was triggered. 1.6 ± 0.0 oocytes were retrieved per aspiration, about two times more than with NC-IVF. The data was broken down according to the age of the women and calculated as the cumulative live birth rate per cycle. Per cycle, 1.4 cleaved embryos were generated in women aged ≤34 years, 1.2 in women aged 35–40 years and 1.0 in women aged >40 years. Thus, approx. one embryo was transferred per cycle, which means that this data can be compared approximately with that in Figs. 19.5 and 19.6.

A flattening of the success curve was already evident at about the third cycle and a plateau was reached after about the fifth cycle. After five cycles, the cumulative live birth rate for women aged ≤34 years was 76.1%, for women aged 35–37 years

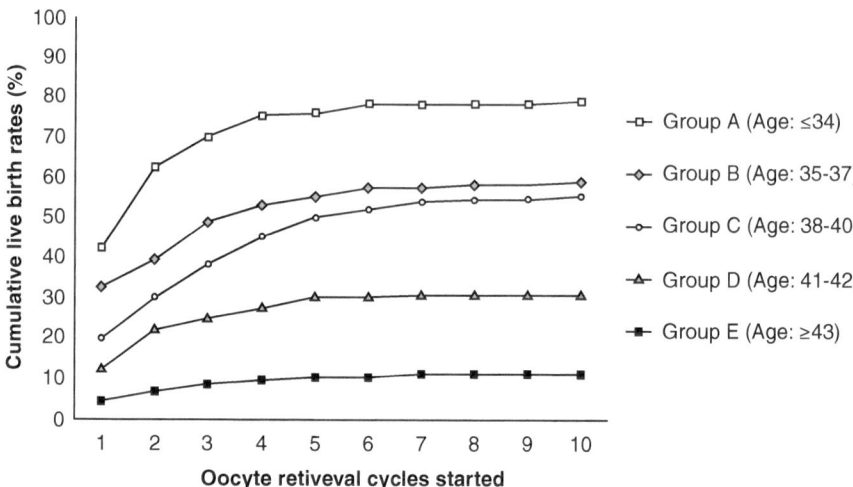

Fig. 19.7 Cumulative live birth rate in 839 women undergoing 2541 minimal stimulation IVF cycles, defined by taking 50–100 mg clomiphene citrate/day. Overall, 1.6 ± 0.0 oocytes were retrieved and 1.2 ± 0.0 cleaved embryos were generated per oocyte retrieval cycle (reprinted with permission from [18])

55.3%, for women aged 38–40 years 50.4% and for women aged 41–42 years 30.5% (Fig. 19.7).

Therefore, regardless of the type of IVF therapies, the success rate increasingly declines after the transfer of approx. four to five day 2–3 embryos.

Because of this, a change to IVF therapies with a higher oocyte yield should be considered not later than after five embryo transfers without a pregnancy. If the ovarian reserve is high, conventional IVF should be considered in normal or high responders and minimal stimulation IVF or mild IVF (150 IE gonadotropins/day) in expected poor responders. Only in women with very low ovarian reserve, NC-IVF can be continued as the oocyte yield cannot be increased by gonadotropin stimulation.

Furthermore, an evaluation of recurrent implantation failure (RIF) should be considered in such cases. However, the evidence regarding the effect of an evalua- tion of RIF is limited. Assuming that RIF is due to the same causes as habitual miscarriages, the following parameters should be evaluated or considered according to international guidelines [19]:

- Screening for lupus anticoagulant, anticardiolipin antibodies, β2 glycoprotein antibodies,
- Screening for thyroid stimulatory hormone (TSH) and thyroid peroxidase anti- bodies (TPO),
- Assessment of uterine anatomy (3D ultrasound, possibly office hysteroscopy),
- Possibly parental karyotyping,
- Possibly endometrial biopsy (exclusion of pathologies and plasma cells).

19.5 Practical Conclusions

- Monthly and consecutive NC-IVF or minimal stimulation IVF therapies are similarly successful as conventional IVF therapy, but only if the transfer rate per cycle is high.
- The success rate depends on the number of transferred embryos. Additional or a higher stimulation dosage should be considered in women with a low transfer rate and if ovarian reserve is still high.
- If the prognostic factors are good (female age <35–37 years, short duration of infertility, severe andrological infertility), three cycles of NC-IVF therapy can be started with. If the transfer rate is high, a further three cycles of NC-IVF therapy can be performed. However, if the transfer rate is low, minimal stimulation IVF should be considered if ovarian reserve is high.
- If the prognostic factors are poor (female age >35–37 years, long duration of infertility, idiopathic infertility), minimal stimulation IVF should be started or, if the prognostic factors are very poor (female age >40 years), conventional IVF should be started directly if the ovarian reserve is high.
- A flattening of the success rate becomes apparent after the transfer of approx. four to five day 2–3 embryos. Additional or stronger stimulation and embryo selection as well as analysis of RIF should then be considered.

References

1. Reig A, Franasiak J, Scott RT Jr, Seli E. The impact of age beyond ploidy: outcome data from 8175 euploid single embryo transfers. J Assist Reprod Genet. 2020;37:595–602.
2. Franasiak JM, Forman EJ, Hong KH, Werner MD, Upham KM, Treff NR, Scott RT Jr. The nature of aneuploidy with increasing age of the female partner: a review of 15,169 consecutive trophectoderm biopsies evaluated with comprehensive chromosomal screening. Fertil Steril. 2014;101:656–63.e1.
3. von Wolff M, Magaton IM. Klassische IVF vs. natural-cycle und minimal-stimulation-IVF. Gynakologe. 2020;53:588–95.
4. von Wolff M, Rohner S, Santi A, Stute P, Popovici R, Weiss B. Modified natural cycle in vitro fertilization an alternative in vitro fertilization treatment with lower costs per achieved pregnancy but longer treatment time. J Reprod Med. 2014;59:553–9.
5. Mitter VR, Grädel F, Kohl Schwartz AS, von Wolff M. Gonadotropin stimulation reduces the implantation and live birth but not the miscarriage rate – a study based on the comparison of gonadotropin stimulated and unstimulated IVF. Hum Reprod. 2021;36(Suppl 1):i452.
6. De Marco MP, Montanari G, Ruscito I, Giallonardo A, Ubaldi FM, Rienzi L, Costanzi F, Caserta D, Schimberni M, Schimberni M. Natural cycle results in lower implantation failure than ovarian stimulation in advanced-age poor responders undergoing IVF: fertility outcomes from 585 patients. Reprod Sci. 2021;28(7):1967–73.
7. Silber SJ, Kato K, Aoyama N, Yabuuchi A, Skaletsky H, Fan Y, Shinohara K, Yatabe N, Kobayashi T. Intrinsic fertility of human oocytes. Fertil Steril. 2017;107:1232–7.
8. von Wolff M, Schwartz AK, Bitterlich N, Stute P, Fäh M. Only women's age and the duration of infertility are the prognostic factors for the success rate of natural cycle IVF. Arch Gynecol Obstet. 2019;299:883–9.

 9. van Loendersloot LL, van Wely M, Limpens J, Bossuyt PM, Repping S, van der Veen F. Predictive factors in in vitro fertilization (IVF): a systematic review and meta-analysis. Hum Reprod Update. 2010;16:577–89.
10. González-Foruria I, Peñarrubia J, Borràs A, Manau D, Casals G, Peralta S, Creus M, Ferreri J, Vidal E, Carmona F, Balasch J, Fàbregues F. Age, independent from ovarian reserve status, is the main prognostic factor in natural cycle in vitro fertilization. Fertil Steril. 2016;106:342–7.
11. Kasius A, Smit JG, Torrance HL, Eijkemans MJ, Mol BW, Opmeer BC, Broekmans FJ. Endometrial thickness and pregnancy rates after IVF: a systematic review and meta-analysis. Hum Reprod Update. 2014;20:530–41.
12. von Wolff M, Fäh M, Roumet M, Mitter V, Stute P, Griesinger G, Kohl SA. Thin endometrium is also associated with lower clinical pregnancy rate in unstimulated menstrual cycles: a study based on natural cycle IVF. Front Endocrinol (Lausanne). 2018;9:776.
13. Magaton IM, Helmer A, Roumet M, Stute P, von Wolff M. High dose gonadotropn stimulation increases endometrial thickness but this gonadotropin induced thickening does not have an effect on implantation. J Gynecol Obstet Hum Reprod, in press.
14. Magaton I, Helmer A, Roumet M, Stute P, von Wolff M. Clomiphene citrate stimulated cycles - additional gonadotrophin stimulation increases endometrium thickness without increasing implantation rate. Facts Views Vis Obgyn. 2022; 4:77–81.
15. Garrido N, Bellver J, Remohí J, Simón C, Pellicer A. Cumulative live-birth rates per total number of embryos needed to reach newborn in consecutive in vitro fertilization (IVF) cycles: a new approach to measuring the likelihood of IVF success. Fertil Steril. 2011;96:40–6.
16. Nargund G, Waterstone J, Bland J, Philips Z, Parsons J, Campbell S. Cumulative conception and live birth rates in natural (unstimulated) IVF cycles. Hum Reprod. 2001;16:259–62.
17. von Wolff M, Nitzschke M, Stute P, Bitterlich N, Rohner S. Low-dosage clomiphene reduces premature ovulation rates and increases transfer rates in natural-cycle IVF. Reprod Biomed Online. 2014;29:209–15.
18. Abe T, Yabuuchi A, Ezoe K, Skaletsky H, Fukuda J, Ueno S, Fan Y, Goldsmith S, Kobayashi T, Silber S, Kato K. Success rates in minimal stimulation cycle IVF with clomiphene citrate only. J Assist Reprod Genet. 2020;37:297–304.
19. ESHRE guideline recurrent pregnancy loss. Hum Reprod Open. 2018;2018(2):hoy004.

Part V
Children's Health

Chapter 20
IVF-Related Children's Health Risks

Michael von Wolff

20.1 Background

Data on malformation rates in children have been published many times and clearly show a slightly increased risk of organic malformations in children after IVF therapy (Table 20.1). However, the risk of functional changes cannot be clearly quantified and is controversial. It is also not entirely clear what part of the increased risk maternal and paternal factors have, and what part IVF therapy as such has. Finally, the question arises as to what extent the risks have decreased in recent years thanks to the advances in IVF therapies. The following data is based on systematic literature research, published 2020 [1] and is relevant to possibly reduce risks (see Chap. 21).

20.2 Malformations in IVF Children

20.2.1 General Risk of Malformation

In a meta-analysis, Qin et al. [2] included 57 cohort studies with predominantly IVF children and children after spontaneous conception (Table 20.1). The relative risk (RR) of a congenital malformation was 1.33 (95% CI 1.24–1.43) in the IVF children.

The generally increased risk persisted when only singletons were studied (RR 1.38; 95% CI 1.30–1.47), when only major malformations were considered (RR

M. von Wolff (✉)
Division of Gynecological Endocrinology and Reproductive Medicine, University Women's Hospital, University of Bern, Bern, Switzerland
e-mail: Michael.vonwolff@insel.ch

© The Author(s), under exclusive license to Springer Nature Switzerland AG 2022   199
M. von Wolff (ed.), *Natural Cycle and Minimal Stimulation IVF*,
https://doi.org/10.1007/978-3-030-97571-5_20

Table 20.1 Risk of child health changes after IVF* treatments according to current meta-analyses (modified by von Wolff and Haaf [1])

Risk factors	References	Included studies	Statistical significant risk increase	Absolute risk changes (absolute numbers and calculations based on RR and OR)
General risk of malformations	Qin et al. [2]	57 studies	RR 1.33 (95% CI 1.24–1.43)	Increase from approx. 4.6% [3] to approx. 6.1% (based on RR (×1.33))
Risk of heart defects	Giorgione et al. [4]	8 studies	OR 1.45 (95% CI 1.20–1.76)	Increase from approx. 0.7% [5] to approx. 1.0% (based on OR (×1.45))
Risk of high blood pressure	Guo et al. [6]	19 studies	Increase in systolic pressure: +1.88 mm Hg (95% CI 0.27–3.49)	Increase in systolic blood pressure: +1.88 mm Hg [7]
			Increase in diastolic pressure: +1.51 mm Hg (95% CI 0.34–2.70)	Increase in diastolic blood pressure: +1.51 mm Hg [7]
Risk of preterm birth (<37 weeks of pregnancy) and low birth weight (<2500 g)	Hoorsan et al. [3]	30 studies	Premature birth: OR 1.79 (95% CI 1.21–2.63)	Increase from approx. 7% (Switzerland, [8]) to approx. 12.5% (based on OR (×1.79))
			Low birth weight: OR 1.89 (95% CI 1.36–2.62)	Increase from approx. 6.5% (Switzerland, [8]) to approx. 12.3% (based on OR (×1.89))
Risk for malformation of specific organ systems	Hoorsan et al. [3]	30 studies	Urogenital tract: OR 1.58 (95% CI 1.28–1.94)	Increase from approx. 1.7% [9] to approx. 2.7% (based on OR (×1.58))
			Musculoskeletal system: OR 1.35 (95% CI 1.12–1.64)	Increase from approx. 1.6% [9] to approx. 2.2% (based on OR (×1.35))
			Central nervous system: RR 1.36 (95% CI 1.10–1.70)	Increase from approx. 0.4% [9] to approx. 0.54% (based on OR (×1.36))

Table 20.1 (continued)

Risk of premature birth, low birth weight after transfer of cryopreserved embryos and macrosomia	Maheshwari et al. [10]	20 studies	Premature birth: RR 0.90 (95% CI 0.84–0.97)	Changes from approx. 9.4% [11] to approx. 8.5% [11] (based on RR (×0.9))
			Low birth weight: RR 0.72 (95% CI 0.67–0.77)	Changes from approx. 8.8% [11] to approx. 6.3% [11] (based on RR (×0.72))
			Macrosomia (>4000 g): RR 1.85 (95% CI 1.46–2.33)	Changes from approx. 6.2% [11] to approx. 11.5% [11] (based on RR (×1.85))

ICSI intracytoplasmic sperm injection, *IVF* in vitro fertilisation, *CI* confidence interval, *OR* odds ratio, *RR* relative risk

*IVF treatments—unless otherwise described—are defined as all IVF technologies, i.e. in vitro fertilisations, irrespective of the technology used (insemination or intracytoplasmic sperm injection) and irrespective of whether the embryos had been cryopreserved or not

1.47; 95% CI 1.29–1.68) and when only high-quality studies were considered (RR 1.40; 95% CI 1.27–1.55). The increased risk was lower but still significant when IVF twins (RR 1.18; 95% CI 1.06–1.32) were compared with spontaneous twins.

A meta-analysis by Zheng et al. [12] also largely confirmed the latter result. However, Zheng et al. [12] also found an increased risk of chromosomal aberrations in multiple pregnancies (RR 1.36; 95% CI 1.04–1.77).

Hoorsan et al. [3] investigated the risk of specific malformations. They found an increased risk of central nervous system malformations (OR 1.36; 95% CI 1.10–1.70), urogenital malformations (RR 1.58; 95% CI 1.28–1.94) and musculoskeletal malformations (OR 1.35; 95% CI 1.12–1.64), but not of chromosomal aberrations (RR 1.14; 95% CI 0.90–1.44).

20.2.2   Risk of Congenital Heart Defects

Giorgione et al. [4] included eight cohort studies with children after IVF and children after spontaneous conception in a meta-analysis (Table 20.1). Single and multiple pregnancies were considered. 1.3% of IVF children had a heart defect compared to 0.68% of children after a spontaneous pregnancy (pooled OR 1.45, 95% CI 1.20–1.76). The increased risk persisted when only singleton pregnancies were included (OR 1.55, 95% CI 1.21–1.99) and when multiple adjustments were performed (pooled OR 1.29, 95% CI 1.03–1.60).

20.3 Obstetric Risks in IVF Children

20.3.1 General Obstetric Risks

Hoorsan et al. [3] included 30 studies of predominantly IVF infants and children after spontaneous conception in a meta-analysis (Table 20.1). The risk of preterm birth (<37 weeks gestation) was found to be OR 1.79 (95% CI 1.21–2.63), and the risk of low birth weight (<2500 g) was found to be OR 1.89 (95% CI 1.36–2.62).

20.3.2 Obstetric Risks of Singletons and Multiples

52 cohort studies with 181,741 IVF singles were compared in a meta-analysis published in 2017 with 4,636,508 spontaneous single pregnancies [5]. The prevalence of preterm birth in IVF pregnancies compared to spontaneous pregnancies was 10.9% (95% CI 10.0–11.8) and 6.4% (95% CI 5.8–7.0) and was thus around 1.7 times higher. The prevalence of low birth weight was 8.7% (95% CI 7.4–10.2) and 5.8% (95% CI 4.8–6.9) and was thus about 1.5 times higher.

Obstetric risks were also increased in multiple pregnancies, although less so than in singleton pregnancies. Qin et al. [8] included 39 cohort studies of multiple pregnancies with 38,053 children after IVF and 107,955 children after spontaneous conception in a meta-analysis. The increased risk of preterm birth after IVF was found to be RR 1.08 (95% CI 1.03–1.14) and the increased risk of low birth weight was found to be RR 1.04 (95% CI 1.01–1.07).

20.4 Risks from IVF-Specific Techniques

20.4.1 Obstetric Risks After the Transfer of Cryopreserved Embryos

Maheshwari et al. [10] compared almost 80,000 singletons after IVF thawing cycles, i.e. embryo transfers of previously cryopreserved embryos, with around 200,000 singletons after IVF fresh cycles in 26 studies (Table 20.1). The risks of preterm birth (RR 0.90; 95% CI 0.84–0.97) and low birth weight (RR 0.72; 95% CI 0.67–0.77) were lower in thawing cycles, but the risks of large for gestational age,

LGA (birth weight >90th percentile) (RR 1.54; 95% CI 1.48–1.61) and macrosomia (>4000 g) (RR 1.85; 95% CI 1.46–2.33) were higher.

20.4.2   Risk of Malformation After Fertilisation with ICSI

Massaro et al. [13] compared children after IVF with ICSI and with children after IVF without ICSI in a meta-analysis of 22 studies. ICSI was associated with an increased risk of genitourinary malformations (OR 1.27; 95% CI 1.02–1.59). However, when only studies with a low risk of bias (IVF with ICSI $n = 7727$, IVF without ICSI $n = 14,308$) were analysed, there was still a trend towards an increased risk of genitourinary malformations, but the difference was just short of statistical significance (OR 1.28, 95% CI 1.00–1.64). A sub-analysis showed that the risks of hypospadias (OR 1.21, 95% CI 0.87–1.69) and cryptorchidism (OR 1.39, 95% CI 0.97–2.00) were increased, but the increase was not significant.

20.5   Functional Disorders in IVF Children

20.5.1   Blood Pressure

Catford et al. [7] carried out a meta-analysis of 19 studies in which 2112 IVF children and young adults were compared with 4096 individuals after spontaneous conception (Table 20.1). The systolic blood pressure of the IVF offspring increased by 1.88 mm Hg (95% CI 0.27–3.49) and the diastolic blood pressure by 1.51 mm Hg (95% CI 0.34–2.70). Furthermore, according to five studies with 402 IVF children compared to 382 spontaneous conception children, the cardiac diastolic function was suboptimal, and the thickness of the vessels was higher.

20.5.2   Glucose Metabolism

To study glucose metabolism, seven studies with 477 IVF children were compared with 1852 children after spontaneous conception [6, 13]. The fasting insulin values of the IVF children were significantly higher (0.38 mIU/L; 95% CI 0.08–0.68), but not the fasting glucose concentrations (−0.03 mM; 95% CI −0.13–0.06) and the HOMA index determined insulin resistance (0.02; 95% CI −0.06–0.12). Overall, there was only a tendency towards impaired glucose metabolism.

20.5.3   Obesity and Lipid Metabolism

A higher birth weight or a relevant change in lipid metabolism could not be clearly demonstrated.

20.5.4   Cognitive Development

Rumbold et al. [11] carried out a systematic review of seven studies on the cognitive development of IVF children. The cognitive development of the children after IVF therapy without fertilisation by ICSI was not impaired. The data situation was less clear for IVF therapies with fertilisation via ICSI. In three studies, IVF and IVF/ ICSI children were compared. One study showed a significant increase in the risk of mental retardation in IVF/ICSI children, one study showed an intelligence quotient that was three points lower in IVF/ICSI children, and one study showed no difference.

Catford et al. [7] came to a similar conclusion in a systematic review in which psychosocial health was specifically examined in IVF children without and with ICSI fertilisation. Fourteen studies examined the neurological development of children aged 2 months to 7.5 years. In 14 studies, children after spontaneous conception served as a comparative collective. ICSI children appeared to have a higher risk of intellectual impairment (5/14 studies) and autism (2 studies). The risk of autism was particularly high when sperm were used after testicular sperm extraction (RR 3.29; 95% CI 1.58–6.87) and was also increased when ICSI was performed without an andrological factor (RR 1.57; 95% CI 1.10–2.09). However, this effect was no longer significant in both collectives when only singletons were included in the analysis.

20.6   Epigenetic Risks

20.6.1   Epigenetic Changes and Their Causes

In the germline and in early embryos, two epigenetic reprogramming waves take place in which (almost) the entire genome is first demethylated and subsequently re-methylated (Fig. 20.1). With the exception of 100–200 imprinted genes, the germline methylation patterns are deleted again in the early embryo and replaced by somatic patterns. During these reprogramming processes, the epigenome is particularly susceptible to external factors. The plasticity of the epigenome decreases continuously during development from fertilisation to the death of the individual [9, 14].

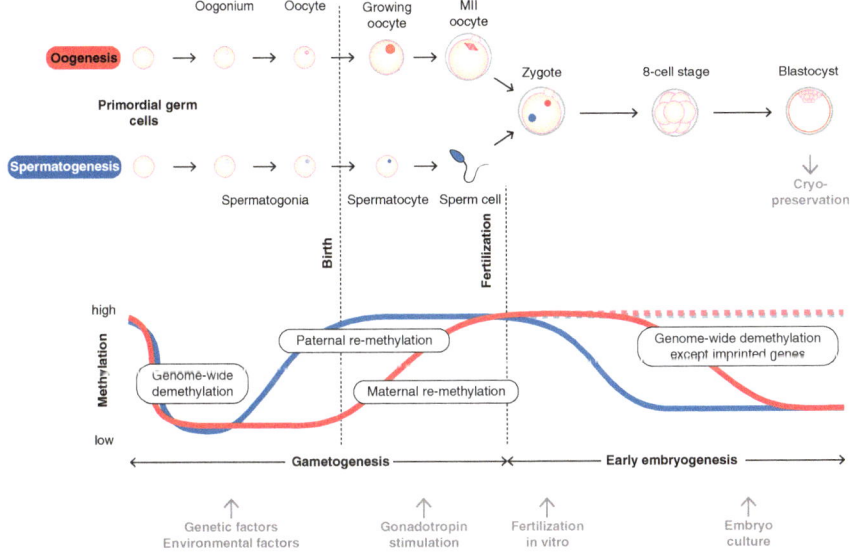

Fig. 20.1 Germ cell development and temporal association of genetic and environmental factors and IVF processes on de- and re-methylation [1]

The various IVF techniques interfere with sensitive stages of germline reprogramming, especially late stages of oocyte maturation, and postzygotic reprogramming. Thus, adverse exposures may occur at the earliest possible stage of development, which may lead to persistent epigenetic changes. The fact that children show a higher overall blood pressure and a tendency to impaired glucose metabolism after IVF therapy, as shown above, is well compatible with the Barker hypothesis proposed in 1990 by the Britisch epidemiologist David Barker.

Numerous studies in mouse and large animal models show that IVF is associated with aberrant DNA methylation and expression patterns in developmentally relevant areas, e.g., imprinted genes in oocytes, embryos, foetuses, which can influence the development and behaviour of the resulting offspring [15–20]. Although epigenetic effects can be demonstrated/estimated in the animal model for each individual IVF step (Fig. 20.1), these studies can only be transferred to humans to a limited extent.

Epigenetic changes are in principle reversible. It has been impressively shown in animal models that the long-term consequences of adverse exposures can be reduced by relatively simple interventions, e.g., certain supplements to the maternal diet [21, 22]. In humans, too, the intake of such supplements in the periconceptional period has specific effects on the epigenome of the offspring [23].

In IVF/ICSI children, methylation changes were detected both at the candidate gene level and genome-wide [24–26], but the observed effect sizes were consistently small. This argues for a threshold model in which a metabolic or cardiovascular phenotype manifests when a certain threshold of unfavourable genetic, epigenetic and environmental factors is exceeded. It is possible that IVF-induced epigenetic modifications are occasionally the last straw to "break the camel's back" [24]. Because of the multitude of other modulating factors that appear as pronounced background noise when IVF-induced methylation changes are examined, the effects of IVF on the epigenome of children can be detected as group differences, but not at an individual level.

20.6.2   Epigenetic Changes in Children After IVF Therapies

In the normal newborn population as well as in IVF children, there are only very rarely highly penetrative (comparable to a pathogenic mutation) epigenetic changes in imprinted genes that are associated with certain imprinting diseases. According to a meta-analysis by Lazaraviciute et al. [27], epigenetic diseases, a group of 12 rare congenital diseases, occur more frequently after IVF therapy (OR 3.67; 95% CI 1.39–9.74). However, this is of little practical relevance, as Beckwith-Wiedemann syndrome is rare, even with a 10-fold increased risk in IVF infants, at 1 per 1126 [28] infants born. Hiura et al. [15] found mosaics of methylation changes in IVF children with imprinting diseases, suggesting emergence during the first cell divisions that occur during the several days of embryo culture.

Epigenetic changes with a possible association with IVF therapies have also been found in human gametes and embryos [16]. A meta-analysis of 24 studies showed significant hypomethylation of the imprinted H19 gene, as well as hypermethylation of SNRPN and MEST, in sperm from men with idiopathic infertility compared to fertile controls [17]. Reduced H19 methylation has also been found in the placenta of IVF/ICSI children [18]. There are only a few studies on a very limited number of human IVF oocytes that suggest epigenetic effects, particularly hormonal stimulation on the methylation of imprinted genes [19]. The placenta appears to be more susceptible than the embryo/foetus to the induction of epigenetic abnormalities by parental and environmental factors. Significant differences have been demonstrated in the placental methylome between in vivo and in vitro conceived pregnancies of infertile couples, including in numerous developmentally relevant genes/pathways [20].

In summary, it can be assumed that the risk of epigenetic changes is increased with IVF therapies. Possible causes are gonadotropin stimulation, fertilisation in vitro, embryo culture and cryopreservation. However, it is not yet clear whether such changes really have a health effect on the children and later adults.

20.7 Which of the Risks Are Maternal or Paternal and Which Are IVF-Induced?

There are two possible study approaches to tentatively answer this question. First, IVF children can be compared with children after spontaneous conception whose parents had subfertility (e.g., duration until pregnancy >1 year). Or siblings of the same mother born after IVF and spontaneous conception are compared.

For the first approach, two of six multiple-adjusted studies by Pinborg et al. [29] were combined into a meta-analysis. The risk of preterm birth was increased in IVF infants with an aOR of 1.55 (95% CI 1.30–1.85) compared to infants of spontaneous pregnancies when subfertility was present.

Luke et al. [30] compared 10,149 IVF singletons with 8054 subfertile singletons. The risk of preterm birth and low birth weight was increased in IVF singletons with an aRR of 1.26 (95% CI 1.14–1.39) and an aRR of 1.21 (95% CI 1.08–1.36), respectively, compared to the subfertile population, defined as women who took medication to improve fertility, but did not undergo IVF.

For the second approach, the comparison of siblings, Pinborg et al. [29] combined two studies, adjusted for maternal age, parity and year of birth, among other factors, into a meta-analysis. The proportion of spontaneously conceived children born before and after IVF was approximately equal. The IVF children had an increased risk of preterm birth with an aOR of 1.27 (95% CI 1.08–1.49).

Westvik-Johari et al. [31] performed a registry-based cohort study with nationwide data from Denmark (1994–2014), Norway (1988–2015) and Sweden (1988–2015) consisted of 4,510,790 live-born singletons, 4,414,703 from natural conception, 78,095 from fresh embryo transfer (ET) and 17,990 from frozen ET. They identified 33,056 offspring sibling groups with the same mother, conceived by at least two different conception methods.

Singletons born after fresh-ET had lower mean birthweight of −51 g (95% CI −58 to −45) and increased odds of small for gestational age (OR 1.20; 95% CI 1.08–1.34), while those born after frozen ET had higher mean birthweight of 82 g (95% CI 70–94) and increased odds of large for gestational age (OR 1.84; 95% CI 1.56–2.17), compared to naturally conceived siblings. Compared to naturally conceived siblings, mean gestational age was 1.0 days lower after fresh-ET (95% CI −1.2 to −0.8), but only borderline lower after frozen ET (0.3 days, 95% CI 0.0–0.6, $p = 0.028$). There were increased odds of preterm birth after fresh ET (OR 1.27; 95% CI 1.17–1.37), and in most models after frozen ET, versus naturally conceived siblings, with somewhat stronger associations in population analyses. For very preterm birth, increased odds were found for fresh ET (OR 1.18; 95% CI 1.0–1.41) but not for frozen ET (OR 0.92; 95% CI 0.67–1.27) compared with natural conception.

In summary, both study approaches show that the risks of an unfavourable peripartum outcome are increased even when choosing control groups that are as identical as possible. This means that both, infertility and the IVF technique seem to be a risk factor.

20.8 Have the Risks Decreased in Recent Years?

To answer this question, Henningsen et al. [32] compared the obstetric outcome of 62,379 IVF singletons with 362,215 singletons after spontaneous conception in Sweden, Denmark, Finland and Norway from 1988 to 2007 over time. Among singletons, the likelihood of preterm birth and of low birth weight infants compared with infants after spontaneous conception decreased from aOR 2.47 (95% CI 2.09–2.92) and aOR 2.94 (95% CI 2.44–3.54), respectively, in 1988–1992 to aOR 1.50 (95% CI 1.43–1.58) and aOR 1.49 (95% CI 1.40–1.58), respectively, in 2003–2007.

Guo et al. [6] took a similar approach when examining blood pressure over time. Although systolic and diastolic blood pressure were elevated overall in IVF children compared to children after spontaneous pregnancies (see above), a separate examination of the 1990–1999 and 2000–2009 cohorts showed that blood pressure was significantly elevated in the older cohorts, but no longer in the younger cohorts (systolic RR −0.19; 95% CI −1.38–1.00; diastolic RR 0.17; 95% CI −0.95–1.30). This was independent of the proportion of ICSI fertilisation and the age of the children studied.

In summary, the risk of some IVF-induced health impairments seems to have decreased over time. The causes are largely speculative. It could be due to a change in the patient population as well as a change in IVF techniques. Treatment approaches such as natural cycle and minimal stimulation IVF can possibly reduce some of the risks (see Chap. 21).

References

1. von Wolff M, Haaf T. In vitro fertilization technology and child health. Dtsch Arztebl Int. 2020;117:23–30.
2. Qin J, Sheng X, Wang H, Liang D, Tan H, Xia J. Assisted reproductive technology and risk of congenital malformations: a meta-analysis based on cohort studies. Arch Gynecol Obstet. 2015;292:777–98.
3. Hoorsan H, Mirmiran P, Chaichian S, Moradi Y, Hoorsan R, Jesmi F. Congenital malformations in infants of mothers undergoing assisted reproductive technologies: systematic review and meta-analysis study. J Prev Med Public Health. 2017;50:347–60.
4. Giorgione V, Parazzini F, Fesslova V, Cipriani S, Candiani M, Inversetti A, Sigismondi C, Tiberio F, Cavoretto P. Congenital heart defects in IVF/ICSI pregnancy: systematic review and meta-analysis. Ultrasound Obstet Gynecol. 2018;51:33–42.
5. Qin JB, Sheng XQ, Wu D, Gao SY, You YP, Yang TB, Wang H. Worldwide prevalence of adverse pregnancy outcomes among singleton pregnancies after in vitro fertilization/intra-

cytoplasmic sperm injection: a systematic review and meta-analysis. Arch Gynecol Obstet. 2017;295:285–301.

6. Guo XY, Liu XM, Jin L, Wang TT, Ullah K, Sheng JZ, Huang HF. Cardiovascular and metabolic profiles of offspring conceived by assisted reproductive technologies: a systematic review and meta-analysis. Fertil Steril. 2017;107:622–31.

7. Catford SR, McLachlan RI, O'Bryan MK, Halliday JL. Long-term follow-up of intracytoplasmic sperm injection-conceived offspring compared with in vitro fertilization-conceived offspring: a systematic review of health outcomes beyond the neonatal period. Andrology. 2017;5:610–21.

8. Qin J, Wang H, Sheng X, Liang D, Tan H, Xia J. Pregnancy-related complications and adverse pregnancy outcomes in multiple pregnancies resulting from assisted reproductive technology: a meta-analysis of cohort studies. Fertil Steril. 2015;103:1492–508.e1–7.

9. El Hajj N, Schneider E, Lehnen H, Haaf T. Epigenetics and life-long consequences of an adverse nutritional and diabetic intrauterine environment. Reproduction. 2014;148:R111–20.

10. Maheshwari A, Pandey S, Amalraj Raja E, Shetty A, Hamilton M, Bhattacharya S. Is frozen embryo transfer better for mothers and babies? Can cumulative meta-analysis provide a definitive answer? Hum Reprod Update. 2018;24:35–58.

11. Rumbold AR, Moore VM, Whitrow MJ, Oswald TK, Moran LJ, Fernandez RC, Barnhart KT, Davies MJ. The impact of specific fertility treatments on cognitive development in childhood and adolescence: a systematic review. Hum Reprod. 2017;32:1489–507.

12. Zheng Z, Chen L, Yang T, Yu H, Wang H, Qin J. Multiple pregnancies achieved with IVF/ICSI and risk of specific congenital malformations: a meta-analysis of cohort studies. Reprod Biomed Online. 2018;36:472–82.

13. Massaro PA, MacLellan DL, Anderson PA, Romao RL. Does intracytoplasmic sperm injection pose an increased risk of genitourinary congenital malformations in offspring compared to in vitro fertilization? A systematic review and meta-analysis. J Urol. 2015;193(5 Suppl):1837–42.

14. Gluckman PD, Hanson MA, Buklijas T, Low FM, Beedle AS. Epigenetic mechanisms that underpin metabolic and cardiovascular diseases. Nat Rev Endocrinol. 2009;5:401–8.

15. Hiura H, Okae H, Miyauchi N, Sato F, Sato A, Van De Pette M, John RM, Kagami M, Nakai K, Soejima H, Ogata T, Arima T. Characterization of DNA methylation errors in patients with imprinting disorders conceived by assisted reproduction technologies. Hum Reprod. 2012;27:2541–8.

16. El Hajj N, Haaf T. Epigenetic disturbances in in vitro cultured gametes and embryos: implications for human assisted reproduction. Fertil Steril. 2013;99:632–41.

17. Santi D, De Vincentis S, Magnani E, Spaggiari G. Impairment of sperm DNA methylation in male infertility: a meta-analytic study. Andrology. 2017;5:695–703.

18. Nelissen EC, Dumoulin JC, Daunay A, Evers JL, Tost J, van Montfoort AP. Placentas from pregnancies conceived by IVF/ICSI have a reduced DNA methylation level at the H19 and MEST differentially methylated regions. Hum Reprod. 2013;28:1117–26.

19. Fauque P. Ovulation induction and epigenetic anomalies. Fertil Steril. 2013;99:616–23.

20. Choufani S, Turinsky AL, Melamed N, et al. Impact of assisted reproduction, infertility, sex and paternal factors on the placental DNA methylome. Hum Mol Genet. 2019;28:372–85.

21. Lillycrop KA, Slater Jefferies JL, Hanson MA, Godfrey KM, Jackson AA, Burdge GC. Induction of altered epigenetic regulation of the hepatic glucocorticoid receptor in the offspring of rats fed a protein-restricted diet during pregnancy suggests that reduced DNA methyltransferase-1 expression is involved in impaired DNA methylation and changes in histone modifications. Br J Nutr. 2007;97:1064–73.

22. Waterland RA, Travisano M, Tahiliani KG, Rached MT, Mirza S. Methyl donor supplementation prevents transgenerational amplification of obesity. Int J Obes (Lond). 2008;32:1373–9.

23. Khulan B, Cooper WN, Skinner BM, et al. Periconceptional maternal micronutrient supplementation is associated with widespread gender related changes in the epigenome: a study of a unique resource in the Gambia. Hum Mol Genet. 2012;21:2086–101.

24. Hiura H, Okae H, Chiba H, Miyauchi N, Sato F, Sato A, Arima T. Imprinting methylation errors in ART. Reprod Med Biol. 2014;13:193–202.
25. Estill MS, Bolnick JM, Waterland RA, Bolnick AD, Diamond MP, Krawetz SA. Assisted reproductive technology alters deoxyribonucleic acid methylation profiles in bloodspots of newborn infants. Fertil Steril. 2016;106:629–39.
26. El Hajj N, Haertle L, Dittrich M, Denk S, Lehnen H, Hahn T, Schorsch M, Haaf T. DNA methylation signatures in cord blood of ICSI children. Hum Reprod. 2017;32:1761–9.
27. Lazaraviciute G, Kauser M, Bhattacharya S, Haggarty P, Bhattacharya S. A systematic review and meta-analysis of DNA methylation levels and imprinting disorders in children conceived by IVF/ICSI compared with children conceived spontaneously. Hum Reprod Update. 2014;20:840–52.
28. Mussa A, Molinatto C, Cerrato F, Palumbo O, Carella M, Baldassarre G, Carli D, Peris C, Riccio A, Ferrero GB. Assisted reproductive techniques and risk of Beckwith-Wiedemann syndrome. Pediatrics. 2017;140:e20164311.
29. Pinborg A, Wennerholm UB, Romundstad LB, Loft A, Aittomaki K, Söderström-Anttila V, Nygren KG, Hazekamp J, Bergh C. Why do singletons conceived after assisted reproduction technology have adverse perinatal outcome? Systematic review and meta-analysis. Hum Reprod Update. 2013;19:87–104.
30. Luke B, Gopal D, Cabral H, Stern JE, Diop H. Pregnancy, birth, and infant outcomes by maternal fertility status: the Massachusetts Outcomes Study of Assisted Reproductive Technology. Am J Obstet Gynecol. 2017;217:327.e1–327.e14.
31. Westvik-Johari K, Romundstad LB, Lawlor DA, Bergh C, Gissler M, Henningsen AA, Håberg SE, Wennerholm UB, Tiitinen A, Pinborg A, Opdahl S. Separating parental and treatment contributions to perinatal health after fresh and frozen embryo transfer in assisted reproduction: a cohort study with within-sibship analysis. PLoS Med. 2021;18:e1003683.
32. Henningsen AA, Gissler M, Skjaerven R, Bergh C, Tiitinen A, Romundstad LB, Wennerholm UB, Lidegaard O, Nyboe Andersen A, Forman JL, Pinborg A. Trends in perinatal health after assisted reproduction: a Nordic study from the CoNARTaS group. Hum Reprod. 2015;30:710–6.

Chapter 21
Natural Cycle and Minimal Stimulation IVF-Related Children's Health Risks

Michael von Wolff

21.1 Background

The risk of malformations, functional disorders and obstetric risks is increased with IVF (see Chap. 20). The causes are maternal and paternal factors, but also the IVF technique itself. In IVF, the causes include gonadotropin stimulation, the fertilisation technique, embryo culture and cryopreservation. With natural cycle-IVF (NC-IVF) or minimal stimulation IVF, the influence of these risk factors is less or even non-existent (Table 21.1). Because of this, it is possible that the risks are lower. However, the data is limited.

21.2 Birth Weight and Risk of Preterm Birth After IVF Fresh Cycles

After conventional IVF, the birth weight is reduced, and the risk of premature birth is increased (see Chap. 20). The question therefore arises of whether these risks are lower with NC-IVF or minimal stimulation IVF.

Three studies directly compared the peripartum outcome between NC-IVFs and conventional IVFs (Table 21.2). Sunkara et al. [2] found no differences after adjustment, whereas Mak et al. [3] and Kohl Schwartz et al. [4] found a higher birth weight and fewer children with a small gestational age (SGA) after NC-IVF. The same was described by Pelinck et al. [1] when comparing minimal stimulation IVF

M. von Wolff (✉)
Division of Gynecological Endocrinology and Reproductive Medicine, University Women's Hospital, University of Bern, Bern, Switzerland
e-mail: Michael.vonwolff@insel.ch

Table 21.1 Risk factors of IVF therapy and possible therapeutic consequences to reduce health risks for IVF children

Possible risk factors	Risks for the children	Epigenetic effects	Risk reduction with NC-IVF/ minimal stimulation IVF?
Gonadotropin stimulation	Lower birth weight	Possible	Yes (as no/less gonadotropin stimulation required)
	Higher proportion of small gestational age (SGA) infants		
	Premature birth		
Fertilisation using ICSI	Increased risk of genitourinary malformations	Possible	No (ICSI is also required for NC-IVF in the case of an andrological factor)
	Poorer sperm quality in the offspring		
	Unclear whether these risks also occur with ICSI in men with normal semen analysis		
Embryo culture	Increased birth weight with transfer of vitrified 6-day versus 5-day blastocysts	Possible	Possibly (embryo culture can be shortened to 2–3 days because there is usually no embryo selection)
	Risks of prolonged embryo culture are largely unclear		
Cryopreservation and thawing of embryos	Increased birth weight	Possible	Yes (cryopreservation is usually not necessary)
	Higher proportion of large gestational age (LGA) infants		
	Premature birth		
	Increased preeclampsia in thawing cycles with hormone replacement		

with conventional IVF. Mitter et al. [5] found, compared to all Swiss singletons, lower birth weight rates in children after conventional IVF but not after NC-IVF.

A meta-analysis by Kamath et al. [6] showed overall a slightly but significantly higher probability of premature birth (RR 1.27; 95% CI: 1.03–1.58) (Table 21.3) and a low birth weight (RR 1.95; 95% CI: 1.03–3.67) (Table 21.4) after conventional IVF versus NC-IVF and minimal stimulation IVF.

The cause of the reduced birth weight and the premature births is likely to be the supraphysiological estradiol (E2) concentrations in conventional IVF. These lead to dysfunction of the endometrium and placenta. In animal models, it has been shown that high E2 concentrations have a negative effect on the invasion of the spiral arteries into the placenta [7] and lead to an oedematous endometrium with the consequence of disturbed trophoblast invasion and placentation [8].

Table 21.2 Studies comparing birth weight after NC-IVF and minimal stimulation IVF therapies with conventional IVF therapies

Study	Patients	Design	Effect
Pelinck et al. [1]	2001–2006: 158 **minimal stimulation IVF** singletons versus 161 conventional fresh transfer cycles IVF singletons	Single Centre, retrospective	Birth weight: Adjusted: +88 g
Sunkara et al. [2]	1991–2011: 262 **NC-IVF** singletons versus 98,667 conventional IVF fresh transfer cycles singletons	Registry analysis, U.K.	No differences after adjustment
Mak et al. [3]	2007–2013: 190 **NC-IVF** singletons versus 174 conventional IVF fresh transfer cycles singletons	Single Centre, retrospective	Birth weight: 3436 ± 420 g versus 3273 ± 574 g, $p < 0.05$. Risk of low birth weight <2500 g: Adjusted OR 0.07 (95% CI: 0.014–0.35)
Kohl Schwartz et al. [4]	2007–2013: 70 **NC-IVF** singletons versus 85 conventional IVF fresh transfer cycle singletons	Single Centre, retrospective	Small gestational age ($\leq$5th percentile): 2% versus 2.86%, $p < 0.05$. Significant association of birth weight with E2 concentration
Mitter et al. [5]	2010–2018: 144 **NC-IVF** singletons or 144 conventional IVF fresh transfer singletons (Bern IVF cohort) versus 633,996 singletons (Swiss live birth registry, SLBR)	Single Centre, retrospective and registry analysis, Switzerland	Conventional IVF versus SLBR: Low birth weight: aRR: 1.72, 95% CI: 1.01–2.93. Small gestational age ($\leq$5th percentile): RR 1.31, 95% CI: 1.05–2.14, aRR 1.31, 95% CI: 0.92–1.87. NC-IVF versus SLBR: No increased risks

Table 21.3 Risk of preterm birth (<37 weeks gestation) in children born after NC-IVF and minimal stimulation IVF and conventional IVF (summary of a meta-analysis [6])

Included studies	Conventional IVF: events/total, n	NC-IVF: events/total, n	Risk ratio (95% CI)	Heterogeneity, I^2
Conventional IVF versus NC-IVF				
2 studies	9296/96,724	79/450	1.32 (1.05–1.66)	0%[a]
Conventional IVF versus modified NC-IVF (= minimal stimulation IVF)				
2 studies	20/272	19/252	0.98 (0.52–1.87)	8%[a]
Overall result	9316/96,996	98/702	1.27 (1.03–1.58)	0%[a]

[a]Indicates low heterogeneity of studies (www.handbook-5-1.cochrane.org)

Pereira et al. [9] impressively confirmed the relationship between supraphysiological E2 concentrations and birth weight in 4071 patients with a singleton birth after conventional IVF. The incidence proportion of low birth weight rose from 6.4% in women with an E2 serum concentration of 2001–2500 pg/mL at the time of

Table 21.4 Risk of low birth weight (<2500 g) in children born after NC-IVF and minimal stimulation IVF and conventional IVF (summary of a meta-analysis [6])

Included studies	Conventional IVF: events/total, n	NC-IVF: events/total, n	Risk ratio (95% CI)	Heterogeneity, I^2
Conventional IVF versus NC-IVF				
2 studies	9100/96,302	19/448	2.98 (0.54–16.29)	80%[a]
Conventional IVF versus modified NC-IVF (= minimal stimulation IVF)				
2 studies	18/272	10/256	1.72 (0.81–3.65)	0%[a]
Overall result	9118/96,574	29/704	1.95 (1.03–3.67)	44%[a]

[a]Indicates moderate heterogeneity of studies (www.handbook-5-1.cochrane.org)

ovulation triggering, to 20.7% with an E2 concentration of 3501–4000 pg/mL. The odds of term low birth weight with E2 >2500 pg/mL were 6.1–7.9 times higher compared to the reference E2 group. Multivariable logistic regression analysis revealed that E2 was an independent predictor for term low birth weight, even after multiple adjustments (adjusted odds ratio 10.8, 95% CI: 9.2–12.5).

It can therefore be assumed that children born after NC-IVF or minimal stimulation IVF have a higher body weight and therefore a lower risk of small gestational age (SGA) and a lower risk of premature birth.

Since lower birth weight and preterm birth are associated with multiple health risks and multiple increases in infant mortality [10], this raises the question of whether infants after NC-IVF or minimal stimulation IVF also have a lower health risk due to their higher birth weight and lower preterm birth rate. However, this question cannot be answered. On the one hand, no data is available, and on the other hand, the health risks also depend on the cause of the reduced birth weight and the premature birth, so that the generally known risks cannot or can only partially be transferred to the IVF-induced changes. The extent of the risk factors also plays a role. Since the birth weight is only slightly changed after IVF therapy and since the preterm births are usually not very early, the effect on the health of the children is probably rather low.

Furthermore, a recent small Swiss study analysing 139 singletons [4] revealed that growth of children conceived after NC-IVF compared to gonadotropin stimulated IVF did not differ between both groups. The median birth weight in NC-IVF children was 3.4 kg (0.1 standard deviation score, SDS) and in conventional IVF 3.3 kg (−0.3 SDS) ($p = 0.53$). Median length at birth in NC-IVF was 50 cm (−0.5 SDS) and did not differ from conventional IVF children 50 cm (−0.8 SDS) ($p = 0.52$). At age 12 months, the median weight was 9.3 kg (0.0 SDS) for NC-IVF children compared to 9.0 kg (−1.7 SDS) for conventional IVF children ($p = 0.44$). Median lengths was 75 cm (0.1 SDS) in NC-IVF versus 71 cm (−1.6 SDS) in conventional IVF children ($p = 0.89$). At age 24 months, median weight in NC-IVF children was 12.3 kg (0.3 SDS) versus 10.5 kg (−1.2 SDS) in conventional IVF

($p = 0.72$) and median lengths 87.5 cm (0.1 SDS) in NC-IVF versus 87.6 cm (0.1 SDS) in conventional IVF children.

In summary, the birth weight tends to be higher and the risk of SGA and premature birth to be lower after NC-IVF or minimal IVF stimulation compared to conventional IVF. However, it is unclear whether this is associated with better children's health.

21.3   Birth Weight and Risk of Preterm Birth After Thawing Cycles

Birth weight is increased after a thawing cycle (see Chap. 20). A meta-analysis by Elias et al. [11] showed an increased risk of preterm birth (pooled ORs 1.39; 95% CI: 1.34–1.44) (Table 21.5) and large gestational age (LGA) (pooled OR 1.57; 95% CI: 1.48–1.68) in singletons after a thawing cycle (Table 21.6).

Since embryos are not usually cryopreserved after NC-IVF or minimal stimulation IVF and therefore no thawing cycles are carried out, this health risk does not apply to most NC-IVF or minimal stimulation IVF treatments.

Some centres cryopreserve embryos after NC-IVF or minimal stimulation IVF for later transfer. However, it needs to be questioned if the systematic performance of prolonged embryo culture and the cryopreservation of blastocysts contradicts the philosophy of natural cycle IVF to minimise IVF risks (see Chap. 2).

In summary, birth weight and thus the risk of LGA and preterm birth are increased after thawing cycles. However, it is still unclear whether this is associated with the health of the children.

Table 21.5 Risk of preterm birth (<37 weeks gestation) in children born after thawing cycles versus spontaneous conceptions (summary of a meta-analysis [11])

Included studies	Thawing cycles: events/total, n	Spontaneous conceptions: events/total, n	Odds ratio (95% CI)	Heterogeneity, I^2
6 studies, overall result	3245/39,054	190,585/3,120,303	1.39 (1.34–1.44)	0%[a]

[a]Indicates very low heterogeneity of studies (www.handbook-5-1.cochrane.org)

Table 21.6 Risk of large gestational age (LGA) in children born after thawing cycles versus spontaneous conceptions (summary of a meta-analysis [11])

Included studies	Thawing cycles: events/total, n	Spontaneous conceptions: events/total, n	Odds ratio (95% CI)	Heterogeneity, I^2
5 studies, overall result	4545/38,097	244,343/3,114,503	1.57 (1.48–1.68)	22%[a]

[a]Indicates low heterogeneity of studies (www.handbook-5-1.cochrane.org)

21.4   Effects of Embryo Culture

If only one embryo develops after fertilisation of the oocytes, it can be transferred after 2–3 days. This avoids a 5–6 day embryo culture, which could lead to epigenetic modifications (see Chap. 20). The neonatal outcome after day 2/3 and day 5/6 transfer has been investigated in several studies. However, the overall data situation is controversial, which is explained in particular by the low study quality or the small patient populations studied [12].

The situation is clearer when comparing previously vitrified day 5 and day 6 embryos. Zeng et al. [13] included eight retrospective studies in a meta-analysis. Compared with vitrified-warmed day 5 blastocyst transfer, vitrified-warmed day 6 blastocyst transfer was associated with increased birth weight (weight mean difference −80.39 g; 95% CI: −151.8 to −8.97). Thus, a greatly prolonged embryo culture appears to have an effect on the embryos. According to the discussion in the Chap. 20, a prolonged embryo culture could have epigenetic effects on the embryos. Ultimately, however, it cannot be ruled out that other embryonic factors that lead to delayed blastocyst development and thus to day 6 transfer are the cause.

In summary, a negative health effect of prolonged embryo culture has not yet been proven. Nevertheless, it must be noted that prolonged embryo culture takes place during the sensitive phases of post-zygotic germline reprogramming.

21.5   Effects of Fertilisation Using ICSI

In the Chap. 20 it was shown that the risk of genitourinary malformations is increased (OR 1.27; 95% CI: 1.02–1.59) [14]. However, it was also shown that if only studies with a low risk of bias were analysed, there was still a trend towards an increased risk of genitourinary malformations, but the difference was no longer statistically significant (OR: 1.28; 95% CI: 1.00–1.64).

Belva et al. [15] studied for the first time the sperm quality of the 18–22 year old sons of couples who had undergone ICSI, and found that their sperm quality was significantly reduced.

Thus, there seems to be an association of ICSI with genitourinary malformations and sperm quality.

In summary, ICSI is associated with an increased risk of genitourinary malformations and poorer semen analyses. Although it is unclear whether these malformations and other ICSI-associated functional changes may only occur in fathers with poor sperm quality [16], fertilisation via ICSI with normal semen analyses should be avoided due to the insufficient data.

References

1. Pelinck MJ, Keizer MH, Hoek A, Simons AH, Schelling K, Middelburg K, Heineman MJ. Perinatal outcome in singletons after modified natural cycle IVF and standard IVF with ovarian stimulation. Eur J Obstet Gynecol Reprod Biol. 2010;148:56–61.
2. Sunkara SK, LaMarca A, Polyzos NP, Seed PT, Khalaf Y. Live birth and perinatal outcomes following stimulated and unstimulated IVF: analysis of over two decades of a nationwide data. Hum Reprod. 2016;31:2261–7.
3. Mak W, Kondapalli LA, Celia G, Gordon J, DiMattina M, Payson M. Natural cycle IVF reduces the risk of low birthweight infants compared with conventional stimulated IVF. Hum Reprod. 2016;31:789–94.
4. Kohl Schwartz AS, Mitter VR, Amylidi-Mohr S, Fasel P, Minger MA, Limoni C, Zwahlen M, von Wolff M. The greater incidence of small-for-gestational-age newborns after gonadotropin-stimulated in vitro fertilization with a supraphysiological estradiol level on ovulation trigger day. Acta Obstet Gynecol Scand. 2019;98:1575–84.
5. Mitter VR, Fasel P, Berlin C, Amylidi-Mohr S, Mosimann B, Zwahlen M, von Wolff M, Kohl Schwartz AS. Perinatal outcomes in singletons after IVF/(ICSI - results of two cohorts and the birth registry. Reprod Biomed online. 2022;44:689–98.
6. Kamath MS, Kirubakaran R, Mascarenhas M, Sunkara SK. Perinatal outcomes after stimulated versus natural cycle IVF: a systematic review and meta-analysis. Reprod Biomed Online. 2018;36:94–101.
7. Bonagura TW, Pepe GJ, Enders AC, Albrecht ED. Suppression of extravillous trophoblast vascular endothelial growth factor expression and uterine spiral artery invasion by estrogen during early baboon pregnancy. Endocrinology. 2008;149:5078–87.
8. Mainigi MA, Olalere D, Burd I, Sapienza C, Bartolomei M, Coutifaris C. Peri-implantation hormonal milieu: elucidating mechanisms of abnormal placentation and fetal growth. Biol Reprod. 2014;90:26.
9. Pereira N, Elias RT, Christos PJ, Petrini AC, Hancock K, Lekovich JP, Rosenwaks Z. Supraphysiologic estradiol is an independent predictor of low birth weight in full-term singletons born after fresh embryo transfer. Hum Reprod. 2017;32:1410–7.
10. Mathews TJ, MacDorman MF. Infant mortality statistics from the 2004 period linked birth/infant death data set. Natl Vital Stat Rep. 2007;55:1–32.
11. Elias FTS, Weber-Adrian D, Pudwell J, Carter J, Walker M, Gaudet L, Smith G, Velez MP. Neonatal outcomes in singleton pregnancies conceived by fresh or frozen embryo transfer compared to spontaneous conceptions: a systematic review and meta-analysis. Arch Gynecol Obstet. 2020;302:31–45.
12. De Vos A, Santos-Ribeiro S, Van Landuyt L, Van de Velde H, Tournaye H, Verheyen G. Birthweight of singletons born after cleavage-stage or blastocyst transfer in fresh and warming cycles. Hum Reprod. 2018;33:196–201.
13. Zeng M, Su Qin S, Wen P, Xu C, Duan J. Perinatal outcomes after vitrified-warmed day 5 blastocyst transfers compared to vitrified-warmed day 6 blastocyst transfers: a meta analysis. Eur J Obstet Gynecol Reprod Biol. 2020;247:219–24.
14. Massaro PA, MacLellan DL, Anderson PA, Romao RL. Does intracytoplasmic sperm injection pose an increased risk of genitourinary congenital malformations in offspring compared to in vitro fertilization? A systematic review and meta-analysis. J Urol. 2015;193(5 Suppl):1837–42.
15. Belva F, Bonduelle M, Roelants M, Michielsen D, Van Steirteghem A, Verheyen G, Tournaye H. Semen quality of young adult ICSI offspring: the first results. Hum Reprod. 2016;31:2811–20.
16. Rumbold AR, Sevoyan A, Oswald TK, Fernandez RC, Davies MJ, Moore VM. Impact of male factor infertility on offspring health and development. Fertil Steril. 2019;111:1047–53.

Chapter 22
Asthma and Breastfeeding After IVF

Michael von Wolff

22.1 Background

IVF therapies are associated with an increased risk of malformations and premature births. The risk of childhood asthma is also increased. The health risks can be countered by preventive measures. One measure is breastfeeding for a long enough period, especially for the prevention of asthma.

22.2 Asthma in Children Born After IVF

In addition to the risks of malformations and functional changes clearly demonstrated in meta-analyses (see Chaps. 20 and 21), there are several studies that also indicate an increased risk of asthma in children.

- In the UK, data from 104 IVF children in the Millennium Cohort Study was studied at the age of 5 years. The incidence of asthma, wheezing within the last year and taking anti-asthmatics in these children was compared with children after a planned pregnancy without infertility therapy with a time to conception <12 months. The risk of asthma, wheezing and taking anti-asthmatics was significantly higher (aOR: 2.65, 95% CI: 1.48–4.76; OR: 1.97 95% CI: 1.10–3.53; OR: 4.67 95% CI: 2.20–9.94, respectively). The absolute risk of asthma increased from 13.2 to 23.7%, for wheezing from 14.3 to 22.4% and for taking anti-asthmatics from 3.2 to 11.8% [1].

M. von Wolff (✉)
Division of Gynecological Endocrinology and Reproductive Medicine, University Women's Hospital, University of Bern, Bern, Switzerland
e-mail: Michael.vonwolff@insel.ch

- In Sweden, registry data from 31,918 IVF children with asthma born 1982–2007 were studied up to 2009. An increased risk of asthma was found in children conceived by IVF (aOR 1.28, 95% CI: 1.23–1.34), increasing the absolute risk from 4.4 to 5.6%. The risk increase for asthma was the same in boys and girls, in singletons and twins, and after caesarean section and vaginal delivery. The risk was higher for preterm than term singletons [2].
- In the Netherlands, 213 IVF children from the Groningen assisted reproductive techniques (ART) cohort study and the preimplantation genetic screening (PGS) trial were studied at the age of 4 years, including three groups of children born following conventional IVF ($n = 81$), natural cycle IVF (NC-IVF) ($n = 53$) and spontaneous conception in subfertile couples ($n = 79$). The rate of asthma medication use was higher in the conventional IVF than in the spontaneous conception group (aOR: 1.96, 95% CI: 1.00–3.84). The absolute proportion of children diagnosed asthma was 15% for conventional IVF, 11% for NC-IVF and 8% for spontaneous conceptions. The corresponding numbers for taking anti-asthmatic drugs were 14, 9 and 5% [3].
- In Norway, registry data from 8368 IVF children in the Norwegian birth registries and 1391 IVF children in the Norwegian Mother and Child Cohort Study were studied at the age of 8 years. IVF children had greater risk of asthma in the birth registry (aRR 1.20; 95% CI: 1.09–1.32) and in the prescription database (aRR 1.42; 95% CI: 1.14–1.76). A sibling analysis yielded similar associations, but the results were not significant [4].

The studies show a generally increased risk of asthma in children born after IVF. This raises the question of whether the increased risk is maternal, paternal or a consequence of the IVF treatment itself (see Chap. 20). The question also arises of whether the risk after NC-IVF is lower than after conventional IVF, as the study from the Netherlands described above suggests.

The above-mentioned Dutch IVF cohort [3] was therefore followed up with regard to possible causes of the increased risk of asthmatic diseases [5]. A validated Dutch version of an asthma questionnaire was used in the follow-up study, which was conducted on children aged 9 years (preliminary study: 4 years). Due to the older age, the authors interpreted the follow-up study as more valid. The questionnaire was filled out by the parents of the children conceived with conventional IVF ($n = 95$), with NC-IVF ($n = 48$) and spontaneously. Asthma prevalence in the groups did not differ: Adjustment for confounders did not alter the results. Accordingly, neither ovarian stimulation nor the in vitro culture procedure was associated with asthma and rhinitis. It needs to be noted that the groups of children were very small [5].

In summary, children born after IVF treatment seem to have a higher risk of asthmatic diseases in childhood. However, it is not known if the increased risk persists in adulthood, nor is it known if the risk is lower with NC-IVF.

Table 22.1 Risk of wheeze/asthma at the age of 5–18 years after more versus less breastfeeding (summary of a meta-analysis [6])

Included studies	Odds ratio (95% CI)	Heterogeneity, I^2
13 cohort studies	0.94 (0.80,1.11)	77.0% ($p = 0.000$)[a]
14 cross-sectional studies	0.93 (0.87–0.99)	25.9% ($p = 0.175$)[a]
2 case-control studies	0.68 (0.50–0.91)	0.0% ($p = 0.381$)[a]
Overall result	0.90 (0.84–0.97)	62.9% ($p = 0.000$)[a]

[a]Indicates substantial and highly significant heterogeneity of studies (www.handbook-5-1.cochrane.org)

22.3 Breastfeeding to Reduce the Risk of Asthma

Breast milk is an immunologically complex solution, facilitating development of the infant's immune system. It contains bioactive components such as secretory IgA and IgG which have an effect on passive immunity and factors that actively stimulate the immune system. Accordingly, breast milk can be assumed to have a protective effect against the development of allergic diseases which are increasingly found worldwide and also in children born after IVF treatments.

Indeed, most but not all studies found a protective effect of breastfeeding on allergic diseases. A very large meta-analysis confirmed such an effect. In this meta-analysis, asthma was defined as physician-diagnosed asthma, parent or self-reported asthma or wheeze, spirometrically diagnosed asthma or asthma recorded on health-related databases. A meta-analysis [6] revealed a positive association of longer breastfeeding duration with reduced risk of asthma for children at the age of 5–18 years (Table 22.1). This was particularly found in medium-/low-income countries. A weak association was also found between breastfeeding and eczema ≤2 years, and allergic rhinitis ≤5 years of age.

In summary, breastfeeding has some protective effect on the development of asthmatic diseases in childhood.

22.4 Breastfeeding in Children Born After Infertility Treatments and IVF

Several studies on breastfeeding following infertility treatment have been published.

- An Australian prospective cohort study with 183 women who gave birth in 2001 showed lower percentages of women breastfeeding at 6 weeks and 8 months in the ART group [7].
- A US cohort study with 1361 women who gave birth in 2008–2010 found that mothers who had undergone fertility treatments were more likely to cease breastfeeding before the 12th month after birth. The study was adjusted for confounders such as preterm birth but not for twins [8].

- An Italian retrospective case-control study with 188 women who gave birth in 2010–2013 found that a lower percentage of women after fertility treatment were breastfeeding at 6 weeks postpartum compared to women after spontaneous conception, but at 6 months postpartum breastfeeding rates no longer differed [9].
- Another US cross-sectional study of 1056 women who gave birth in 2012–2015 reported lower odds of breastfeeding at 8 weeks postpartum among women who conceived through infertility treatments, but this difference was no longer significant after adjustment for multiples and preterm birth [10].
- A Chinese prospective cohort study with 935 women who gave birth in 2015 found lower breastfeeding rates at 6 months postpartum in the infertility treatment group compared to a spontaneous conception group, but similar breastfeeding rates at 12 months postpartum. The study was adjusted for confounding factors such as maternal BMI or infant's birthweight [11].

None of the studies described an increased breastfeeding rate after infertility treatment. Most studies even found lower breastfeeding rates.

These studies grouped all kind of infertility treatments without specifically addressing children after IVF treatment. A recent study therefore specifically addressed children after IVF treatments:

- A Swiss study with 198 women who gave birth in 2010–2016 specifically addressed children conceived after IVF treatments and performed multiple adjustments [12]. Furthermore, a comparison between conventional and NC-IVF was made. The IVF children were compared with a representative registry-based Swiss population. This population also included children after IVF treatments, which account for around 2.5% of all Swiss children. The study did not find a difference between IVF treatments and the general population (Fig. 22.1). Furthermore, no difference was found between conventional and NC-IVF treatments (Fig. 22.2).

In summary, breastfeeding habits do not seem to be different in women who conceived after different IVF treatments.

This is contrast to the increased risk of asthmatic diseases in children conceived by IVF. Mothers should therefore be encouraged to breastfeed their IVF children for a sufficient period of time.

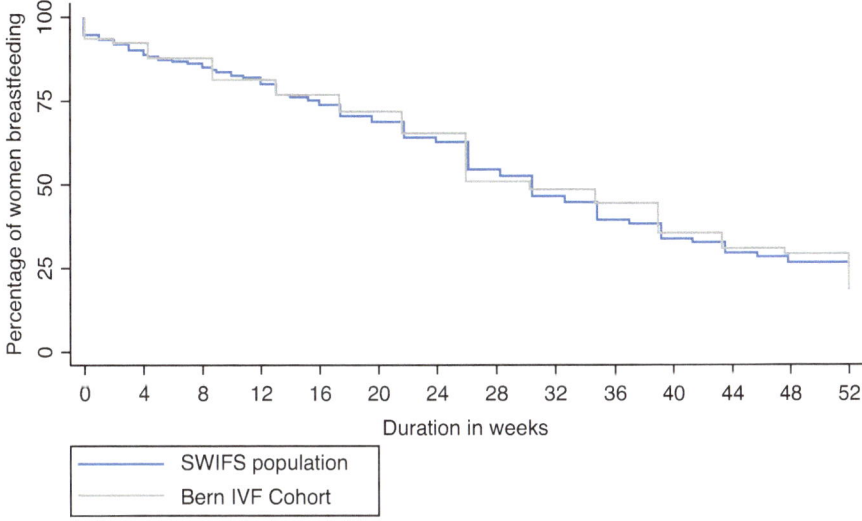

Fig. 22.1 Kaplan–Meier estimates of women breastfeeding in women after all kind of IVF treatments (Bern IVF cohort) compared to a representative Swiss population (SWIFS population) (adapted according to [12])

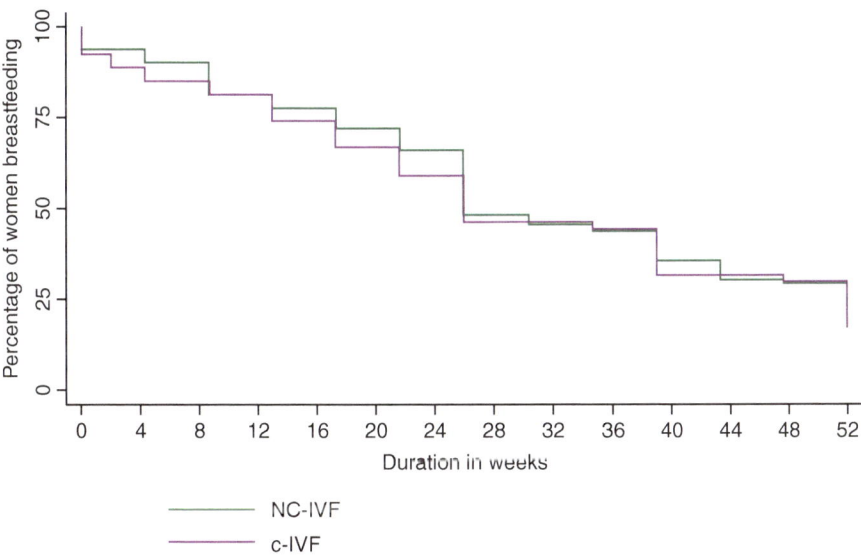

Fig. 22.2 Kaplan–Meier estimates of women breastfeeding after natural cycle IVF (NC-IVF) treatments compared to women after conventional gonadotropin stimulated IVF (c-IVF) (kindly provided by V. Mitter and according to [12])

References

1. Carson C, Sacker A, Kelly Y, Redshaw M, Kurinczuk JJ, Quigley MA. Asthma in children born after infertility treatment: findings from the UK Millennium Cohort Study. Hum Reprod. 2013;28:471–9.
2. Källén B, Finnström O, Nygren KG, Olausson PO. Asthma in Swedish children conceived by in vitro fertilization. Arch Dis Child. 2013;98:92–6.
3. Kuiper DB, Seggers J, Schendelaar P, Haadsma ML, Roseboom TJ, Heineman MJ, Hadders-Algra M. Asthma and asthma medication use among 4-year-old offspring of subfertile couples–association with IVF? Reprod Biomed Online. 2015;21:711–4.
4. Magnus MC, Karlstad Ø, Parr CL, Page CM, Nafstad P, Magnus P, London SJ, Wilcox AJ, Nystad W, Håberg SE. Maternal history of miscarriages and measures of fertility in relation to childhood asthma. Thorax. 2019;74:106–13.
5. Kuiper DB, Koppelman GH, la Bastide-van GS, Seggers J, Haadsma ML, Roseboom TJ, Hoek A, Heineman MJ, Hadders-Algra M. Asthma in 9-year-old children of subfertile couples is not associated with in vitro fertilization procedures. Eur J Pediatr. 2019;178:1493–9.
6. Lodge CJ, Tan DJ, Lau MX, Dai X, Tham R, Lowe AJ, Bowatte G, Allen KJ, Dharmage SC. Breastfeeding and asthma and allergies: a systematic review and meta-analysis. Acta Paediatr. 2015;104:38–53.
7. Hammarberg K, Fisher JRW, Wynter KH, Rowe HJ. Breastfeeding after assisted conception: a prospective cohort study. Acta Paediatr. 1992;2011(100):529–33.
8. Michels KA, Mumford SL, Sundaram R, Bell EM, Bello SC, Yeung EH. Differences in infant feeding practices by mode of conception in a United States cohort. Fertil Steril. 2016;105:1014–1022.e1.
9. Cromi A, Serati M, Candeloro I, Uccella S, Scandroglio S, Agosti M, Ghezzi F. Assisted reproductive technology and breastfeeding outcomes: a case-control study. Fertil Steril. 2015;103:89–94.
10. Barrera CM, Kawwass JF, Boulet SL, Nelson JM, Perrine CG. Fertility treatment use and breastfeeding outcomes. Am J Obstet Gynecol. 2019;220:261.e1–7.
11. Sha T, Yan Y, Gao X, Liu S, Chen C, Li L, He Q. Association of assisted reproductive techniques with infant feeding practices: a community-based study in China. Breastfeed Med. 2019;14:654–61.
12. Purtschert LA, Mitter VR, Zdanowicz JA, Minger MA, Spaeth A, von Wolff M, Kohl Schwartz AS. Breastfeeding following in vitro fertilisation in Switzerland - does mode of conception affect breastfeeding behaviour? Acta Paediatr. 2021;110:1171–80.

Part VI
Miscellaneous

Chapter 23
Biopsychosocial Aspects of Natural Cycle IVF/Minimal Stimulation IVF

Annemarie Schweizer-Arau

23.1 Background

Infertility can become a great psychological burden and strain on partnership for couples, comparable to other severe illnesses [1]. Feelings of loss of control, anxiety, and depression are reported worldwide from a majority of couples undergoing Artificial Reproductive Techniques (ART) especially after failed treatment.

For a long time, most publications regarded infertility simply as an organic issue and reported success only by biochemical pregnancy rates/cycle or "Time to pregnancy" (TTP) (see Chap. 19 for detail). The increasing trend to report ART outcomes in terms of cumulative live birth rates (CLBR)/patient has highlighted the importance of dropouts and the direct correlation between felt stress during ART treatment and discontinuing treatment [2].

23.2 Dropout Rates in IVF Therapies

Dropout rates can be regarded as an adverse outcome of infertility treatment, as they lower the chances of cumulative success rates [3]. High dropout rates are even made responsible for the huge discrepancy between real observed cumulative live birth rates (CLBR) per patient and estimated cumulative pregnancies and deliveries per woman [4] (Fig. 23.1).

According to a retrospective German study 39.9% of couples discontinued treatment after their first cIVF cycle and 62% by the fourth IVF-cycle, and therefore instead of expected 53.3% only 31.2% couples became pregnant after four cIVF

A. Schweizer-Arau (✉)
Insula-Institut, Hannover, Germany
e-mail: a.schweizer-arau@insula-institut.org

227
M. von Wolff (ed.), *Natural Cycle and Minimal Stimulation IVF*,
https://doi.org/10.1007/978-3-030-97571-5_23

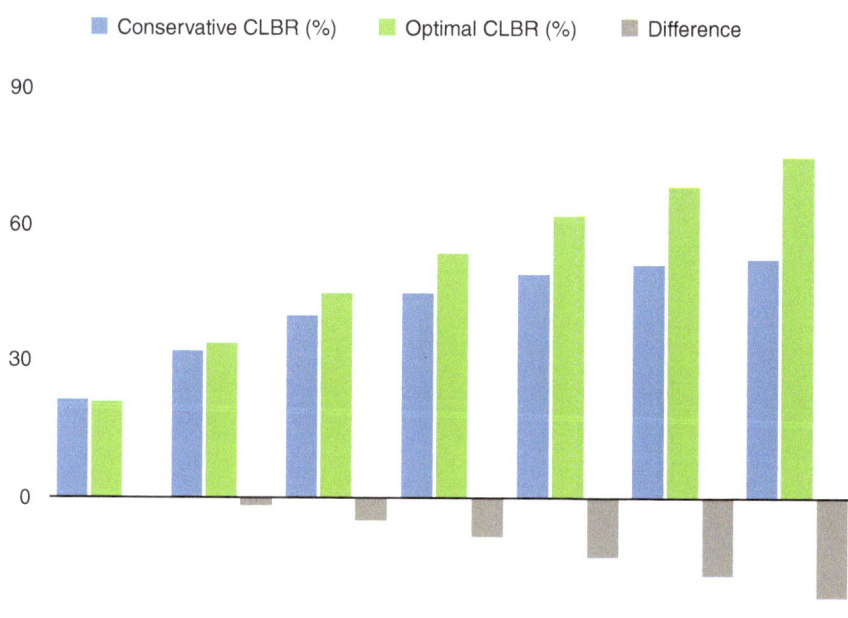

Fig. 23.1 Data obtained from the Belgian IVF Registry. The figure shows the conservative (blue) and optimal estimates of CLBRs (green) after six fresh and thawing transfer cycles. CLBRs of conservative estimate of CLBR (blue) after six fresh and thawing transfer cycles reach a level of 54.1% and would be 76.3% according to the optimal estimated (green). The negative columns (gray) show the difference CLBRs after six cycles. All CLBRs decrease with increasing age for both conservative (62.2% <35 years to 17,7% for women 41–42 years of age) and optimal estimates (85.63% <35 years, 6.4% for women 41–42 years of age). Due to dropouts, there is an increasing difference between conservative and optimal estimated CLBRs reaching more than 20% after six fresh and attached frozen-thawed embryo transfer cycles. Conditional LBR decline from 29% after the first, to 24.8% after the second, 21.8% after the third, 20.7% after the fourth, to 17.6% after the fifth to 12.5% after the sixth cycle (modified according to [5])

cycles [6]. This data corresponds to most publications reporting dropout rates well above 50% [2].

To be able to show impressive probabilities of cumulative clinical live birth rates (CLBR) 89%, statistical methods like the Kaplan–Meier method (see Chap. 19, Fig. 19.5) are used to consult patients. These extrapolations try to reduce the complex biopsychosocial mind-body system to one variable (the number of transferred embryos per cycles or started cycles and to circumvent the issue of dropout rates) (Table 23.1).

As primary reason for discontinuing cIVF treatment, 28–40% of couples cite the physical and psychological distress [7]. Beside anxiety and depressive mood changes, the short- and long-term side effects of hyperstimulation, anesthesia, and possible epigenetic effects on the offsprings are predominant [3].

Table 23.1 Expected CLBR/patient and real observed (CLBR) per patient after more than four cIVF treatment cycles

Study	Patients n	Number of started cycles or transferred embryos (n)	Estimated CLBR/ patient %	Real CLBR/ patient %
Olivius et al. [8]	974	4 started cycles	65.5	53.9
Witsenburg et al. [9]	750	5 started cycles	80.5	59.3[a]
Elizur et al. [10]	1928	14 started cycles	87	35.7
Malizia et al. [11]	6164	6 started cycles	72	50.7
Garrido et al. [12]	11,429	8 transferred embryos	70.0	45.7
Luke et al. [4][a]	246,740	7 started cycles	89.9	57[a]
Smith et al. [13]	156,947	9 started cycles	87.5	44.7
McLernon et al. [14]	107,347	8 started cycles	82.4	43.9

[a]Data including donor egg cycles

A systematic review from 2012 including 22 studies with a total of 21,453 patients from eight countries [15] (Fig. 23.1) found as the most common reasons for discontinuation of IVF treatment to be:

- postponement of treatment or unknown reason (39.2%),
- psychological burden (14.0%),
- physical burden (6.3%),
- relational and personal problems (16.7%),
- treatment rejection (13.2%).

Dropout rates can be seen as a marker for the quality of IVF therapy and can be used to calculate CLBR and cost-effectiveness of IVF treatment [2].

23.3 Treatment Stress Related to IVF Therapies

One huge advantage of NC-IVF or mild stimulation strategies IVF is a patient friendly approach with reduced treatment-related stress in comparison to conventional cIVF therapies with high doses of gonadotropins. Women that have experience with both methods describe the NC-IVF often with words like "incomparably smooth," "mild and soft," "less disturbing to the inner balance," "far easier to be integrated in daily life." Other patients express regret: "If I had known that there is the possibility to do IVF in a natural cycle, I would not have hesitated so long to do an IVF."

The results of the few studies comparing dropout rates of milder therapy strategies with single embryo transfer and cIVF are consistent with these statements, emphasizing an association between lower dropout rates in mild treatment groups compared with the conventional IVF groups (OR 0.53; 95% CI, 0.28–0.98) due to less stress [2].

Haemmerli Keller et al. [16] reported that even three NC-IVF cycles are felt significantly less stressful than one single cIVF cycle. This study compared psychological distress and treatment-related satisfaction and quality of life, using validated psychological questionnaires, before and NC-IVF and cIVF treatments (Table 23.2). To avoid different pregnancy rates in the two treatment groups, one cIVF was compared with three NC-IVF therapies, resulting in the same cumulative pregnancy rate. NC-IVF patients had a significantly lower level of depression (CES-D, 13.4 vs. 15.7, $p < 0.05$) and a higher degree of satisfaction with the treatment (Treatment FertiQoL, 67.9 vs. 62.9, $p < 0.05$) compared with cIVF patients. The level of psychological distress increased during cIVF treatment and decreased during NC-IVF treatment. In contrast, during NC-IVF treatment, there was a significant increase in satisfaction with the treatment, whereas satisfaction with treatment in the cIVF patients was decreased.

It has been controversial for many years whether treatment-related stress and stress reactions due to cIVF treatment have a negative impact on success rates or if high levels of preexisting anxiety and depression influence the outcome, failure und dropout. Studies which implemented structured psychiatric interviews found depression and anxiety in 40% of infertile women [17]. Later studies from Denmark and Sweden confirmed this data [18].

In the course of infertility treatment, each new failure can trigger individual vulnerability of the couple and augment distress leading to the termination of treatment [15, 19].

Failures can trigger negative emotions, rooting in deep, unconscious negative life-events as studies in patients suffering from endometriosis, chronic pelvic pain or

Table 23.2 Test scores of validated psychological tests after up to three cycles of natural cycle IVF (NC-IVF) or one cycle of conventional IVF (cIVF) treatment (modified according to [16])

Skala	NC-IVF		cIVF	
	Mean	SD	Mean	SD
BSI	0.43	0.46	0.41	0.35
BSI depression	0.74	0.87	0.72	0.71
BSI obsession	0.61	0.64	0.51	0.48
CES-D	13.4*	10.9	15.7*	7.9
Total FertiQol	68.1	14.5	68.5	11.0
Core FertiQol	68.1	16.9	70.9	13.5
Treatment FertiQol	67.9*	13.8	62.9*	12.8
IDS	20.4	6.7	21.7	6.2
WHO Qol brief	71.1*	17.8	77.3*	15.0

BSI Brief symptom inventory, *CES-D* Centre for Epidemiologic Studies Depression Score, *FertiQol* Fertility Quality of Life Questionnaire, *GSI* Global Severity Index, *IDS* Infertility Distress Scale, *WHOQuol* World health Organization Quality of Life
*Significant difference $p \leq 0.05$

post-miscarriage have demonstrated [20–22]. Early adverse childhood experiences of failure, neglect, and abuse on the other hand stimulate anxiety and negative expectations regarding pregnancy and delivery, functioning like a self-fulfilling prophecy.

But, nevertheless, patients should not be blamed for not being favorable (having anxiety or depression) as in the conclusion of the renowned study of Luke et al. 2004 in New England: "*Our results indicate that live-birth rates approaching natural fecundity can be achieved by means of assisted reproductive technology when there are favorable patient and embryo characteristics*" [4].

Awareness of the preexisting stress of infertility patients should lead one to focus on stress reduction before, during, and after IVF, and to less demanding, mild IVF approaches. Furthermore: The popular habit of presenting impressive figures of pregnancy rates/cycle or *Time to pregnancy* should be disposed of as it is a well-known fact that 67% of cIVF cycles do not result in a live birth of a healthy baby [23]. Real CLBR per patient are certainly more realistic and do not exploit the pressure and illusions of patients yearning to become pregnant as quickly as possible, especially as success rates in cIVF and minimal stimulation IVF in defined groups of patients are comparable [24].

Success of IVF treatment must also take into account the impact of quality of life of the less fortunate couples. These couples should not be left with feelings of defeat, blame, and guilt. Follow-up studies investigating the aftermath of unsuccessful infertility treatments found that for couples, failed fertility treatments usually bring on intense feelings of failure, guilt, and shame with prolonged grief reactions [25–29], suicide risk [30], and lasting depression and anxiety for longer than 20 years [31].

23.4 Reduction of Treatment Stress by NC-IVF or Minimal Stimulation IVF Treatments

As patients describe their experience with NC-IVF normally as less stressful, there are different components that contribute to this impression. Some women find it pleasant to skip daily injections, others are relieved that they do not need anesthesia during follicle puncture. Other women find NC-IVF more in accordance with their own personal beliefs, others appreciate that processes like follicle development are not disturbed by high doses of hormones. Many patients report that their inner balance remains stable during a NC-IVF cycle without great mood changes, irritability, and weight gain. There is no need for anxiety to develop an ovarian hyperstimulation syndrome (OHSS) and or twin pregnancy with a risk for preterm delivery resulting in low birth weight or very preterm delivery (<32 weeks) and very low birth weight (<2500 g) [32]. In the course of several attempts, women improve their understanding of their inner physiological processes and are able to predict their ovulation. If feelings of anxiety and frustration do arise, one will normally find that they root in earlier experiences and can be treated by an integrated holistic treatment (Table 23.3).

Table 23.3 Direct comparison of risks, outcomes, and treatment stress factors in NC-IVF and cIVF

Burden	NC-IVF	cIVF
Costs of stimulation medication	Low	High
Daily hormonal injections	No	Yes
Risk of ovarian hyperstimulation syndrome	No	Yes
Side effects of stimulation	No	Often
Mood changes	Rarely	Often
Follicle aspiration under anesthesia	No	Mostly
Embryo selection	No	Yes
Freezing of remaining embryos	Not necessary	Often
Risk of low birth weight	Low	High
Cumulative live birth rate (CLBR)	Comparable	Comparable

23.5 Holistic Infertility Treatments

Modern organic minded attitude favors, beside NC-IVF-therapy, integrative holistic treatment approaches (see Foreword) of complementary and alternative medicine (CAM). Up to 47% of couples worldwide are trying to improve their chances of achieving parenthood through CAM [33–37].

The number of investigations regarding the effect of acupuncture—without doubt the most popular CAM modality—has become almost unsurveyable [33, 38, 39], with more than a thousand randomized controlled trials [40], but with inconclusive and contradictory results regarding the effects on infertility. Most of these trials were not based on tradition Chinese medicine (TCM) pattern diagnosis and had no individual holistic treatment approach, rather standardized needle applications. Meta-analyses [41–43] of controlled randomized CAM trials therefore have come to contradicting conclusions; some found no statistically significant pooled benefits with few sessions of fixed acupuncture adjuvant to cIVF. The efficiency and effect of CAM procedure on NC-IVF have rarely been investigated.

Holistic treatment approaches can prepare or accompany woman in NC-IVF cycles, especially for pain symptoms and menstrual irregularity, depression, and anxiety [44, 45]. Regarding the preexisting emotional imbalances of infertile patients, it seems recommended to support patients individually during their NC-IVF treatments with every kind of stress reduction and well-being promoting interventions. Some studies pinpointed benefit on women's psychological state after acupuncture through increased relaxation, reduced psychological stress, and enhanced well-being and self-efficacy [46, 47], some also with significant effects on pregnancy rates [48] and CLBR [49]. A meta-analysis suggested that the probability of achieving a pregnancy with Chinese herbal medicine (CHM) is 1.74 higher than with Western therapy alone [50]. There is a proof that treatment independent CLBRs of 10–24% are reported in long-term follow-ups of unsuccessful ART, suggesting a fertility enhancing effect of stress reduction after treatment discontinuation [7, 51–53].

23.6   Neurophysiology of Stress and Infertility

The potential impact of psychological stress factors and stress reducing interventions on infertility treatment outcome was usually seen as a controversial topic [54] with conflicting study results [55]. The main goal of stress response is to maintain homeostasis in real or perceived stress [56]. Compelling new evidence of animal models indicates that stress-induced levels of glucocorticoids result in profound reproductive dysfunction with the molecular mechanisms still to be fully understood [57].

The different effects of stress on the biopsychosocial body system are shown in Fig. 23.2.

As shown besides cortisol, alpha-amylase, cytokines, prolactin, and inflammation mediators are secreted as stress response [58]. In one prospective study, high alpha-amylase levels, a potent biomarker of sympathetic stress, were correlated with an 29% increase of infertility and Time to Pregnancy but not cortisol levels [59]. Even during pregnancy, IVF mothers expressed different stress markers and anxiety levels than natural conception mothers. IVF mothers had in one study higher cortisol levels with a sharp prepartum decrease ($P = 0.059$, $\Delta\log(\text{cortisol}) = -0.94$), and no sharp prepartum alpha-amylase level decreases as after natural conception [60]. These results show the complex stress reactions at different times of treatment and pregnancy and may even indicate an increased risk in the fetal neurodevelopment. Other studies showed that successful ART treatments are associated with significantly lower levels of stress hormones like adrenaline at the time of oocyte retrieval and ET (embryo transfer) and lower levels of noradrenaline at the time of ET [61–64].

Therefore, it cannot be concluded that maternal stress does not affect IVF outcome negatively as previous studies have wanted to derive by using only stress biomarkers of the hypothalamus–pituitary–adrenal (HPA) axis as salivary cortisol level and not using markers of the sympathetic stress reaction as alpha-amylase, adrenaline or noradrenaline levels [65].

23.7   Impact of Biopsychosocial Interventions

The neurophysiological mechanisms by which psychological interventions may work were examined in a recent review [66], concluding that the application of these techniques was associated with a reduction of stress biomarkers and that, hypothetically, these interventions may thereby attenuate the stress-induced effects on IVF outcomes.

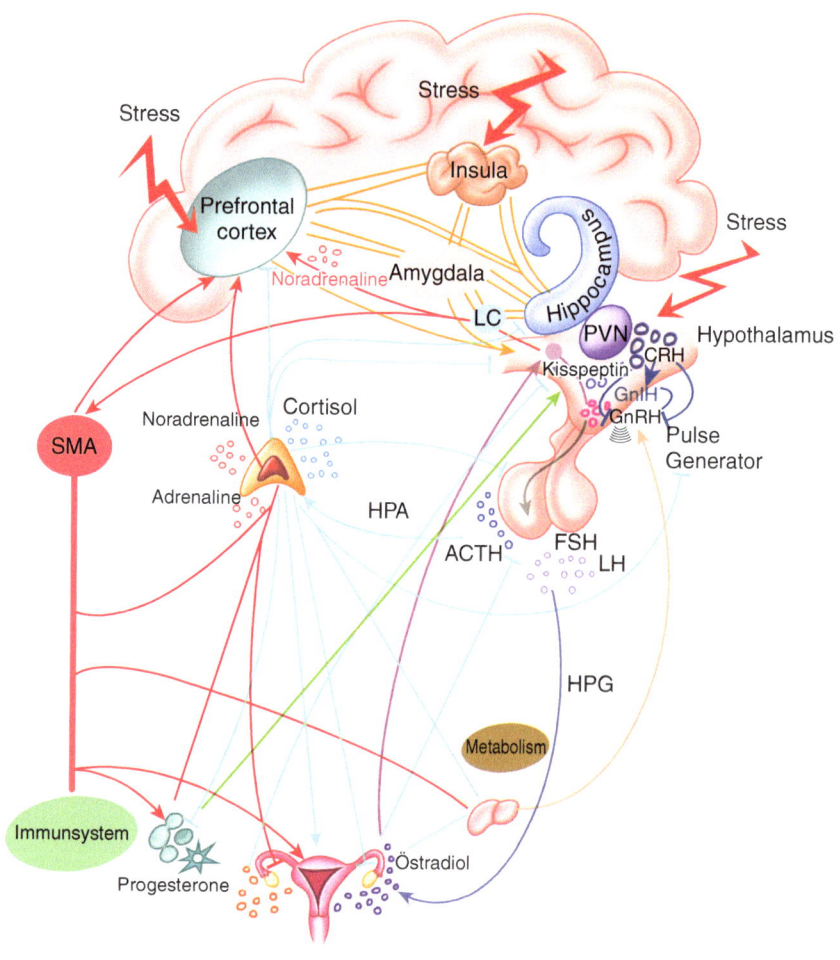

inhibitory ▲ and stimulating ← pathways, ⚡ stress, PVN =Paraventricular Nucleus, LH= Luteinizing Hormone,
FSH=Follicle Stimulating Hormone, red Sympathetic Nervous System SNS (Adrenaline, Noradrenaline), blue HPA (CRH,
Cortisol) purple reproductive circuits , green immune function,   central brain circuits. (drawing A.Schweizer-Arau))

Fig. 23.2 Schematic model for stress-induced modulation of reproductive function. The hypothalamus receives stress signals from different brain areas that influence the hypothalamic pituitary
adrenal axis (HPA) and sympatho-adrenomedullary activity (SMA). Cortico releasing hormone
(CRH) coordinates the behavioral and physiologic sequela. CRH inhibits gonadotropin releasing
hormone (GnRH) and the suppresses GnRH pulse generator and activates the hypothalamus–pituitary–adrenal axis (HPA). CRH modulates immune functions (green) and metabolism (brown) via
adrenocorticotropin hormone (ACTH) that stimulates cortisol release from the adrenal gland. CRH
stimulates gonadotropin inhibiting hormone (GnIH) and inhibits kisspeptin (KISS1). Stress
response and somatic characteristics are a result of descending sympathetic fibers from locus coe-
ruleus (LC). There is an intricate relationship between the brain and reproductive functioning

In patients with endometriosis Meissner et al. [67] could show that Sinosomatics, a holistic intervention, combining hypnotherapy and East asian medicine, treatment reduced stress, anxiety, and pain scores while promoting quality of life. In the concurrent functional magnetic brain scans of these patients Beissner et al. [68] could demonstrate changes of functional connectivity patterns of different hippocampal subregions, giving first hints on the mechanism of Sinosomatics. In a recent analysis of registry data (2014–2016) of 212 unselected patients treated with Sinosomatics, the author found that this complementary treatment led to a live birth in 71,4% patients (147 out of 206). CLBR was 80.8% for women ≤36 years, 61.2% for women between 37 and 39 years, and 66.6% for women ≥40 years. Mild treatment strategies were sufficient in 62,6% as the main method of conception was NC-IVF (34%) (50/147), followed by natural conception (27%) (39/147), egg donation (17%) (26/147), cIVF (17,7%) (26/147) and IUI 2% (3/147) (3 unknown). Among this cohort were mostly "unfavorbale patients:" 53 patients (34.9%) with endometriosis, 33 (21.7%) with poor egg quality, and 21 (13.8%) with recurrent pregnancy loss, and most of them 133 (63%) had experienced prior unsuccessful cIVF treatment cycles (72.7%; mean 4 (2–7) failed cycles).

These registry data indicate that cIVF is often not necessary and NC-IVF together with an integrated holistic treatment can help a high percentage of patients to continue treatment (dropout rate 17% in 3 years) and reach parenthood, even after prior unsuccessful cIVF treatment cycles (see Foreword).

In conclusion, NC-IVF treatments flanked by holistic interventions and support services seem to be a feasible way to develop coping strategies and a sense of controllability in infertility treated women. This approach lowers treatment burden by inducing relaxation, well-being, and positive thoughts as well as emotional balance and mindfulness. Holistic interventions can reduce burden of stress, pain, and despair, resulting in lower dropout rates.

References

1. Cousineau TM, Domar AD. Psychological impact of infertility. Best Pract Res Clin Obstet Gynaecol. 2007;21(2):293–308.
2. Verberg MF, et al. Why do couples drop-out from IVF treatment? A prospective cohort study. Hum Reprod. 2008;23(9):2050–5.
3. Domar AD, et al. Burden of care is the primary reason why insured women terminate in vitro fertilization treatment. Fertil Steril. 2018;109(6):1121–6.
4. Luke B, et al. Cumulative birth rates with linked assisted reproductive technology cycles. N Engl J Med. 2012;366(26):2483–91.
5. De Neubourg D, et al. How do cumulative live birth rates and cumulative multiple live birth rates over complete courses of assisted reproductive technology treatment per woman compare among registries? Hum Reprod. 2016;31(1):93–9.
6. Schroder AK, et al. Cumulative pregnancy rates and drop-out rates in a German IVF programme: 4102 cycles in 2130 patients. Reprod Biomed Online. 2004;8(5):600–6.
7. Brandes M, et al. The relative contribution of IVF to the total ongoing pregnancy rate in a subfertile cohort. Hum Reprod. 2010;25(1):118–26.

8. Olivius K, Friden B, Lundin K, et al. Cumulative probability of live birth after three in vitro fertilization/intracytoplasmic sperm injection cycles. Fertil Steril. 2002;77(3):505–10

9. Witsenburg C, Dieben S, Van der Westerlaken L et al. Cumulative live birth rates in cohorts of patients treated with in vitro fertilization or intracytoplasmic sperm injection. Fertil Steril. 2005;84:99–107. https://doi.org/10.1016/j.fertnstert.2005.02.013

10. Elizur SE, Lerner-Geva L, Levron J, Shulman A, Bider D, Dor J, et al. Cumulative live birth rate following in vitro fertilization: study of 5,310 cycles. Gynecol Endocrinol. 2006;22:25–30

11. Malizia B, Hacker M, Penzias A. Cumulative live-birth rates after in vitro fertilization. N Engl J Med. 2009;360:236–43

12. Garrido N, Bellver J, Remohi J, Simon C, Pellicer A. Cumulative live-birth rates per total number of embryos needed to reach newborn in consecutive in vitro fertilization (IVF) cycles: a new approach to measuring the likelihood of IVF success. Fertil Steril 2011;96:40–6.

13. Smith A. et al. Live-birth rate associated with repeat in vitro fertilization treatment cycles. JAMA. 2015;314(24);2654–62.

14. McLernon D, Steyerberg EW, Egbert R te Velde, 2 Amanda J Lee, 1 Siladitya Bhattacharya. Predicting the chances of a live birth after one or more complete cycles of in vitro fertilisation: population based study of linked cycle data from 113 873 women BMJ. 2016;355:i5735

15. Gameiro S, et al. Why do patients discontinue fertility treatment? A systematic review of reasons and predictors of discontinuation in fertility treatment. Hum Reprod Update. 2012;18(6):652–69.

16. Haemmerli Keller K, Alder G, Loewer L, Faeh M, Rohner S, von Wolff M. Treatment-related psychological stress in different in vitro fertilization therapies with and without gonodatropin. Acta Obstet Gynecol Scand. 2018;97:269–76.

17. Chen TH, et al. Prevalence of depressive and anxiety disorders in an assisted reproductive technique clinic. Hum Reprod. 2004;19(10):2313–8.

18. Volgsten H, et al. Prevalence of psychiatric disorders in infertile women and men undergoing in vitro fertilization treatment. Hum Reprod. 2008;23(9):2056–63.

19. Gameiro S, et al. Women's adjustment trajectories during IVF and impact on mental health 11-17 years later. Hum Reprod. 2016;31(8):1788–98.

20. Liebermann C, et al. Maltreatment during childhood: a risk factor for the development of endometriosis? Hum Reprod. 2018;33(8):1449–58.

21. Demakakos P, Linara-Demakakou E, Mishra GD. Adverse childhood experiences are associated with increased risk of miscarriage in a national population-based cohort study in England. Hum Reprod. 2020;35(6):1451–60.

22. Ebbesen SMS, Zachariae R, Mehlsen MY, Thomsen D, Hojgaard A, Ottosen L, et al. Stressful life events are associated with a poor in-vitro fertilization (IVF) outcome: a prospective study. Hum Reprod. 2009;24:2173–82

23. Dhillon RK, et al. Predicting the chance of live birth for women undergoing IVF: a novel pre-treatment counselling tool. Hum Reprod. 2016;31(1):84–92.

24. Abe T, et al. Success rates in minimal stimulation cycle IVF with clomiphene citrate only. J Assist Reprod Genet. 2020;37(2):297–304.

25. Volgsten H, Svanberg AS, Olsson P. Unresolved grief in women and men in Sweden three years after undergoing unsuccessful in vitro fertilization treatment. Acta Obstet Gynecol Scand. 2010;89(10):1290–7.

26. Gameiro S, Finnigan A. Long-term adjustment to unmet parenthood goals following ART: a systematic review and meta-analysis. Hum Reprod Update. 2017;23(3):322–37.

27. Gonzalez LO. Infertility as a transformational process: a framework for psychotherapeutic support of infertile women. Issues Ment Health Nurs. 2000;21(6):619–33.

28. Wirtberg I, et al. Life 20 years after unsuccessful infertility treatment. Hum Reprod. 2007;22(2):598–604.

29. Koert E, Daniluk JC. When time runs out: reconciling permanent childlessness after delayed childbearing. J Reprod Infant Psychol. 2017;35(4):342–52.

30. Shani C, et al. Suicidal risk among infertile women undergoing in-vitro fertilization: incidence and risk factors. Psychiatry Res. 2016;240:53–9.
31. Vikstrom J, et al. Mental health in women 20-23 years after IVF treatment: a Swedish cross-sectional study. BMJ Open. 2015;5(10):e009426.
32. Mak W, et al. Natural cycle IVF reduces the risk of low birthweight infants compared with conventional stimulated IVF. Hum Reprod. 2016;31(4):789–94.
33. Smith JF, et al. The use of complementary and alternative fertility treatment in couples seeking fertility care: data from a prospective cohort in the United States. Fertil Steril. 2010;93(7):2169–74.
34. Smith CA, Bateson DJ, Weisberg E. A survey describing the use of complementary therapies and medicines by women attending a family planning clinic. BMC Complement Altern Med. 2013;13:224.
35. Domar AD, et al. Lifestyle behaviors in women undergoing in vitro fertilization: a prospective study. Fertil Steril. 2012;97(3):697–701 e1.
36. Miner SA, et al. Evidence for the use of complementary and alternative medicines during fertility treatment: a scoping review. BMC Complement Altern Med. 2018;18(1):158.
37. Huang CW, et al. The utilization of complementary and alternative medicine in Taiwan: an internet survey using an adapted version of the international questionnaire (I-CAM-Q). J Chin Med Assoc. 2019;82(8):665–71.
38. Coulson C, Jenkins J. Complementary and alternative medicine utilisation in NHS and private clinic settings: a United Kingdom survey of 400 infertility patients. J Exp Clin Assist Reprod. 2005;2(1):5.
39. Zhang Y, et al. The effect of complementary and alternative medicine on subfertile women with in vitro fertilization. Evid Based Complement Alternat Med. 2014;2014:419425.
40. Kong J, et al. Expectancy and treatment interactions: a dissociation between acupuncture analgesia and expectancy evoked placebo analgesia. NeuroImage. 2009;45(3):940–9.
41. Zheng CH, et al. Effects of acupuncture on pregnancy rates in women undergoing in vitro fertilization: a systematic review and meta-analysis. Fertil Steril. 2012;97(3):599–611.
42. Manheimer E, et al. The effects of acupuncture on rates of clinical pregnancy among women undergoing in vitro fertilization: a systematic review and meta-analysis. Hum Reprod Update. 2013;19(6):696–713.
43. Cheong YC, et al. Acupuncture and assisted reproductive technology. Cochrane Database Syst Rev. 2013;7:CD006920.
44. Yang H, et al. Systematic review of clinical trials of acupuncture-related therapies for primary dysmenorrhea. Acta Obstet Gynecol Scand. 2008;87(11):1114–22.
45. Manheimer E, et al. Evidence from the Cochrane collaboration for traditional Chinese medicine therapies. J Altern Complement Med. 2009;15(9):1001–14.
46. de Lacey S, Sanderman E, Smith CA. IVF, acupuncture and mental health: a qualitative study of perceptions and experiences of women participating in a randomized controlled trial of acupuncture during IVF treatment. Reprod Biomed Soc Online. 2021;12:22–31.
47. LoGiudice JA, Massaro J. The impact of complementary therapies on psychosocial factors in women undergoing in vitro fertilization (IVF): a systematic literature review. Appl Nurs Res. 2018;39:220–8.
48. Wang X, Wang Y, Wei S, He B, Cao Y, Zhang N, Li M. An overview of systematic reviews of acupuncture for infertile women undergoing in vitro fertilization and embryo transfer. Front Public Health. 2021;20(9):651811. https://doi.org/10.3389/fpubh.2021.651811. PMID: 33959581; PMCID: PMC8096176
49. Quan K, Yu C, Wen X, Lin Q, Wang N, Ma H. Acupuncture as treatment for female infertility: a systematic review and meta-analysis of randomized controlled trials. Evid Based Complement Alternat Med. 2022;2022:3595033.https://doi.org/10.1155/2022/3595033. PMID: 35222669; PMCID: PMC8865966.
50. Ried K. Chinese herbal medicine for female infertility: an updated meta-analysis. Complement Ther Med. 2015;23(1):116–28.

51. Osmanagaoglu K, et al. Spontaneous pregnancies in couples who discontinued intracytoplasmic sperm injection treatment: a 5-year follow-up study. Fertil Steril. 2002;78(3):550–6.
52. Troude P, et al. Seven out of 10 couples treated by IVF achieve parenthood following either treatment, natural conception or adoption. Reprod Biomed Online. 2016;33(5):560–7.
53. ElMokhallalati Y, et al. Treatment-independent live birth after in-vitro fertilisation: a retrospective cohort study of 2, 133 women. Hum Reprod. 2019;34(8):1470–8.
54. Rooney KL, Domar AD. The relationship between stress and infertility. Dialogues Clin Neurosci. 2018;20(1):41–7.
55. Peaston G, et al. The impact of emotional health on assisted reproductive technology outcomes: a systematic review and meta-analysis. Hum Fertil (Camb). 2020:1–12.
56. Russell G, Lightman S. The human stress response. Nat Rev Endocrinol. 2019;15(9):525–34.
57. Whirledge S, Cidlowski JA. A role for glucocorticoids in stress-impaired reproduction: beyond the hypothalamus and pituitary. Endocrinology. 2013;154(12):4450–68.
58. Dhama K, et al. Biomarkers in stress related diseases/disorders: diagnostic, prognostic, and therapeutic values. Front Mol Biosci. 2019;6:91.
59. Lynch CD, et al. Preconception stress increases the risk of infertility: results from a couple-based prospective cohort study--the LIFE study. Hum Reprod. 2014;29(5):1067–75.
60. Garcia-Blanco A, et al. Anxiety and depressive symptoms, and stress biomarkers in pregnant women after in vitro fertilization: a prospective cohort study. Hum Reprod. 2018;33(7):1237–46.
61. Demyttenaere K, et al. Coping style and depression level influence outcome in in vitro fertilization. Fertil Steril. 1998;69(6):1026–33.
62. Smeenk JM, et al. The effect of anxiety and depression on the outcome of in-vitro fertilization. Hum Reprod. 2001;16(7):1420–3.
63. Smeenk JM, et al. Stress and outcome success in IVF: the role of self-reports and endocrine variables. Hum Reprod. 2005;20(4):991–6.
64. Turner K, et al. Stress and anxiety scores in first and repeat IVF cycles: a pilot study. PLoS One. 2013;8(5):e63743.
65. Miller N, et al. Does stress affect IVF outcomes? A prospective study of physiological and psychological stress in women undergoing IVF. Reprod Biomed Online. 2019;39(1):93–101.
66. Raad G, et al. Neurophysiology of cognitive behavioural therapy, deep breathing and progressive muscle relaxation used in conjunction with ART treatments: a narrative review. Hum Reprod Update. 2020;
67. Meissner K, et al. Psychotherapy with somatosensory stimulation for endometriosis-associated pain: a randomized controlled trial. Obstet Gynecol. 2016;128(5):1134–42.
68. Beissner F, Preibisch C, Schweizer-Arau A, Popovici RM, Meissner K. Psychotherapy with somatosensory stimulation for endometriosis-associated pain: the role of the anterior hippocampus. Biol Psychiatry. 2018;84(10):734–42. https://doi.org/10.1016/j.biopsych.2017.01.006

Chapter 24
Future Aspects of Natural Cycle and Minimal Stimulation IVF

Michael von Wolff

24.1 Background

Although natural cycle IVF (NC-IVF) and minimally stimulated IVF are already an integral part of the IVF treatment spectrum in some centres, there are still many questions that need to be addressed in the future. This becomes particularly evident when centres consider these techniques as the last straw in frustrated IVF therapies with conventional high-dose gonadotropin stimulation and when the logistics of conventional IVF are transferred to NC-IVF and minimally stimulated IVF without any adaptations. Such a transfer may lead to inadequate treatment, painful follicular aspirations, and high costs. Accordingly, it is of importance to teach IVF centres about NC-IVF and minimal stimulation IVF in the future, so that these techniques are used in the right way and for the correct indication. Such knowledge transfer is based on precise knowledge of the physiology and endocrinology as well as the technical requirements, risks, costs, efforts, and success rates. A major goal would also be to make NC-IVF and minimal stimulation IVF reimbursable by the health care system, since almost all reimbursement models worldwide were developed at a time when the goal was still to obtain as many oocytes as possible, which has now proven counterproductive in many cases.

Future challenges and tasks regarding NC-IVF and minimal stimulation IVF treatments:

- Sharpen the indications
- Evaluating efficacy of different treatment protocols

M. von Wolff (✉)
Division of Gynecological Endocrinology and Reproductive Medicine, University Women's Hospital, University of Bern, Bern, Switzerland
e-mail: Michael.vonwolff@insel.ch

- Evaluating the success rates of different treatment protocols
- Evaluating the risks of the different treatment protocols
- Evaluating the costs per treatment cycle and per achieved pregnancy
- Simplifying treatments
- Reimbursing NC-IVF and minimal stimulation IVF treatments by the health system
- Educating IVF centres
- Introducing NC-IVF and minimal stimulation IVF treatments worldwide

24.2   Sharpen the Indications

An essential key to the success of a medical therapy is its correct indication. This also applies to the various IVF therapies and thus also to NC-IVF and minimal stimulation IVF. The known indications for or against these treatments are presented in the Chap. 3.

The aim will be to further refine the indications in order to offer couples the treatment that is most successful for them (see Chap. 19).

The IVF-Naturelle® network centres have been conducting a prospective data collection of all their NC-IVF and minimal stimulation IVF described in the Chap. 15 and of conventional IVF therapy cycles since January 2022 (clinical.trials.gov: NCT05125497) for 12 months. Not only pregnancy and birth rates are recorded, but also data on ovarian reserve, duration of infertility, causes of infertility, number of previous embryo transfers as well as on treatment related information such as number of consultations and pain score of follicle aspiration, etc. are collected. It is estimated that around 5000 IVF cycles with a fresh transfer will be recorded and compared. Since this register is set up prospectively, as it is a representative multicentre study and because the register will be set up and evaluated with an institute for statistics, the data promises to sharpen the indications. It is planned to use this data as a basis to develop a mobile App that will allow couples, but also physicians, to individually identify the ideal treatment protocol.

24.3   Evaluating of Treatment Protocols Regarding Efficacy, Risks, and Costs

In addition to the success rate, other factors play a role in the choice of IVF therapy. If NC-IVF or minimal stimulation IVF treatment is carried out instead of conventional gonadotropin-stimulated therapy, more therapy cycles are required. This makes it difficult to compare these IVF treatments. Because of this, it is important to collect data on the therapeutic effort of the treatments, their complication rate and pregnancy complications as well as to calculate the costs per cycle and per pregnancy achieved. All this has already been rudimentarily carried out in smaller studies (see Chaps. 17, 18, 20, 21). However, it is necessary to carry out such an evaluation in a large study involving a large number of centres in order to obtain reliable data. The above-mentioned registry will collect all these parameters and promises answers to the still largely unanswered questions.

24.4 Simplifying Treatments

NC-IVF and minimal stimulation IVF treatments are very popular with couples, partly because they are very simple and not very complex (see Chap. 15). Injections are also hardly necessary. Accordingly, one goal is to further simplify the treatments.

A study is being prepared, based on the Kato Ladies Clinic in Tokyo (see Chap. 28), using GnRH analogue nasal spray for ovulation induction (clinical.trials.gov: NCT04850261). The aim is to avoid any injections (short name of the study: "Injection free IVF") to reduce treatment related stress.

24.5 Reimbursing NC-IVF and Minimal Stimulation IVF Treatments by the Health System

Most reimbursement systems were introduced many years ago when the aim was still to obtain as many oocytes as possible. Accordingly, three to four IVF cycles with conventional high-dose gonadotropin stimulation are usually reimbursed. If a couple wishes to have NC-IVF performed, then the NC-IVF cycle is considered a full IVF cycle. Accordingly, couples usually first perform several conventional IVF cycles and only then consider to undergo NC-IVF or minimal stimulation IVF treatment.

The aim should be to modify the reimbursement systems in such a way that it is possible for the couple and the reproductive health professional to perform three NC-IVF or minimal stimulation IVF therapies instead of one conventional gonadotropin-stimulated IVF. Three NC-IVF or minimal stimulation IVF treatments cost about the same as one conventional IVF (see Chap. 18) and have a similar overall success rate (see Chap. 19).

In Switzerland, the Swiss Society of Reproductive Medicine, SGRM, has applied for the introduction of an IVF reimbursement system which covers conventional as well as NC-IVF and minimal stimulation IVF treatments. If approved, this application would be a model for reimbursement systems in other countries.

24.6 Educating Other IVF Centres and Introducing NC-IVF and Minimal Stimulation IVF Treatments Worldwide

This is certainly one of the most difficult tasks ahead. A lot of patience, perseverance and enthusiasm is needed to spread the benefits of these techniques.

The professional societies have a special role to play in dissemination. The International Society for Mild Approaches in Assisted Reproduction, ISMAAR (www.ismaar.org) successfully informs about the benefits of mild IVF approaches at international congresses. It also publishes position papers on the techniques (see Chap. 4).

Another effective tool for the dissemination of NC-IVF and minimal stimulation IVF is the association of centres specialising in these techniques. One such example is the IVF-Naturelle® network (www.IVF-Naturelle.com) as well as the network of the Kato Ladies clinic in Tokyo, Japan and the New Hope Fertility Center in New York, U.S. (see Chaps. 25–28). With the help of a good website and using modern media, information about these techniques can be effectively disseminated and can arouse interest among infertile couples. Couples then approach their fertility specialists about NC-IVF and minimal stimulation IVF, thus putting pressure on fertility centres to look into these techniques (see Chap. 4).

Accordingly, specialised fertility centres should be encouraged to join forces and thus benefit from the advantages of networks for themselves and for the couples.

Part VII
Worldwide Programs

Chapter 25
Natural Cycle IVF and Minimal Stimulation IVF Worldwide

Michael von Wolff

25.1 Background

Although natural cycle IVF (NC-IVF) and minimal stimulation IVF therapies are now promoted by many centres, it is unclear how often they are performed worldwide and if the number of cycles is increasing. However, a separate evaluation should be carried out in registers, since a change in the number of NC-IVF and minimal stimulation IVF therapies leads to a distortion of the register data, because the oocyte numbers and thus also the subordinate numerical values are very different for these IVF therapies.

25.2 Natural Cycle IVF and Minimal Stimulation IVF Cycles According to National and International Registers

The latest annual report in 2013 from the International Committee for Monitoring Assisted Reproductive Technologies (ICMART), which records IVF cycles worldwide, does not show any natural cycle IVF or minimal stimulation IVF cycles [1].

The same is true for the latest 2016 annual report from the European IVF-Monitoring Consortium (EIM) for the European Society of Human Reproduction and Embryology (ESHRE) [2], which also does not report NC-IVF or minimal stimulation IVF cycles.

M. von Wolff (✉)
Division of Gynecological Endocrinology and Reproductive Medicine, University Women's Hospital, University of Bern, Bern, Switzerland
e-mail: Michael.vonwolff@insel.ch

© The Author(s), under exclusive license to Springer Nature Switzerland AG 2022   245
M. von Wolff (ed.), *Natural Cycle and Minimal Stimulation IVF*,
https://doi.org/10.1007/978-3-030-97571-5_25

Some national registers now report the proportion of NC-IVF cycles. However, it is not always clear whether the data is correct.

Sunkara et al. [3] analysed the data from the Human Fertilisation and Embryology Authority (HFEA), U.K. from 1991 to 2011. A total of 591,003 fresh IVF cycles involving 584,835 stimulated IVF cycles and 6168 unstimulated IVF cycles were analysed. According to these numbers, around 1% of IVF cycles were performed as unstimulated cycles. However, 0 oocytes were found in 44.2% of cycles, 1 oocyte in around 37%, 2 oocytes in around 9%, 3 oocytes in around 5% and ≥3 oocytes in around 6% of cycles. Overall, >1 oocyte was found in 20% of cycles. These numbers seem to be unrealistic for unstimulated cycles, and it can be assumed that several stimulated cycles were classified as unstimulated IVF cycles.

The data from the infertility centre in Bern can be used to determine in how many unstimulated, i.e. NC-IVF cycles 0, 1 or 2 oocytes can be expected. In 2016–2019, 1267 NC-IVF treatment cycles were carried out. No oocytes were found in 35% of cycles, 1 oocyte in 62% and 2 oocytes in 3% of cycles. Three or more oocytes were never found. Overall, >1 oocyte was found in 3% of cycles. This number can be assumed to be realistic, questioning the validity of the HEFA data published by Sunkara et al.

In 2019, a total of around 100,000 cycles were documented in the German IVF Register (https://www.deutsches-ivf-register.de/ivf-international.php) around 70,000 stimulated fresh cycles, around 30,000 frozen cycles and around 3,800 NC-IVF cycles. Thus, the proportion of NC-IVF cycles among fresh cycles in Germany is around 5%. It should be noted that a total of three fresh cycles are reimbursed in Germany. It does not matter whether these are stimulated cycles or NC-IVF cycles. Accordingly, NC-IVF cycles are usually only carried out after three stimulated cycles have been performed, i.e. when these have to be paid for by the couples themselves.

In 2020, an overall total of around 12,000 IVF cycles were documented in the Swiss IVF register (www.fivnat-registry.ch): Around 6,000 stimulated fresh cycles, around 5,000 frozen cycles and around 600 NC-IVF cycles.

The register is designed in such a way that stimulated cycles cannot accidentally be classified as natural cycles. Thus, the proportion of NC-IVF cycles among fresh cycles in Switzerland can be assumed to be correct and is around 10%. However, it should be noted that in Switzerland 4 of the 33 IVF centres belong to the IVF-Naturelle® network (see Chap. 26), so the philosophy of NC-IVF and minimal stimulation IVF is widespread in Switzerland. It should also be noted that IVF treatment is not reimbursed in Switzerland, making natural cycle IVF therapies financially attractive to many couples.

Japan is a country with a large number of minimal stimulation IVF cycles. According to the national registers, around 10% of the cycles are NC-IVF cycles and around 30% are minimal stimulation IVF cycles (see Chap. 28).

Overall, it can be assumed that in most countries, the proportion of NC-IVF treatments is rather low and in the range of 1 to 5%, but in individual countries such as Switzerland and Japan, it can reach 10%.

The proportion of NC-IVF treatments seems to depend strongly on the national reimbursement system, the initiative and influence of individual large centres and networks, and also on the national culture.

Data on minimal IVF stimulation can hardly be collected from the registers since it is usually not possible to separate low and high gonadotropin stimulation doses.

25.3   Natural Cycle IVF and Minimal Stimulation IVF in Large Centres or Networks

According to the national register, the proportion of NC-IVF and minimal stimulation IVF cycles performed in the total number of registered IVF cycles is low. However, there are some centres that perform a very large number of NC-IVF and minimal stimulation IVF cycles (Table 25.1). This suggests that these therapies are preferably performed in a few specialised centres and then in very large numbers, but that these techniques are not yet offered by most centres.

NC-IVF and minimal stimulation IVF therapies are often promoted as low-cost IVF techniques [4, 5], which is likely to lead to their widespread use in low-income countries. However, reliable data on the dissemination of these or similar IVF therapies as low-cost IVF is not yet available.

In low-income countries, various projects have been launched to make IVF therapies more cost-effective and therefore also available to low-income couples [6]. However, it is doubtful whether these techniques are really widespread in low-income countries, as the average costs per pregnancy achieved are hardly lower than for conventional IVF with high-dose gonadotropin stimulation (see Chap. 18). Only if the pregnancy occurs in the first or second NC-IVF or minimal stimulation IVF cycles are the costs relevantly lower. It remains to be seen whether the dissemination will increase through a simplification of the laboratory technique, as is being attempted in the "Walking Egg" project [7].

Table 25.1 Natural cycle IVF (NC-IVF) and minimal stimulation IVF cycles in large centres or networks worldwide

Centre/network	Characteristics of the centre/networks	Number of natural cycle IVF and minimal stimulation IVF cycles in 2020
IVF-Naturelle®; Germany, Switzerland, Austria (see Chap. 26)	Network of 13 independent centres, organised by the infertility Centre, Bern, Switzerland	Infertility Centre, Bern: $n = 568$. IVF-Naturelle® network: $n = \approx3,000$
Kato Ladies Clinic; Tokyo, Japan (see Chap. 28)	Single Centre. The Centre has trained around 11 other centres in NC-IVF and minimal stimulation IVF	Kato Ladies Clinic: $n = 17,584$
New Hope Fertility Centre; New York, United States (see Chap. 27)	Single Centre. The Centre has trained around 5 other centres in NC-IVF and minimal stimulation IVF	New Hope Fertility Centre: $n = 4,300$

References

1. Banker M, Dyer S, Chambers GM, Ishihara O, Kupka M, de Mouzon J, Zegers-Hochschild F, Adamson GD. International Committee for Monitoring Assisted Reproductive Technologies (ICMART): world report on assisted reproductive technologies, 2013. Fertil Steril. 2021;116(3):741–56.
2. European IVF-monitoring Consortium (EIM)‡ for the European Society of Human Reproduction and Embryology (ESHRE); Wyns C, Bergh C, Calhaz-Jorge C, De Geyter C, Kupka MS, Motrenko T, Rugescu I, Smeenk J, Tandler-Schneider A, Vidakovic S, Goossens V. ART in Europe, 2016: results generated from European registries by ESHRE. Hum Reprod Open. 2020;2020:hoaa032.
3. Sunkara SK, LaMarca A, Polyzos NP, Seed PT, Khalaf Y. Live birth and perinatal outcomes following stimulated and unstimulated IVF: analysis of over two decades of a nationwide data. Hum Reprod. 2016;31:2261–7.
4. Teoh PJ, Maheshwari A. Low-cost in vitro fertilization: current insights. Int J Women's Health. 2014;6:817–27.
5. Inhorn MC, Patrizio P. Infertility around the globe: new thinking on gender, reproductive technologies and global movements in the 21st century. Hum Reprod Update. 2015;21:411–26.
6. Chiware TM, Vermeulen N, Blondeel K, Farquharson R, Kiarie J, Lundin K, Matsaseng TC, Ombelet W, Toskin I. IVF and other ART in low- and middle-income countries: a systematic landscape analysis. Hum Reprod Update. 2021;27:213–28.
7. Ombelet W, Goossens J. The Walking Egg Project: how to start a TWE centre? Facts Views Vis Obgyn. 2016;8:119–24.

Chapter 26
Germany, Switzerland, Austria—IVF-Naturelle® Network

Michael von Wolff

26.1 Background

IVF-Naturelle® is a trademark registered, founded and co-ordinated by Michael von Wolff since 2010 which includes all kind of natural cycle IVF (NC-IVF) and minimal stimulation IVF treatments. It is a network (www.IVF-Naturelle.com) of 15 independent infertility centres that offer all kind of IVF treatments but which are also specialised in NC-IVF and minimal stimulation IVF. The aim is to evaluate and optimise NC-IVF and minimal stimulation IVF treatments based on scientific and clinical studies, and thus to offer a high standard of quality to couples.

26.2 Definitions Used by the IVF-Naturelle® Network

IVF-Naturelle® is defined as IVF therapies without (NC-IVF) or with very low dose (minimal stimulation IVF) gonadotropin stimulation.

NC-IVF is defined as IVF therapy without stimulation of folliculogenesis and without luteal phase support. Adjuvants such as ibuprofen or single injections of a GnRH antagonist may be used to better control ovulation, which is triggered by human chorionic gonadotropin (HCG).

M. von Wolff (✉)
Division of Gynecological Endocrinology and Reproductive Medicine, University Women's Hospital, University of Bern, Bern, Switzerland
e-mail: Michael.vonwolff@insel.ch

© The Author(s), under exclusive license to Springer Nature Switzerland AG 2022   249
M. von Wolff (ed.), *Natural Cycle and Minimal Stimulation IVF*,
https://doi.org/10.1007/978-3-030-97571-5_26

Minimal stimulation IVF is defined as IVF therapies with very low dose stimulation of folliculogenesis with clomiphene citrate, letrozole or a maximum of 75–100 IU gonadotropins, alone or in combination (see Chap. 2).

26.3 Philosophy of the IVF-Naturelle® Network

The philosophy of IVF-Naturelle® (www.IVF-Naturelle.com) is to perform IVF therapy as naturally as possible, but also as effectively as possible (Fig. 26.1).
This means:

- If the individual chance of success with NC-IVF is high, NC-IVF therapy should be chosen as the primary treatment. How to proceed is revaluated after three NC-IVF therapies (Fig. 26.2).
- NC-IVF does not involve stimulation of folliculogenesis or luteal phase suppression; however, adjuvants are given if needed to prevent premature ovulation (Fig. 26.3).
- A broad spectrum of minimal stimulation IVF treatments can be offered if a larger number of oocytes is required (Fig. 26.4) (see Chap. 15).
- The therapies do not require anaesthesia, embryo selection and cryopreservation of embryos.
- If it is beneficial for the couple conventional IVF therapy with high-dose gonadotropin stimulation should be offered.
- NC-IVF, minimal stimulation IVF and conventional IVF therapies should not compete, but should be seen as complementary forms of treatment.
- The different therapies contribute to an individualised and patient-oriented IVF treatment.

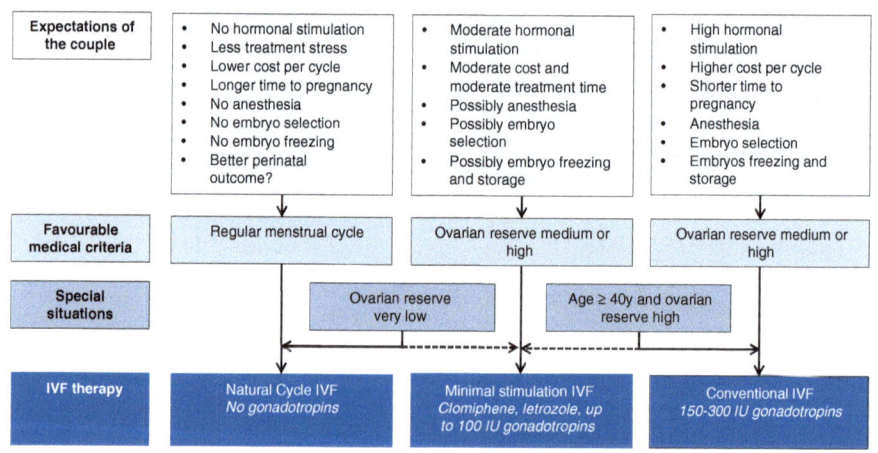

Fig. 26.1 Different IVF treatment options, characteristics and indications (adapted from von Wolff [1])

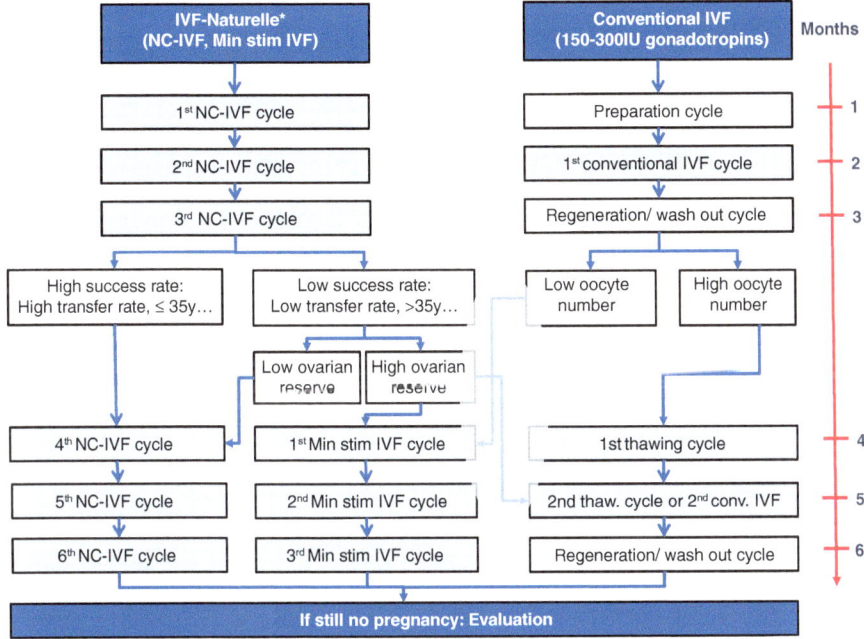

* IVF-Naturelle = IVF without gonadotropin stimulation (NC-IVF) and IVF with minimal gonadotropin stimulation (Min stim IVF)

Fig. 26.2 Orientating flow chart of IVF treatment strategy (adapted from von Wolff and Magaton [2])

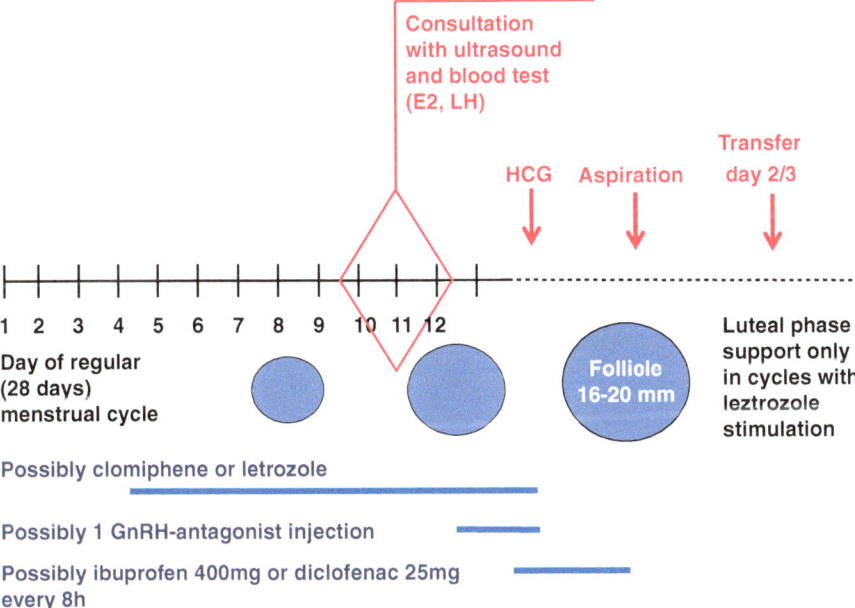

Fig. 26.3 Treatment principle of NC-IVF in IVF-Naturelle® centres

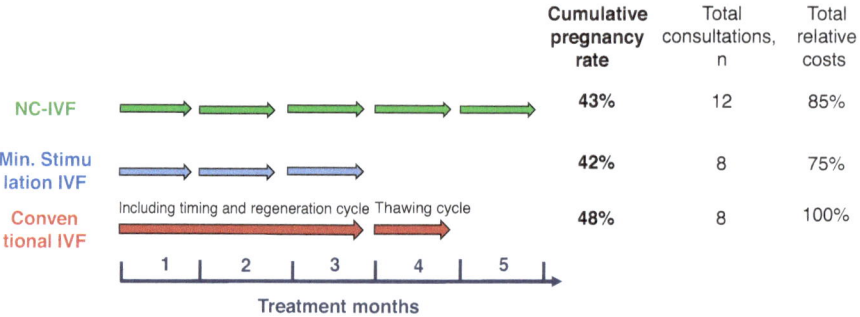

Fig. 26.4 Overview of IVF treatment modalities and its characteristics (adapted from von Wolff and Magaton [2])

26.4   History and Structure of the IVF-Naturelle® Network

The IVF-Naturelle® network comprises eight centres in Germany, four in Switzerland, two in Austria and one centre in Barcelona, Spain (as of April 2022) (Fig. 26.5). Approximately, 3000 IVF-Naturelle® cycles are performed every year.

The IVF-Naturelle® network is a network of various independent infertility centres that offer all kind of IVF therapies including NC-IVF and minimal stimulation IVF. It is coordinated by M. von Wolff, chief physician of the Division of Gynaecological Endocrinology and Reproductive Medicine at the University Women's Hospital in Berne, Switzerland. The aim is to evaluate and optimise IVF-Naturelle® treatments based on scientific and clinical studies. The network runs a website (www.IVF-Naturelle.com) in 4 languages, organises clinical studies, annual working meetings (Fig. 26.6), joint publications, media relations and a joint register.

The multilingual website, international publications and this book are intended to make knowledge about natural cycle and minimal stimulation IVF available to an international audience.

26.5   Reimbursement in Germany, Switzerland and Austria

To better understand the IVF-Naturelle® network and the techniques offered, the reimbursement policy in these countries is briefly described. In Germany around 5% of fresh IVF cycles performed are NC-IVF treatments and in Switzerland around 10%.

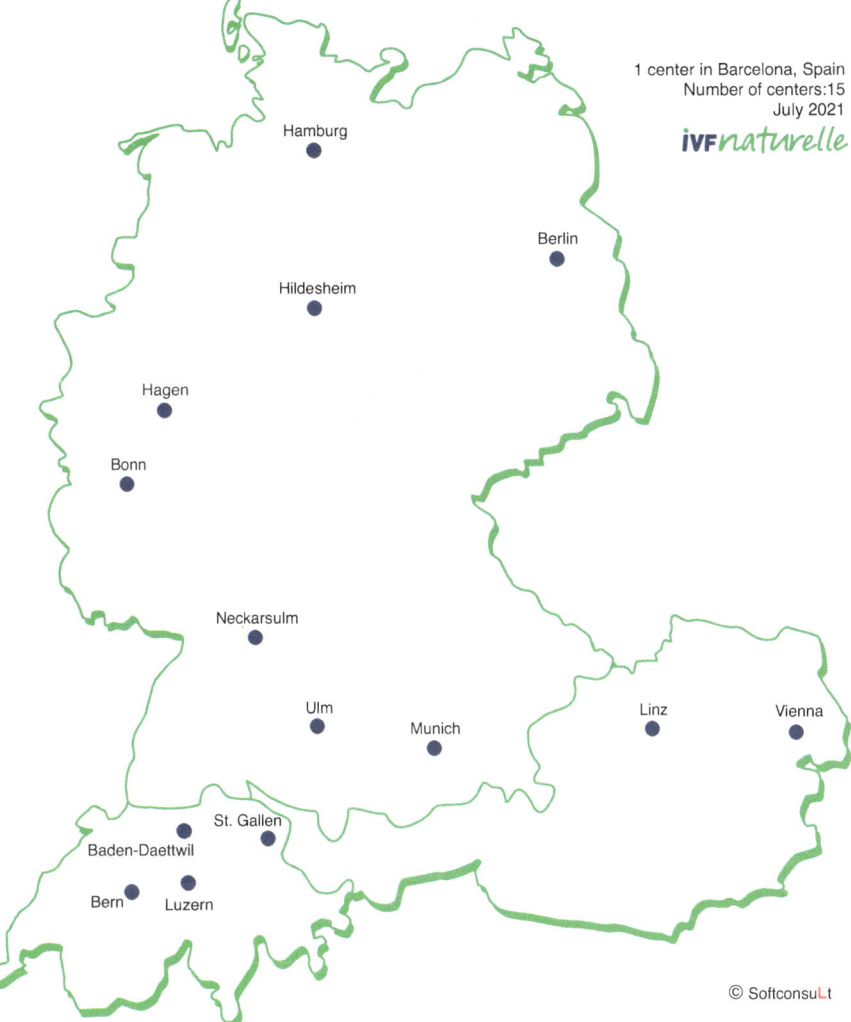

1 center in Barcelona, Spain
Number of centers:15
July 2021

Fig. 26.5 IVF-Naturelle® centres in Germany, Switzerland and Austria (April 2022)

26.5.1   *Germany*

Around 50% of the costs of three fresh IVF cycles are reimbursed in married couples (ages: females 25–40 years, males 25–50 years). The number of reimbursed cycles is independent from the IVF technique (NC-IVF, minimal stimulation IVF, conventional IVF). Accordingly, three cycles are partially reimbursed, irrespective whether it is a NC-IVF, minimal stimulation IVF or a conventional IVF treatment. Some private insurance companies reimburse 100% of the costs of four IVF cycles.

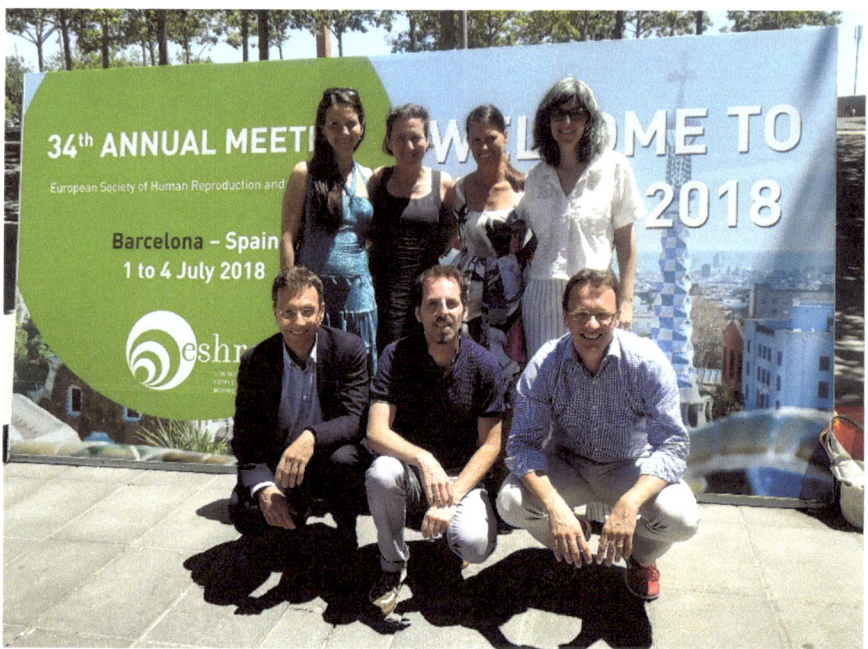

Fig. 26.6 The IVF-Naturelle® meeting at the ESHRE Congress in Barcelona in 2018 with five IVF-Naturelle® members. Front: From left to right: Michael von Wolff, Bern Switzerland; Oliver Ernst, Barcelona, Spain; Mischa Schneider, Baden, Switzerland. Back: From left to right: Mónica Redondo Ania, Barcelona, Spain; Roxana Popovici, Munich, Germany; Eva-Maria Boogen, Bonn, Germany; Esther Ibarrola Torres, Barcelona, Spain

26.5.2 Switzerland

IVF treatments are not reimbursed. Accordingly, the calculated relative costs of the different IVF treatment protocols as shown in Fig. 26.4 are roughly the costs the patients need to pay to the IVF centres. Reimbursement is currently applied to the authorities, including reimbursement of three conventional IVF or (as in poor responders) twelve NC-IVF or minimal stimulation IVF treatment cycles. The decision of the authorities is expected in 2023.

26.5.3 Austria

Around 70% of the costs of four fresh IVF, ICSI or thawing cycles are reimbursed (female age: maximum 40 years). The number of reimbursed cycles is independent from the IVF technique (NC-IVF, minimal stimulation IVF, conventional IVF). Accordingly, four cycles are partially reimbursed, irrespective whether it is a NC-IVF, minimal stimulation IVF or a conventional IVF treatment.

26.6 Scientific Achievements of the IVF-Naturelle® Networks

Approx. 30 PubMed-referenced publications on NC-IVF have been published or are currently be submitted for publication over the last 10 years. Fundamental science and clinical research projects were carried out.

The most important studies are the following (in chronological order):

Follicular fluid hormone and granulosa cell mRNA concentrations are dysregulated in conventional IVF compared to NC-IVF

Title: "Gonadotrophin stimulation for in vitro fertilization significantly alters the hormone milieu in follicular fluid: a comparative study between natural cycle IVF and conventional IVF". Hum Reprod [3].

Type of study: Cross-sectional study with 76 treatment cycles.

Title: "Gonadotrophin stimulation for in vitro fertilization leads to dissociation of follicular fluid hormone and granulosa cells mRNA concentrations: a comparative study between natural cycle IVF and conventional IVF". Reprod Biomed Online [4].

Type of study: Cross-sectional study with 93 treatment cycles.

NC-IVF can be combined with very low dosages of clomiphene citrate to increase the transfer rate

Title: "Low-dosage clomiphene reduces premature ovulation rates and increases transfer rates in natural-cycle IVF". Reprod Biomed Online [5].

Type of study: Retrospective controlled study with 211 cycles from 112 women.

Treatment-related stress is lower in NC-IVF compared to conventional IVF

Title: "Treatment-related psychological stress in different in vitro fertilization therapies with and without gonadotropin stimulation". Acta Obstet Gynecol Scand [6].

Type of study: Prospective controlled study with 119 women.

Patient's related factors to calculate success rates in NC-IVF

Title: "Only women's age and the duration of infertility are the prognostic factors for the success rate of natural cycle IVF". Arch Gynecol Obstet [7].

Type of study: Retrospective study with 201 embryo transfers from 201 women.

High oestradiol serum concentration is related to lower birth weight

Title: "The greater incidence of small-for-gestational-age newborns after gonadotropin-stimulated in vitro fertilization with a supraphysiological estradiol level on ovulation trigger day". Acta Obstet Gynecol Scand [8].

Type of study: Cohort study with 155 children.

Flushing of the follicles increases oocyte yield in NC-IVF

Title: "Follicular flushing leads to higher oocyte yield in monofollicular IVF: a randomized controlled trial". Hum Reprod [9].

Type of study: Randomised controlled study with 164 women with each one follicle aspiration.

Optimal follicle size and oestrogen concentration for aspiration in NC-IVF

Title: "Optimal timing of ovulation triggering to achieve highest success rates in natural cycles - an analysis based on follicle size and estradiol concentration in natural cycle IVF". Front Endocrinol [10].

Type of study: Retrospective study with 604 treatment cycles from 290 women.

Endometrium thickness but not pregnancy rate is increased by gonadotropin stimulation

Title: "High dose gonadotropin stimulation increases endometrial thickness but this gonadotropin induced thickening does not increase pregnancy rate". Gynecol Obstet Hum Reprod [11].

Type of study: Retrospective study with 851 IVF treatment cycles from 435 women.

Gonadotropin stimulation reduces the implantation and live birth

Title: "Gonadotropin stimulation reduces the implantation and live birth but not the miscarriage rate – a study based on the comparison of gonadotropin stimulated and unstimulated IVF". Hum Reprod. (Suppl) [12].

Type of study: Retrospective study with 977 treatment cycles from 634 women.

Birth weight is reduced in children after conventional IVF but not after NC-IVF

Title: "Perinatal outcomes in singletons after fresh IVF/ICSI – results of two cohorts and the birth registry". Reprod Biomed Online [13].

Type of study: Retrospective and registry study comparing 144 NC-IVF singletons or 144 conventional IVF fresh transfer singletons (Bern IVF cohort) with 633,996 Swiss singletons.

26.7 Future Perspective of the IVF-Naturelle® Network

The goals for the next few years are as follows:

- One goal of the IVF-Naturelle® network is to include more centres to provide comprehensive care nationwide in Germany, Switzerland and Austria for couples interested in NC-IVF and minimal stimulation IVF. However, the focus of the expansion of the network is to include only those centres that are willing to specialise in these techniques.
- The second goal is the prospective analysis of different treatment protocols (see Chap. 15). All IVF-Naturelle® centres are prospectively collecting data on different treatment protocols including conventional IVF to objectively analyse success rates, treatment burden, costs, etc. (see Chap. 24) to improve the techniques and to better define indications for the different therapies. The prospective data analysis is performed in 2022/2023.
- The third goal is to complete the "Injection free IVF" study. This study tests whether a nasally administered GnRH agonist can be used for ovulation induction in NC-IVF without the need for luteal phase support or embryo cryopreser-

vation. Such therapy would further simplify the burden of NC-IVF therapy (see Chap. 24).

- The fourth goal is to implement reimbursement for NC-IVF and minimal stimulation IVF. Based on the activities in Switzerland where such a reimbursement will probably be introduced (political decision expected in 2023), introduction in Germany and possibly also in Austria will be actively pursued.

References

1. von Wolff M. The role of natural cycle IVF in assisted reproduction. Best Pract Res Clin Endocrinol Metab. 2019;33:35–45.
2. von Wolff M, Magaton IM. Klassische IVF vs. Natural-Cycle und Minimal-Stimulation-IVF. Der Gynäkologe. 2020;53:588–95.
3. von Wolff M, Kollmann Z, Flück CE, Stute P, Marti U, Weiss B, Bersinger NA. Gonadotrophin stimulation for in vitro fertilization significantly alters the hormone milieu in follicular fluid: a comparative study between natural cycle IVF and conventional IVF. Hum Reprod. 2014;29:1049–57.
4. von Wolff M, Eisenhut M, Stute P, Bersinger NA. Gonadotrophin stimulation reduces follicular fluid hormone concentrations and disrupts their quantitative association with cumulus cell mRNA. Reprod Biomed Online. 2022;44:193–9.
5. von Wolff M, Nitzschke M, Stute P, Bitterlich N, Rohner S. Low-dosage clomiphene reduces premature ovulation rates and increases transfer rates in natural-cycle IVF. Reprod Biomed Online. 2014;29:209–15.
6. Haemmerli Keller K, Alder G, Loewer L, Faeh M, Rohner S, von Wolff M. Treatment-related psychological stress in different in vitro fertilization therapies with and without gonadotropin stimulation. Acta Obstet Gynecol Scand. 2018;97:269–76.
7. von Wolff M, Schwartz AK, Bitterlich N, Stute P, Fäh M. Only women's age and the duration of infertility are the prognostic factors for the success rate of natural cycle IVF. Arch Gynecol Obstet. 2019;299:883–9.
8. Kohl Schwartz AS, Mitter VR, Amylidi-Mohr S, Fasel P, Minger MA, Limoni C, Zwahlen M, von Wolff M. The greater incidence of small-for-gestational-age newborns after gonadotropin-stimulated in vitro fertilization with a supraphysiological estradiol level on ovulation trigger day. Acta Obstet Gynecol Scand. 2019;98:1575–84.
9. Kohl Schwartz AS, Calzaferri I, Roumet M, Limacher A, Fink A, Wueest A, Weidlinger S, Mitter VR, Leeners B, Von Wolff M. Follicular flushing leads to higher oocyte yield in mono-follicular IVF: a randomized controlled trial. Hum Reprod. 2020;35:2253–61.
10. Helmer A, Magaton I, Stalder O, Surbek D, Stute P, von Wolff M. Optimal timing of ovulation triggering to achieve highest success rates in natural cycles – an analysis based on follicle size and estradiol concentration in natural cycle IVF. Front Endocrinol. 2022, 26 May.
11. Magaton I.M, Helmer A, Roumet M, Stute P, von Wolff M. High dose gonadotropin stimulation increases endometrial thickness but this gonadotropin induced thickening does not have an effect on implantation. J Gynecol Obstet Hum Reprod, in press.
12. Mitter VR, Grädel F, Kohl Schwartz AS, von Wolff M. Gonadotropin stimulation reduces the implantation and live birth but not the miscarriage rate – a study based on the comparison of gonadotropin stimulated and unstimulated IVF. Hum Reprod. 2021;(Suppl 1):i452.
13. Mitter VR, Fasel P, Berlin C, Amylidi-Mohr S, Mosimann B, Zwahlen M, von Wolff M, Kohl Schwartz AS. Perinatal outcomes in singletons after fresh IVF/IVSI: results of two cohorts and the birth registry. Reprod Biomed Online. 2022;44:689–98.

Chapter 27
United States—Mini IVF®

John Zhang

New Hope Fertility Center (NHFC) (www.newhopefertility.com) was founded by Dr. John Zhang in 2004. This was a celebration of friendship, science, and the will to change reproductive medicine and the lives of many people through innovation and the practice of the best medicine possible.

Supported by the late Dr. O. Kato, J. Zhang founded New Hope's first clinic at Park Avenue, New York City and quickly revolutionized the old ways of ovarian stimulation. New Hope offers patients tailor-made stimulation protocols in the form of Dr. Zhang's Mini IVF and state of the art IVF lab technologies. NHFC quickly rose to become one of the major IVF centers in the USA.

With this newly gained reputation, challenging cases quickly populated NHFC.

NHFC quickly adapted and developed new protocols in the form of natural cycles such as luteal phase stimulation and several variations of Mini IVF, which became NHFC's trademark protocol. NHFC eventually developed a patient centered approach which is less invasive in every step of the process including the stimulation, egg retrieval, and the embryo transfer. Today, NHFC has become a pioneer in single embryo transfer, frozen embryo transfer, and oocyte cryopreservation.

In 2007, Dr. Alejandro Chavez-Badiola joined New Hope Fertility Center with the aim to expand the Mini IVF philosophy, to accompany Dr. Zhang in long-standing research projects and to incorporate Mexico into NHFC's global projects. In 2008, New Hope Fertility Center Mexico (Guadalajara) became NHFC's second grand opening which was then followed by NHFC at Columbus Circle, NY (2009), and NHFC Mexico City (2013). The result of these new projects became palpable in the form of scientific collaborations, new research and of course, the first baby ever to be born following a spindle nuclear transfer [1]. This is probably still the most revolutionary technology introduced in the field of IVF, thus far.

J. Zhang (✉)
New Hope Fertility Center, New York, USA

© The Author(s), under exclusive license to Springer Nature Switzerland AG 2022　　259
M. von Wolff (ed.), *Natural Cycle and Minimal Stimulation IVF*,
https://doi.org/10.1007/978-3-030-97571-5_27

Since new times bring new challenges, NHFC has been quick to adapt to the COVID-19 pandemic with new projects and new protocols. We believe if reproductive medicine in the form of IVF is ever to become mainstream, we need to get closer to patients, become less invasive, and to make the best possible use of upcoming technologies. Under the umbrella of innovation and working towards breaking barriers in accessibility, NHFC has developed At-Home IVF, and Needle-Free IVF protocols.

At NHFC, we not only believe the future is brilliant, inclusive, and abundant, but we are working to make sure it becomes such a world. Our current pioneering research focuses on stem cell, synthetic gametes, cryopreservation, artificial intelligence, and automation. NHFC is perhaps the first IVF center in the world to have adopted artificial intelligence assistance for embryo selection as a standard protocol since 2018.

Reference

1. Zhang J, Liu H, Luo S, Lu Z, Chávez-Badiola A, Liu Z, Yang M, Merhi Z, Silber SJ, Munné S, Konstantinidis M, Wells D, Tang JJ, Huang T. Live birth derived from oocyte spindle transfer to prevent mitochondrial disease. Reprod Biomed Online. 2017;34:361–8.

Chapter 28
Japan—Kato Ladies Clinic

Keiichi Kato and Satoshi Ueno

28.1 Definitions Used by Kato Ladies Clinic

The term "Natural cycle" is used when IVF is carried out (NC-IVF) in a spontaneous menstrual cycle without any medication taken at any time during the cycle. The term "Modified natural cycle" is used when exogenous hormones or drugs are applied during a woman's spontaneous menstrual cycle. In our modified natural cycle scenario, the only exogenous hormone given until oocyte retrieval is a gonadotropin-releasing hormone agonist (GnRHa) that triggers final oocyte. Both natural and modified natural cycle IVFs are performed, but the modified natural cycle IVF is more frequent. In our chapter, we refer to the "Modified natural cycle IVF" as the "Natural cycle IVF" as a matter of convenience. Minimal stimulation IVF is defined as IVF treatment with minimal stimulation of folliculogenesis with clomiphene citrate (CC), letrozole, or an injection of gonadotropin (75 or 150 IU/day, maximum dose: 450 IU gonadotropins/cycle).

28.2 Philosophy of the Kato Ladies Clinic

The idea of the NC-IVF and minimal stimulation IVF performed in Kato Ladies Clinic is to minimize the use of fertility drugs as much as possible and utilize endogenous hormones to stimulate the ovaries as naturally as possible. A sufficient understanding of the physiological hormone dynamics is necessary to routinely manage NC-IVF and minimal stimulation. In addition, follicular monitoring and aspiration are offered 365 days/year to handle unpredictable ovulation.

K. Kato (✉) · S. Ueno
Kato Ladies Clinic, Tokyo, Japan
e-mail: k-kato@towako.net

© The Author(s), under exclusive license to Springer Nature Switzerland AG 2022   261
M. von Wolff (ed.), *Natural Cycle and Minimal Stimulation IVF*,
https://doi.org/10.1007/978-3-030-97571-5_28

28.3   Natural Cycle IVF

- All patients with a regular menstrual cycle and spontaneous ovulation can be treated by NC-IVF regardless of age.
- The only pharmaceutical intervention until the follicle aspiration is the final oocyte maturation with nasally applied GnRHa (intranasal application of 3 × 1 hub of 0.15 mg buserelin (Suprecur®) = 0.45 mg in total) (Fig. 28.1).
- The medical examination on day 3 after menstruation is not mandatory and the first visit date can take place on day 10 depending on the patients' menstruation cycle.
- When the leading follicle reaches 18 mm in diameter with a concomitant serum E2 level of 250 pg/mL, oocyte maturation is triggered. Oocyte retrieval is performed 34–35 h later.
- Usually, day 2 cleaved stage embryos are transferred in fresh and blastocysts are vitrified, warmed, and transferred later. The first line regimen of endometrial preparation for vitrified and warmed embryo transfer is natural ovulatory cycle except for patients with PCOS, luteal phase insufficiency and pituitary dysfunction.
- Luteal phase support is performed in case of transfer of day 2 cleaved stage embryos with dydrogesterone (3 × 10 mg/day, orally) starting on the day of embryo transfer for 10 days. In case of blastocyst transfer, progesterone is additionally administered (800 mg/day, intravaginally) along with oral dydrogesterone for 7 days if luteal function is insufficient (progesterone concentration on the

Natural cycle

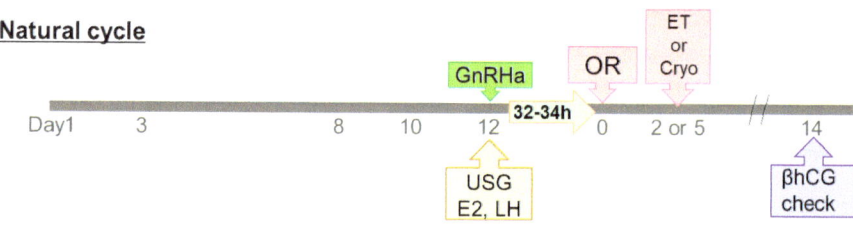

Minimal stimulation cycle

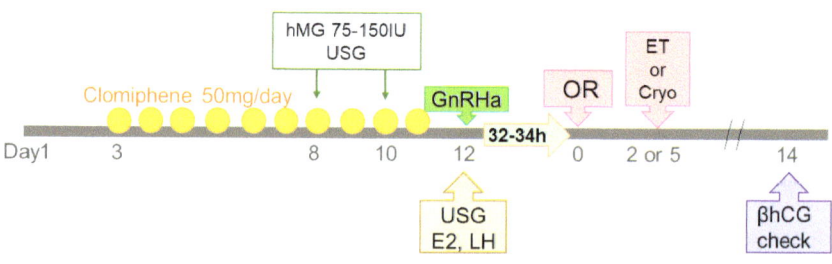

Fig. 28.1 Protocol for natural cycle IVF and minimal stimulation IVF (*USG* Ultrasonography, *OR* Oocyte retrieval, *ET* Embryo transfer)

day of ovulation triggering 8–11 ng/mL). Blastocyst transfer is cancelled if the progesterone concentration is <8 ng/mL.

28.4 Minimal Stimulation IVF

- Clomiphene citrate (CC)-based minimal stimulation IVF is indicated in World Health Organization group II ovulation disorders; thus, this approach is suitable for a large number of patients of different ages.
- The first patient consultation is scheduled on day 3 of the cycle (Fig. 28.1). Administration of CC (50 mg/day) is started on day 3 and continued until right before triggering ovulation. Because CC is started on day 3, ovarian stimulation using CC starts before follicle recruitment. CC is administered for two purposes: for its main effect to promote follicular maturation and to inhibit the luteinizing hormone (LH) surge, which is achieved through its anti-oestrogenic effect.
- For patients with insufficient levels of follicle-stimulating hormone (FSH) because of negative feedback from follicle growth or delayed follicular growth, an appropriate dose of gonadotropins (75–150 IU s.c./day) is administered. Considering the half-life of gonadotropins, alternate-day administration (rather than daily administration) is sufficient.
- Since the pituitary gland is not inhibited, oocyte maturation can be induced prior to retrieval by triggering an endogenous LH surge with GnRHa (3 intranasal hubs of 0.15 mg of buserelin = 0.45 mg in total).
- The criteria for confirming follicular maturation are a dominant follicle diameter of ≥18 mm and sufficient oestradiol (E2) levels relative to the number of growing follicles. Oocyte retrieval is performed 34–35 h later.
- Day 2 cleaved stage embryos are considered to be transferred directly without freezing. The criterion for fresh transfer in clomiphene citrate-based minimal stimulation cycle IVF is an endometrial thickness of ≥8 mm on the day of ovulation triggering [1]. Otherwise, embryos are vitrified either on day 2 or day 5–7 and transferred later in a thawing cycle. The first line regimen of endometrial preparation for thawing cycles is a natural ovulatory cycle except for patients with polycystic ovarian syndrome, luteal phase insufficiency, and pituitary dysfunction.
- Dydrogesterone (3 × 10 mg/day, orally) is administered during the luteal phase after embryo transfer.

28.5 Attempts to Prevent Ovulation

Predicting the LH surge and determining whether the LH surge has already started are the most important factors in oocyte retrieval during NC-IVF and minimal stimulation IVF cycles. Figure 28.2 shows the physiological hormone dynamics and

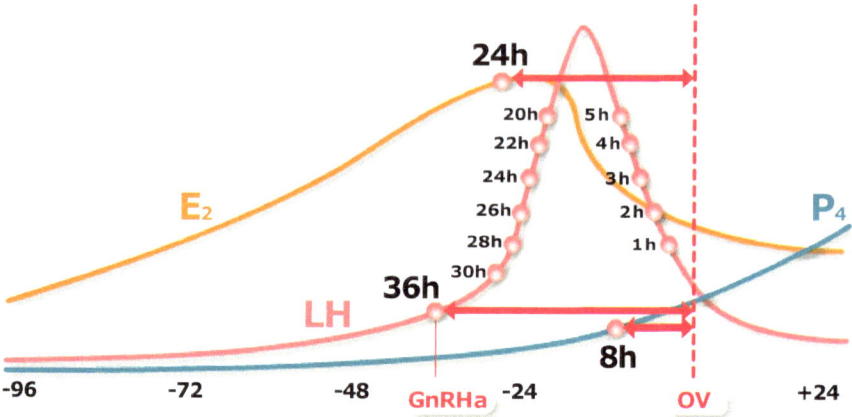

Fig. 28.2 Diagram of LH surge and timing of ovulation (OV)

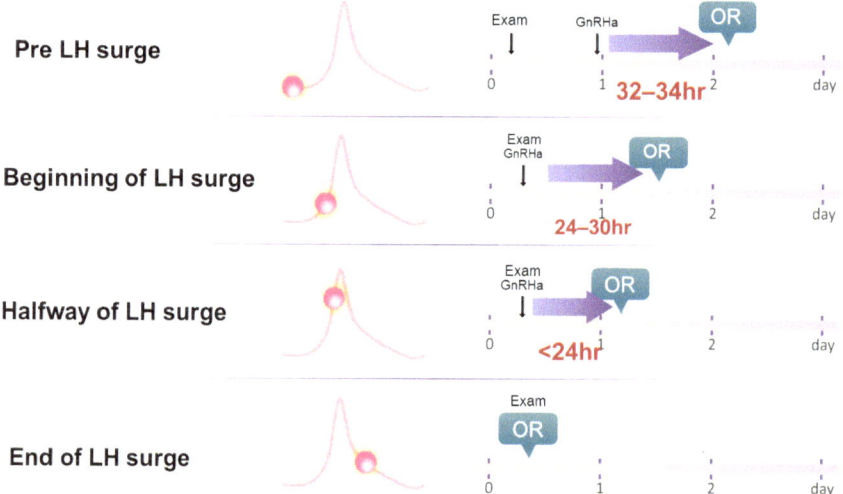

Fig. 28.3 LH surge and appropriate timing of oocyte retrieval (OR)

timing of ovulation. The timing of GnRHa administration and oocyte retrieval according to LH levels is shown in Fig. 28.3. If the LH surge has already begun on the day of follicle monitoring, GnRHa is administered immediately, and oocyte retrieval is performed according to the LH levels. If the LH surge has already ended on the time of follicle monitoring, ovulation is predicted to occur on the same day and oocyte retrieval is performed on that day.

Cyclooxygenase (COX) enzyme-2 is induced by the LH surge in granulosa cells prior to ovulation. Non-steroidal anti-inflammatory drugs (NSAIDs) inhibit COX. Therefore, NSAID administration if LH surge has already started is likely to reduce the rate of premature ovulation.

8 and 14 h before the scheduled oocyte retrieval time, 25 mg of diclofenac is administered as a rectal suppository. We have previously shown [2] that diclofenac reduced the rate of premature ovulation and increased the likelihood of obtaining matured oocytes.

28.6 Centres Specialized in Natural Cycle IVF and Minimal Stimulation IVF in Japan

In 2017, 234,127 egg retrieval cycles were performed in Japan. Among them, NC-IVF and minimal stimulation IVF account for 9.8 and 33.0%, respectively.

Japan has approximately 600 IVF clinics. Members of the "TOWAKO group" (11 centres) and several other centres were trained NC-IVF and minimal stimulation IVF techniques in the Kato Ladies Clinic's; only these centres are familiar with Kato Ladies Clinic method and actively practise NC-IVF and minimal stimulation IVF. This means that these centres mainly carry out NC-IVF and minimal stimulation IVF for most patients. Other institutions also use these techniques, but the treatment protocols are partially different, and the target patients are often poor responders with advanced age and recurrent pregnancy failure (Fig. 28.4).

28.7 Reimbursement in Japan

To better understand the Kato Ladies Clinic and the techniques offered, the reimbursement policy in Japan is briefly described. In Japan, around 10% of IVF cycles performed are NC-IVF treatments.

Three to six IVF cycles are partially reimbursed, depending on the age of the women. Up to the age of 39 years six cycles are reimbursed, in women aged 40-42 years three cycles are covered. The upper limit for women is 42 years, A cycle is defined as any cycle irrespective if it is a fresh or a thawing cycle and irrespective if it is a NC-IVF, minimal stimulation IVF of a conventional IVF cycle.

28.8 Scientific Achievements of the Kato Ladies Clinic

A total of 35 PubMed-referenced publications on NC-IVF and minimal stimulation IVF have been published over the last 15 years. The studies that relate to ovarian stimulation are as follows (in chronological order):

Prolonged, consecutive use of clomiphene citrate is an alternative regimen in minimal stimulation IVF

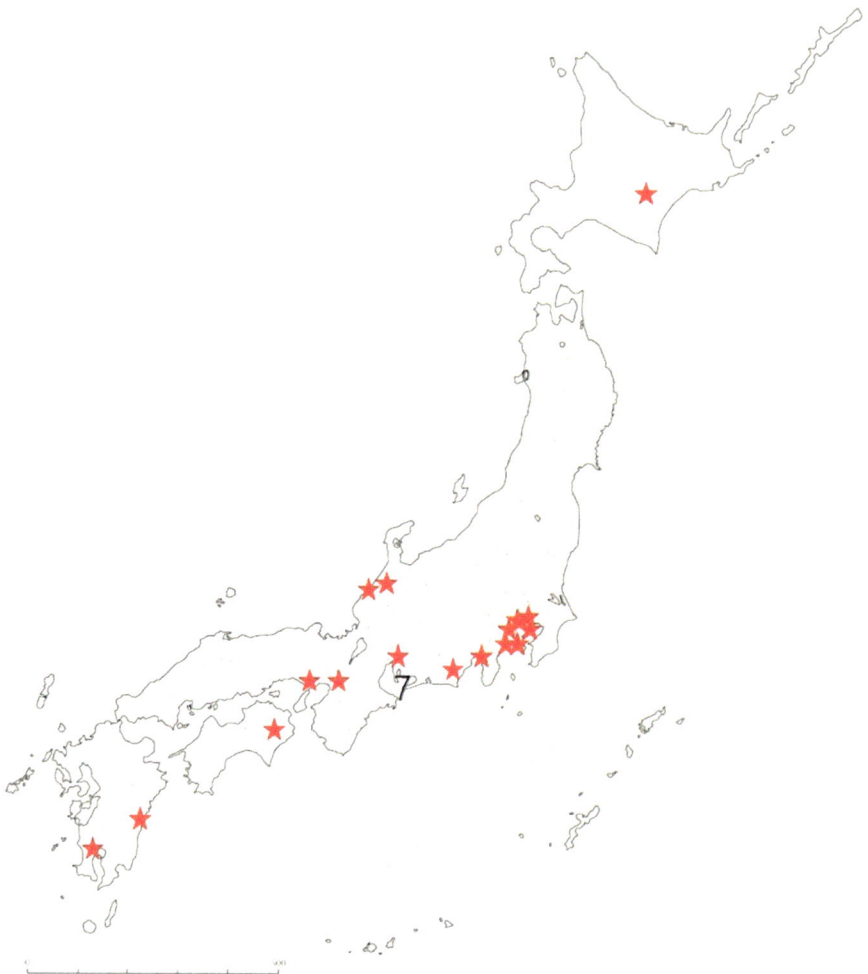

Fig. 28.4 IVF centres specialized in natural cycle IVF and minimal stimulation IVF in Japan

"Minimal ovarian stimulation with clomiphene citrate: a large-scale retrospective study". Reprod Biomed Online [3].

A retrospective cohort study of 44,345 cycles with minimal IVF stimulation cycles. Administration of 50 mg/day of clomiphene citrate was started from day 3 and continued until a day before GnRH agonist was administered as a maturation trigger. Human menopausal gonadotropin (HMG) or recombinant FSH (rFSH; 150 IU) was administered on days 8, 10, and 12. This protocol takes advantage of the antagonistic action of enclomiphene on oestrogen receptors and its short half-life (≤24 h). In addition, this protocol is advantageous for reducing the dose of HMG and rFSH.

Non-steroidal anti-inflammatory drugs (NSAIDs) decrease the rate of premature ovulation

"Short-term, low-dose, non-steroidal anti-inflammatory drug application diminishes premature ovulation in natural-cycle IVF". Reprod Biomed Online [2].

A retrospective cohort study of 1865 patients with natural cycle IVF. The high cancellation rates due to premature LH surge and premature ovulation are considered the main drawbacks of NC-IVF. The administration of 25 mg of NSAID 8 and 14 h before oocyte retrieval was associated with a significantly lower risk of premature ovulation during oocyte retrieval.

An elective single-embryo transfer program based on natural and minimal stimulation IVF can yield acceptable live birth rates per embryo transfer in patients until their mid-40s

"Minimal ovarian stimulation combined with elective single embryo transfer policy: age-specific results of a large, single-centre, Japanese cohort". Reprod Biol Endocrinol [4].

A retrospective cohort study of 7244 infertile patients who underwent 20,244 cycles of NC-IVF and minimal stimulation IVF cycles. Elective single-embryo transfer was performed exclusively. Successful oocyte retrieval, fertilization, and cleavage rates were not age-dependent. Blastocyst formation and live birth rates showed an age-dependent decrease. Overall, acceptable live birth rates can be achieved in infertile patients until their mid-40s.

A novel blastocyst grading system was established using women's age and embryo developmental speed as objective parameters

"Women's age and embryo developmental speed accurately predict clinical pregnancy after single vitrified-warmed blastocyst transfer". Reprod Biomed Online [5].

A retrospective study of 5948 patients who underwent 7321 single vitrified-warmed blastocyst transfer (SVBT) cycles. The morphological evaluation of blastocysts has been widely used in embryology laboratories. However, this morphological evaluation is subjective and observer-dependent. Using women's age and embryo developmental speed as subjective parameters, blastocysts can be successfully stratified into five groups, and each group can accurately predict pregnancy outcomes following blastocyst transfer.

The use of human chorionic gonadotropin (hCG) to trigger oocyte maturation impairs blastocyst implantation and decidualization

"Ovarian stimulation using human chorionic gonadotrophin impairs blastocyst implantation and decidualization by altering ovarian hormone levels and downstream signaling in mice". Mol Hum Reprod [6].

An experimental study using mice. Mice were primed with hCG or equine chorionic gonadotropin (eCG), and uterine receptivity and subsequent implantation and decidualization were assessed. The use of hCG was associated with a failure to develop uterine receptivity, implantation, and decidualization as a result of altering the expression of steroid receptors and their downstream signalling associated with embryo implantation.

Administration of hCG to trigger oocyte maturation may affect patient's fertility during the subsequent menstrual cycle

"Administering human chorionic gonadotropin injections for triggering follicle maturation could impact fertility during the subsequent menstrual cycle". Int J Gynaecol Obstet [7].

A prospective cohort study of 319 patients, including 63 patients who were administered hCG during their preceding cycle and 246 patients who were not exposed to any fertility drugs or hormones. The use of hCG negatively affected the rates of successful oocyte retrieval and live births. In addition, the incidence of empty follicles and degenerated oocytes increased when hCG was used in the preceding cycle.

The intrinsic fertility per oocyte in natural cycles seems to be greater than that reported in conventional IVF with high-dose gonadotropin stimulation

"Intrinsic fertility of human oocytes". Fertil Steril [8].

A retrospective cohort study of 13,949 natural cycle IVF cycles. The live birth rate per oocyte in patients aged ≤35 years and patients aged ≤42 years was 26 and 18%, respectively, which were greater than those reported for hyperstimulated cycles in the literature.

Clomiphene citrate is linked to a lower pregnancy rate after fresh blastocyst transfer, but this effect does not persist in the subsequent natural IVF cycle

"Comparison of pregnancy outcomes following fresh and electively frozen single blastocyst transfer in natural cycle and clomiphene-stimulated IVF cycles". Hum Reprod Open [9].

A retrospective study of 1653 women, including 157 women who underwent natural cycle IVF and 1496 women who underwent minimal stimulation cycle IVF. When fresh blastocyst transfer was performed, the live birth rate in the minimal stimulation group was significantly lower than that in the natural cycle group; however, these negative effects were not observed when a frozen blastocyst transfer was performed in their subsequent natural ovulatory cycle.

The administration of buserelin, a GnRH agonist, does not affect uterine receptivity

"Evaluation of uterine receptivity after gonadotropin releasing hormone agonist administration as an oocyte maturation trigger: a rodent model". Sci Rep [10].

Experimental study using mice. Buserelin, a GnRH agonist, was used to trigger oocyte maturation in our minimal stimulation regimen. This study showed that buserelin administration does not affect uterine receptivity as it has no effect on ovarian steroidogenesis or endometrial steroid signalling.

Minimal stimulation IVF with clomiphene citrate promises to achieve acceptable cumulative live birth rates (CLBR)

"Success rates in minimal stimulation cycle IVF with clomiphene citrate only". J Assist Reprod Genet [11].

A retrospective cohort study of 839 women with 2488 cycles of clomiphene citrate only minimal stimulation cycle. CLBRs were assessed according to the age group of Society of Assisted Reproduction Technology (SART) patients. CLBRs after the first and third cycles in patients aged 35–37 years and 41–42 years were 32.9 and 49.1%, and 12.6 and 25.2%, respectively. Although patient aging was significantly correlated with declining CLBRs, overall CLBRs were acceptable.

28.9   Future Perspectives of the Kato Ladies Clinic

The basic idea remains to treat patients' infertility as naturally as possible. Therefore, a sufficient understanding of the physiological hormone dynamics is required. In principle, it is necessary to establish a system in which oocytes can be retrieved every day (365 days/year). Our clinic established a system when it was opened which allows oocytes to be retrieved 365 days/year since. Although doing so may be difficult due to the capacity of infertility treatment centres and personnel issues, there is a great potential benefit for patients. If clinics wish to carry out a method similar to ours, they should adopt our strategy.

It is necessary to consider appropriate ovarian stimulation methods that can lead to satisfactory success rates with minimal burden on the body. Infertile patients who undergo IVF may have a suitable number of oocytes retrieved. Therefore, the injection of gonadotropins may be an effective option in some cases. The issue that should be considered is how much gonadotropins should be used. The dosage should be individualized, based on AMH concentration and other factors. Furthermore, in the future, the regimen of minimal ovarian stimulation using aromatase inhibitors will also be considered as an alternative option for patients.

We hope that NC-IVF and minimal stimulation cycle IVF will be introduced as basic protocols in a greater number of institutions in the future.

References

1. Nishihara S, Fukuda J, Ezoe K, Endo M, Nakagawa Y, Yamadera R, Kobayashi T, Kato K. Does the endometrial thickness on the day of the trigger affect the pregnancy outcomes after fresh cleaved embryo transfer in the clomiphene citrate-based minimal stimulation cycle? Reprod Med Biol. 2020;19:151–7.
2. Kawachiya S, Matsumoto T, Bodri D, Kato K, Takehara Y, Kato O. Short-term, low-dose, non-steroidal anti-inflammatory drug application diminishes premature ovulation in natural-cycle IVF. Reprod Biomed Online. 2012;24:308–13.
3. Teramoto S, Kato O. Minimal ovarian stimulation with clomiphene citrate a large-scale retrospective study. Reprod Biomed Online. 2007;15:134–48.
4. Kato K, Takehara Y, Segawa T, Kawachiya S, Okuno T, Kobayashi T, Bodri D, Kato O. Minimal ovarian stimulation combined with elective single embryo transfer policy: age-specific results of a large, single-center, Japanese cohort. Reprod Biol Endocrinol. 2012;10:35.
5. Kato K, Ueno S, Yabuuchi A, Uchiyama K, Okuno T, Kobayashi T, Segawa T, Teramoto S. Women's age and embryo developmental speed accurately predict clinical pregnancy after single vitrified-warmed blastocyst transfer. Reprod Biomed Online. 2014;29:411–6.
6. Ezoe K, Daikoku T, Yabuuchi A, Murata N, Kawano H, Abe T, Okuno T, Kobayashi T, Kato K. Ovarian stimulation using human chorionic gonadotrophin impairs blastocyst implantation and decidualization by altering ovarian hormone levels and downstream signaling in mice. Mol Hum Reprod. 2014;20:1101–16.
7. Fukuda J, Abe T, Okuno T, Kobayashi T, Kato K. Administering human chorionic gonadotropin injections for triggering follicle maturation could impact fertility during the subsequent menstrual cycle. Int J Gynaecol Obstet. 2016;132:309–13.

8. Silber SJ, Kato K, Aoyama N, Yabuuchi A, Skaletsky H, Fan Y, Shinohara K, Yatabe N, Kobayashi T. Intrinsic fertility of human oocytes. Fertil Steril. 2017;107:1232–7.
9. Kato K, Ezoe K, Yabuuchi A, Fukuda J, Kuroda T, Ueno S, Fujita H, Kobayashi T. Comparison of pregnancy outcomes following fresh and electively frozen single blastocyst transfer in natural cycle and clomiphene-stimulated IVF cycles. Hum Reprod Open. 2018;2018:hoy006.
10. Ezoe K, Murata N, Yabuuchi A, Kobayashi T, Kato K. Evaluation of uterine receptivity after gonadotropin releasing hormone agonist administration as an oocyte maturation trigger: a rodent model. Sci Rep. 2019;9:12519.
11. Abe T, Yabuuchi A, Ezoe K, Skaletsky H, Fukuda J, Ueno S, Fan Y, Goldsmith S, Kobayashi T, Silber S, Keiichi K. Success rates in minimal stimulation cycle IVF with clomiphene citrate only. J Assist Reprod Genet. 2020;37:297–304.

Part VIII
Case Discussions

Chapter 29
Andrological Infertility—Case Discussion and IVF Treatments Suggested by Different Centres

Michael von Wolff and Keiichi Kato

29.1 Introduction

Natural cycle-IVF (NC-IVF) and minimal stimulation IVF treatments should be understood as complementary therapies in IVF treatment programmes. The success of these treatments depends on the infertility factor and kind of treatment chosen.

Young healthy couples in whom infertility is only due to an andrological factor have the highest IVF treatment success rates. Two centres or networks (IVF-Naturelle® network in Germany, Switzerland and Austria; Kato Ladies Clinic in Japan) specialised in natural cycle and minimal stimulation IVF describe and discuss the treatment they suggest in couples with andrological infertility. The suggested treatments are based on the treatment concepts described in Chaps. 15, 26 and 28.

29.2 Case Description

- Primary infertility for 2 years.
- Healthy couple without any infertility-related lifestyle factors.

M. von Wolff (✉)

Division of Gynecological Endocrinology and Reproductive Medicine, University Women's Hospital, University of Bern, Bern, Switzerland
e-mail: Michael.vonwolff@insel.ch

K. Kato
Kato Ladies Clinic, Tokyo, Japan

- Her: 33 years old, BMI 22 kg/m^2, regular cycle, patent tubes, normal endometrial thickness, normal vaginal ultrasound, no severe discomfort during vaginal ultrasound, AMH 1 ng/mL (7.1 pmol/L).
- Him: 38 years old, BMI 24 kg/m^2, oligoasthenoteratozoospermia (concentration: 1 mill/mL; total motility: 10%; morphology according to Kruger's strict criteria: 1%).

29.3 General Considerations

- Apart from the infertility, the couple is healthy.
- The cause of infertility is low sperm quality, requiring IVF/ICSI treatment.
- The fertility of the women can be assumed to be normal.
- The woman is suitable for NC-IVF or minimal stimulation IVF as the ovaries can easily be reached and aspiration is possible without analgesia.
- As the fertility of the women can be assumed to be normal, the NC-IVF success rate per transferred embryo can be expected to be high (clinical pregnancy rate per transfer of one fresh day 2 embryo in women aged <34 years: 26.3%, live birth rate: 22.4% [1]. Live birth rate per aspirated oocyte in women aged <35 years: 26% [2]) (see Chap. 19).

29.4 Treatment Suggested by the IVF-Naturelle® Network

The couple is basically suitable for any IVF therapy (NC-IVF, minimal stimulation IVF, conventional IVF). Based on their personal wishes (Chap. 26, Figs. 26.1–26.4; Chap. 15, Figs. 15.1–15.6), they can freely choose which kind of IVF treatment they prefer to start with.

If the couple chooses NC-IVF as a first line therapy, they will start with around three treatment cycles. If pregnancy is not achieved after three cycles, the treatment strategy is evaluated.

For NC-IVF, the first consultation (follicle monitoring) takes place around 3 days before the expected day of ovulation. Vaginal ultrasound is performed and concentrations of estradiol (E2) and luteinizing hormone (LH) are analysed. On average, 1.2 consultations are required before follicle aspiration.

If LH concentration is already increased, ibuprofen or diclofenac is given (Chap. 11). If the couple wishes to be aspirated 1 day after the scheduled day, one injection of GnRH antagonists can be offered.

Ovulation is triggered with 5000 IU of urinary hCG, 36 h before aspiration. Aspiration is performed with 19G aspiration needles without any anaesthesia or analgesia. Follicles are flushed five times (Chap. 13).

The embryo is transferred 2–3 days after aspiration. Luteal phase support is only required if luteal phase is <12 days. hCG blood test is performed 14 days after aspiration, and the next cycle is directly started without a break.

Alternatively, NC-IVF can be combined with very low doses of clomiphene citrate (25 mg/day) to reduce the risk of premature ovulation and thereby increase the transfer rate. If the endometrium thickness is substantially reduced under this therapy (reduction of thickness >1 mm compared to unstimulated cycles or thickness <8 mm), treatment with clomiphene citrate should be stopped.

29.5 Treatment Suggested by Kato Ladies Clinic, Japan

The couple is suitable for both NC-IVF and minimal stimulation cycle IVF. However, in this case, minimal stimulation cycle should be the first line of treatment to increase IVF efficiency (see Chap. 15, Fig. 15.8).

In brief, administration of clomiphene citrate (CC; 50 mg/day) is initiated on day 3 of menstruation and continued until application of oocyte maturation trigger. Usually, two to three times of FSH (150 IU) is administered during the follicular phase. Gonadotropin-releasing hormone agonist (GnRHa) is administered intranasally to trigger ovulation when dominant follicle diameter is ≥ 18 mm, and E2 levels relative to the number of growing follicles are sufficiently high. Oocyte retrieval is performed 34–35 h after GnRHa administration. ICSI is chosen due to severe oligoasthenoteratozoospermia.

References

1. von Wolff M, Schwartz AK, Bitterlich N, Stute P, Fäh M. Only women's age and the duration of infertility are the prognostic factors for the success rate of natural cycle IVF. Arch Gynecol Obstet. 2019;299:883–9.
2. Silber SJ, Kato K, Aoyama N, Yabuuchi A, Skaletsky H, Fan Y, Shinohara K, Yatabe N, Kobayashi T. Intrinsic fertility of human oocytes. Fertil Steril. 2017;107:1232–7.

Chapter 30
Idiopathic Infertility—Case Discussion and IVF Treatments Suggested by Different Centres

Michael von Wolff and Keiichi Kato

30.1 Introduction

Natural cycle IVF (NC-IVF) and minimal stimulation IVF treatments should be understood as complementary therapies in IVF treatment programmes. The success of these treatments depends on the infertility factor and kind of treatment chosen.

Couples with idiopathic infertility are a challenge in infertility treatment, as the cause of infertility is unknown. Two centres or networks (IVF-Naturelle® network in Germany, Switzerland and Austria; Kato Ladies Clinic in Japan), specialized in natural cycle and minimal stimulation IVF, describe and discuss the treatment they suggest in couples with idiopathic infertility. The suggested treatments are based on the treatment concepts described in Chaps. 15, 26 and 28.

30.2 Case Description

- Primary infertility for 3–4 years.
- Healthy couple without any infertility-related lifestyle factors.

M. von Wolff (✉)
Division of Gynecological Endocrinology and Reproductive Medicine, University Women's Hospital, University of Bern, Bern, Switzerland
e-mail: Michael.vonwolff@insel.ch

K. Kato
Kato Ladies Clinic, Tokyo, Japan

- Her: 36 years old, BMI 22 kg/m^2, regular cycle, patent tubes, normal endometrial thickness, normal vaginal ultrasound, no severe discomfort during vaginal ultrasound, AMH 2 ng/mL (14.3 pmol/L).
- Him: 38 years old, BMI 24 kg/m^2, normozoospermia

30.3 General Considerations

- Apart from the infertility, the couple is healthy.
- The cause of infertility is unknown.
- The couple has been trying to conceive for 4 years.
- The woman is suitable for NC-IVF or minimal stimulation IVF as the ovaries can easily be reached and aspiration is possible without analgesia.
- The woman is of slightly increased age.
- The infertility might be due to factors which can easily be treated by IVF/ICSI, such as undetected fallopian tube dysfunction, resulting in high success rates. The infertility might also be due to oocyte dysfunction which requires a high number of oocytes, embryo selection and possibly even PGT-A.
- Due to the women's slightly increased age, the IVF success rate per transferred embryo is slightly reduced (clinical pregnancy rate per transfer in women aged 34–37 years: 25.7%, live birth rate 18.9% [1]) (see Chap. 19).
- Due to the longer duration of the patient's infertility (3–4 years), the IVF success rate per transferred embryo is reduced (clinical pregnancy rate per one fresh day 2 embryo in women with a duration of infertility of 3–4 years: 21.8%, live birth rate: 18.9% [1]. Live birth rate per aspirated oocyte in women aged 36 years: 21% [2]) (see Chap. 19).
- Due to the unknown cause of infertility, the woman's slightly increased age and the high ovarian reserve, a few cycles of NC-IVF can be considered. However, if pregnancy is not achieved, the treatment should be switched to minimal stimulation IVF or conventional IVF.

30.4 Treatment Suggested by the IVF-Naturelle® Network

The couple is basically suitable for any IVF therapy (NC-IVF, minimal stimulation IVF, conventional IVF). Based on their personal wishes (Chap. 26, Fig. 26.1), the couple can choose which kind of IVF treatment they would prefer to start with.

If the couple chooses NC-IVF treatment as a first-line therapy, they start with around three treatment cycles. This treatment is described in detail in Chap. 15 and "Treatment protocols by the IVF-Naturelle® centers".

If pregnancy is not achieved after three cycles, the treatment strategy is evaluated. The couple should then either switch to minimal stimulation IVF or directly to conventional IVF, including embryo selection. If pregnancy is still not achieved, PGT-A can be considered.

However, minimal stimulation IVF is also an option as a first-line therapy if two to three oocytes can be collected per cycle. Two embryos could be transferred on day 2/3 after aspiration. Alternatively, embryo culture is prolonged and only one embryo is transferred.

Minimal stimulation IVF can be performed monthly and is therefore equally effective as conventional IVF per treatment time. A protocol combining clomiphene citrate and 75 IU of gonadotropin can be expected to achieve the highest number of oocytes and therefore the highest success rate. If the endometrium thickness is substantially reduced under this therapy (reduction of thickness >1 mm compared to unstimulated cycles or thickness <8 mm), treatment with clomiphene citrate should be stopped. A protocol with low dose gonadotopins and GnRH antagonists might then be required.

30.5 Treatment Suggested by the Kato Ladies Clinic, Japan

Considering the female partner's age and semen analysis data, intrauterine insemination (IUI) could be encouraged before proceeding with IVF. To decide whether this couple can be treated by IUI, the couple undergoes the postcoital test (Huhner test, Sims–Huhner test) and semen examination at their first visit.

If they do not meet the criteria for IUI, clomiphene citrate (CC)-based minimal stimulation IVF is the first-line treatment (see Chap. 15, Fig. 15.8). In brief, administration of CC (50 mg/day) is initiated on day 3 of menstruation and continued until right before the oocyte maturation trigger. The administration of follicle stimulating hormone (FSH) is decided based on follicular growth and FSH and E2 levels. In case there is no FSH administration during the cycle, the woman visits the clinic on or around day 12 of menstruation, and the day of oocyte pick up (OPU) is decided. A gonadotropin-releasing hormone (GnRH) agonist is administered in the form of nasal spray, and OPU is performed 34–35 h after GnRH agonist administration. To prevent premature ovulation, non-steroidal anti-inflammatory drugs (25 mg of diclofenac) are administered 8 and 14 h before scheduled OPU.

References

1. von Wolff M, Schwartz AK, Bitterlich N, Stute P, Fäh M. Only women's age and the duration of infertility are the prognostic factors for the success rate of natural cycle IVF. Arch Gynecol Obstet. 2019;299:883–9.
2. Silber SJ, Kato K, Aoyama N, Yabuuchi A, Skaletsky H, Fan Y, Shinohara K, Yatabe N, Kobayashi T. Intrinsic fertility of human oocytes. Fertil Steril. 2017;107:1232–7.

Chapter 31
Increased Age—Case Discussion and IVF Treatments Suggested by Different Centres

Michael von Wolff and Keiichi Kato

31.1 Introduction

Natural cycle IVF(NC-IVF) and minimal stimulation IVF treatments should be understood as complementary therapies in IVF treatment programmes. The success of these treatments depends on the infertility factor and kind of treatment chosen.

Women with increased age are a challenge in infertility treatment. Two centres or networks (IVF-Naturelle® network in Germany, Switzerland and Austria; Kato Ladies Clinic in Japan), specialised in natural cycle and minimal stimulation IVF, describe and discuss the treatment they suggest in women with increased age. The suggested treatments are based on the treatment concepts described in Chaps. 15, 26 and 28.

31.2 Case Description

- Primary infertility for 2 years.
- Healthy couple without any infertility-related lifestyle factors.
- Her: 40 years old, BMI 22 kg/m², regular cycles, patent tubes, normal endometrial thickness, normal vaginal ultrasound, no severe discomfort during vaginal ultrasound, AMH 1.0 ng/mL (7.1 pmol/L).

M. von Wolff (✉)
Division of Gynecological Endocrinology and Reproductive Medicine, University Women's Hospital, University of Bern, Bern, Switzerland
e-mail: Michael.vonwolff@insel.ch

K. Kato
Kato Ladies Clinic, Tokyo, Japan

- Him: 42 years old, BMI 24 kg/m^2, moderate oligoasthenoteratozoospermia (concentration: 10 mill/mL; total motility: 30%; morphology according to Kruger's strict criteria: 3%).

31.3   General Considerations

- Apart from the infertility, the couple is healthy.
- The cause of infertility is increased age and reduced sperm quality, requiring intrauterine insemination or IVF/ICSI treatment.
- The ovarian reserve is rather low but normal for the patient's age.
- The woman is suitable for NC-IVF or minimal stimulation IVF as the ovaries can easily be reached and aspiration is possible without analgesia.
- Due to the increased age, the NC-IVF success rate per transferred embryo is low (clinical pregnancy rate per one fresh day 2 embryo in women aged 38–42 years 15.7%, live birth rate 3.9% [1]. Live birth rate per aspirated oocyte in women aged 40 years: 9% [2]).

31.4   Treatment Suggested by the IVF-Naturelle® Network

The main problem is the increased age and therefore the reduced oocyte quality with a low live birth rate per oocyte. Furthermore, female fertility and ovarian reserve will rapidly decrease within a short period of time.

The couple should therefore be advised to choose the treatment with the highest efficacy. Intrauterine insemination is one option. However, as the success rate is low in woman aged 40 years [3], the number of cycles should be limited.

If IVF therapy is preferred, the IVF treatment with the highest number of oocytes per month and therefore with the highest success rate per treatment time such as minimal stimulation IVF or conventional IVF (Chap. 26, Fig. 26.4) should be chosen.

As the ovarian reserve is still not too low, conventional IVF with maximum gonadotropin dosage (300 IU gonadotropin) should be the first-line treatment if treatment is performed on a monthly basis.

If, however, one cycle of conventional IVF requires 2–3 months, minimal stimulation IVF might be an alternative if one treatment cycle is performed every month. NC-IVF would only be the first-line therapy if the ovarian reserve was very low (Chap. 15 and "Treatment protocols by the IVF-Naturelle® centers"). Minimal stimulation IVF is described in Chap. 15, Figs. 15.3–15.6.

31.5   Treatment Suggested by Kato Ladies Clinic, Japan

Ovarian reserve is normal for the patient's age but rather low. Minimal stimulation IVF is chosen (see Chap. 15, Fig. 15.8).

In brief, administration of clomiphene citrate (50 mg/day) is initiated on day 3 of menstruation and continued until right before the oocyte maturation trigger. The administration of follicle stimulating hormone (FSH) is decided based on follicular growth and FSH and E2 levels. A gonadotropin-releasing hormone agonist (GnRHa) is administered in the form of nasal spray, and oocyte retrieval is performed 34–35 h after GnRHa administration. ICSI is chosen due to oligoasthenoteratozoospermia.

References

1. von Wolff M, Schwartz AK, Bitterlich N, Stute P, Fäh M. Only women's age and the duration of infertility are the prognostic factors for the success rate of natural cycle IVF. Arch Gynecol Obstet. 2019;299:883–9.
2. Silber SJ, Kato K, Aoyama N, Yabuuchi A, Skaletsky H, Fan Y, Shinohara K, Yatabe N, Kobayashi T. Intrinsic fertility of human oocytes. Fertil Steril. 2017;107:1232–7.
3. Corsan G, Trias A, Trout S, Kemmann E. Ovulation induction combined with intrauterine insemination in women 40 years of age and older: is it worthwhile? Hum Reprod. 1996;11:1109–12.

Chapter 32
Low Ovarian Reserve—Case Discussion and IVF Treatments Suggested by Different Centres

Michael von Wolff and Keiichi Kato

32.1 Introduction

Natural cycle IVF (NC-IVF) and minimal stimulation IVF treatments should be understood as complementary therapies in IVF treatment programmes. The success of these treatments depends on the infertility factor and kind of treatment chosen.

Women with low ovarian reserve are a challenge in infertility treatment. Two centres or networks (IVF-Naturelle® network in Germany, Switzerland and Austria; Kato Ladies Clinic in, Japan) specialized in NC-IVF and minimal stimulation IVF, describe and discuss the treatment they suggest in women with low ovarian reserve. The suggested treatments are based on the treatment concepts described in Chaps. 15, 26 and 28.

32.2 Case Description

- Primary infertility for 2 years.
- Healthy couple without any infertility-related lifestyle factors.
- Her: 34 years old, BMI 22 kg/m², slightly irregular cycles with cycle length of 21–28 days, patent tubes, normal endometrial thickness, normal vaginal ultra-

M. von Wolff (✉)
Division of Gynecological Endocrinology and Reproductive Medicine, University Women's Hospital, University of Bern, Bern, Switzerland
e-mail: Michael.vonwolff@insel.ch

K. Kato
Kato Ladies Clinic, Tokyo, Japan

285

sound with low antral follicle count, no severe discomfort during vaginal ultrasound, AMH 0.5 ng/mL (3.6 pmol/L).
- Him: 38 years old, BMI 24 kg/m², oligoasthenoteratozoospermia (concentration: 1 mill/mL; total motility: 10%; morphology according to Kruger's strict criteria: 1%).

32.3 General Considerations

- Apart from the infertility, the couple is healthy.
- The cause of infertility is the low sperm quality, requiring IVF/ICSI treatment.
- Another cause of infertility is the slightly irregular cycle and possibly LOOP (luteal-out-of-phase).
- The ovarian reserve is low.
- The woman is young; therefore, the oocyte quality can be assumed to be high.
- The woman is suitable for NC-IVF or minimal stimulation IVF as the ovaries can easily be reached and aspiration is possible without analgesia.
- As the fertility of the women can still be assumed to be normal, the NC-IVF success rate per transferred embryo can be expected to be high (clinical pregnancy rate per one fresh day 2 embryo in women aged <34 years 26.3%; live birth rate per aspirated oocyte 22.4% [1]). However, the transfer rate might be decreased due to the irregular cycles. Live birth rate per oocyte in women aged <35 years: 26% [2].
- In NC-IVF, timing of the aspiration might be difficult due to the irregular cycle.
- Conventional IVF will probably result in a poor response.

32.4 Treatment Suggested by the IVF-Naturelle® Network

As conventional IVF with maximum gonadotropin dosage (300 IU gonadotropin) will almost certainly result in a poor response, NC-IVF or minimal stimulation IVF are the treatments of choice (Chap. 26, Figs. 26.1–26.4; Chap. 15, Figs. 15.1–15.6).

NC-IVF can be chosen as first-line therapy, but the couple needs to be counselled that the irregular cycle will possibly require several follicle monitoring consultations and the transfer rate might be lower due to the increased risk of premature LH surge and therefore premature ovulation. NC-IVF plus low dosages of clomiphene citrate might therefore be preferred as first-line treatment. NC-IVF treatment with and without clomiphene citrate is described in detail in Chap. 15 and "Treatment protocols by IVF-Naturelle® centers".

However, minimal stimulation IVF is also an option as a first-line therapy if two to three oocytes can be collected per cycle (described in Chap. 15 and "Treatment protocols by IVF-Naturelle® centers". However, if only one follicle develops in two performed cycles, the therapy should be continued with NC-IVF.

The therapy will be started with three treatment cycles and the treatment strategy will be evaluated after three cycles.

In case, follicular growth already starts in the luteal phase leading to LOOP (luteal out-of-phase) and subsequent desynchronized follicle and endometrial growth, options to inhibit premature follicular growth should be discussed (see Chap. 5).

One option is to administer a combined oral contraceptive pill (i.e., 30 µg ethinyl oestradiol plus levonorgestrel) for around 10–20 days to avoid follicular growth. However, this option is associated with an increased risk of thrombosis and every second cycle is lost.

Another option is to add oestrogen in the luteal phase (i.e., 50–100 µg oestrogen patches) to suppress premature FSH increase.

It should be noted that these options have not been proven in clinical studies.

32.5   Treatment Suggested by Kato Ladies Clinic, Japan

If basal follicle stimulating hormone (FSH) level is increased, hormonal therapy using contraceptive pills is considered before proceeding with IVF. When basal FSH level is normal, minimal stimulation cycle with clomiphene citrate is chosen as the first-line treatment (see Chap. 15, Figs. 15.7 and 15.8).

In case of low levels of basal FSH and high levels of E2 on day 3 of menstruation, NC-IVF is performed. Blood examination and ultrasonography are performed regularly to determine hormonal dynamics (E2, LH, FSH, and progesterone) and follicular growth. When the leading follicle reaches 18 mm in diameter and the E2 level is increased appropriately, ovulation is triggered with gonadotropin-releasing hormone agonist (GnRHa) and oocyte pick-up is performed 34–35 h after administration.

If FSH levels are increased, FSH stimulation is not required. However, the decision for or against FSH stimulation depends on the basal concentrations of FSH and LH and on follicular growth. There is a risk for premature increase of FSH and LH levels and premature luteinization due to slow follicular development. In such cases, contraceptive pills may prevent such a premature increase of FSH and LH.

References

1. von Wolff M, Schwartz AK, Bitterlich N, Stute P, Fäh M. Only women's age and the duration of infertility are the prognostic factors for the success rate of natural cycle IVF. Arch Gynecol Obstet. 2019;299:883–9.
2. Silber SJ, Kato K, Aoyama N, Yabuuchi A, Skaletsky H, Fan Y, Shinohara K, Yatabe N, Kobayashi T. Intrinsic fertility of human oocytes. Fertil Steril. 2017;107:1232–7.

Chapter 33
Endometriosis—Case Discussion and IVF Treatments Suggested by Different Centres

Michael von Wolff and Keiichi Kato

33.1 Introduction

Natural cycle-IVF (NC-IVF) and minimal stimulation IVF treatments should be understood as complementary therapies in IVF treatment programmes. The success of these treatments depends on the infertility factor and kind of treatment chosen.

Women with severe endometriosis are a challenge in infertility treatment. Two centres or networks (IVF-Naturelle® network in Germany, Switzerland and Austria; Kato Ladies Clinic in Japan), specialised in natural cycle and minimal stimulation IVF, describe and discuss the treatment they suggest in couples with endometriosis. The suggested treatments are based on the treatment concepts described in the Chaps. 15, 26 and 28.

33.2 Case Description

- Primary infertility for 2 years.
- Severe endometriosis rASRM stage III, bilateral endometrioma, blocked tubes.
- Otherwise healthy couple without any infertility-related lifestyle factors.

M. von Wolff (✉)
Division of Gynecological Endocrinology and Reproductive Medicine, University Women's Hospital, University of Bern, Bern, Switzerland
e-mail: Michael.vonwolff@insel.ch

K. Kato
Kato Ladies Clinic, Tokyo, Japan

- Her: 33 years old, BMI 22 kg/m², regular cycles, blocked tubes, normal endometrial thickness, vaginal ultrasound with bilateral endometrioma and ovaries close to the vagina, moderate discomfort during vaginal ultrasound, AMH 1.5 ng/mL (10.7 pmol/L).
- Him: 42 years old, BMI 24 kg/m², normozoospermia.

33.3 General Considerations

- Apart from the infertility, the couple is healthy.
- The cause of infertility is severe endometriosis and blocked tubes. Ovarian reserve is slightly decreased.
- The woman seems to be suitable for NC-IVF or minimal stimulation IVF as the ovaries and follicles can probably be reached. However, whether the women is really suitable for aspiration without anaesthesia needs to be re-evaluated after the first aspiration.
- Surgery to remove the endometrioma reduces the ovarian reserve [1].
- Ovarian endometrioma might grow by 10% per IVF stimulation [2].
- The ovum pick-up efficiency and oocyte quality are decreased in patients with endometriosis [3, 4].
- Fertilisation outcomes are affected by endometriosis, and these negative effects are influenced by the degree of severity [5–7].
- The NC-IVF success rate per transferred embryo can be expected to be rather high (clinical pregnancy rate per transfer of one fresh day 2 embryo in women aged <34 years: 26.3%, live birth rate: 22.4% [8]. Live birth rate per apirated oocyte in women aged <35 years: 26% [9]). However, the overall success rate is reduced, and the miscarriage rate is increased in women with endometriosis [10].

33.4 Treatment Suggested by the IVF-Naturelle® Network

The kind of treatment needs to be based on the individual situation. According to the case description above, the couple is suitable for any kind of IVF treatment (NC-IVF, minimal stimulation IVF, conventional IVF) (Chap. 26, Figs. 26.1–26.4; Chap. 15, Figs. 15.1–15.6).

However, several factors need to be considered:

- Can the follicles be reached—without and with anaesthesia?
- Can aspiration really be performed without anaesthesia?
- Which techniques provide the shortest time to pregnancy?
- Which therapy bears the lowest risk of endometriosis progression?

The decision on which treatment should be started with needs to be based on all these factors and the personal wishes of the couple.

According to the case description above, the woman is young and can possibly undergo aspiration without anaesthesia. She only has a slightly reduced ovarian reserve. Therefore, minimal stimulation IVF and conventional IVF are both possible.

Both IVF treatments should be performed without long-lasting interruptions. If the treatment is interrupted, endocrine treatment such as progestogens to prevent progress of the endometriosis is recommended.

In minimal stimulation IVF, a protocol combining clomiphene citrate and 75–100 IU gonadotropin might be the first choice. The protocol provides high oocyte yield and clomiphene citrate (a selective oestrogen receptor modulator, SERM) has anti-estrogenic actions on the endometrium and thereby also on the endometriosis.

In conventional IVF, stimulation can be combined with aromatase inhibitors to reduce oestrogen blood concentration and reduce the risk of endometriosis progression [11].

In all events, treatment needs to be re-evaluated at short intervals and in a multi-disciplinary setting to provide the best care for the patient.

33.5 Treatment Suggested by Kato Ladies Clinic, Japan

A minimal stimulation cycle is recommended for ovarian stimulation method (see Chap. 15, Fig. 15.8).

In brief, administration of clomiphene citrate (50 mg/day) is initiated on day 3 of menstruation and continued until right before the oocyte maturation trigger. The administration of follicle stimulating hormone (FSH) is decided based on follicular growth and FSH and E2 levels. Usually, two to three times of FSH (150 IU) is administered during the follicular phase. A GnRH agonist is administered in the form of nasal spray, and oocyte retrieval is performed 34–35 h after GnRHa administration. When oocyte retrievals are performed, care has to be taken not to puncture endometriotic cysts. Anaesthesia is not necessary during oocyte retrievals. In case of severe endometriosis, all freeze strategy is applied, and surgical treatment is recommended before embryo transfer.

References

1. Hamdan M, Dunselman G, Li TC, Cheong Y. The impact of endometrioma on IVF/ICSI outcomes: a systematic review and meta-analysis. Hum Reprod Update. 2015;21:809–25.
2. Seyhan A, Urman B, Turkgeldi E, Ata B. Do endometriomas grow during ovarian stimulation for assisted reproduction? A three-dimensional volume analysis before and after ovarian stimulation. Reprod Biomed Online. 2018;36:239–44.
3. Goud PT, Goud AP, Joshi N, Puscheck E, Diamond MP, Abu-Soud HM. Dynamics of nitric oxide, altered follicular microenvironment, and oocyte quality in women with endometriosis. Fertil Steril. 2014;102:151–9.e5.

4. Singh AK, Dutta M, Chattopadhyay R, Chakravarty B, Chaudhury K. Intrafollicular interleu-
   kin-8, interleukin-12, and adrenomedullin are the promising prognostic markers of oocyte and
   embryo quality in women with endometriosis. J Assist Reprod Genet. 2016;33:1363–72.
5. Barnhart K, Dunsmoor-Su R, Coutifaris C. Effect of endometriosis on in vitro fertilization.
   Fertil Steril. 2002;77:1148–55.
6. Senapati S, Sammel MD, Morse C, Barnhart KT. Impact of endometriosis on in vitro fertilization outcomes: an evaluation of the Society for Assisted Reproductive Technologies Database.
   Fertil Steril. 2016;106:164–71.e1.
7. Harb HM, Gallos ID, Chu J, Harb M, Coomarasamy A. The effect of endometriosis on in vitro
   fertilisation outcome: a systematic review and meta-analysis. BJOG. 2013;120:1308–20.
8. von Wolff M, Schwartz AK, Bitterlich N, Stute P, Fäh M. Only women's age and the duration
   of infertility are the prognostic factors for the success rate of natural cycle IVF. Arch Gynecol
   Obstet. 2019;299:883–9.
9. Silber SJ, Kato K, Aoyama N, Yabuuchi A, Skaletsky H, Fan Y, Shinohara K, Yatabe N,
   Kobayashi T. Intrinsic fertility of human oocytes. Fertil Steril. 2017;107:1232–7.
10. Kohl Schwartz AS, Wölfler MM, Mitter V, Rauchfuss M, Haeberlin F, Eberhard M, von Orelli
    S, Imthurn B, Imesch P, Fink D, Leeners B. Endometriosis, especially mild disease: a risk fac-
    tor for miscarriages. Fertil Steril. 2017;108:806–14.e2.
11. Kohl Schwartz A, Imboden S, von Wolff M. Endometriosis. In: von Wolff M, Nawroth F, edi-
    tors. Fertility preservation in oncological and non-oncological diseases. 1st ed. Springer; 2020.

Chapter 34
Luteal Phase Minimal Stimulation IVF

John Zhang

34.1 Background

In 2005, New Hope Fertility Center (NHFC) first introduced the concept of luteal phase stimulation. This approach aimed to make the most of stimulation cycles in patients with low ovarian reserve and also reduced stimulation time. This innovative idea came from observing ovarian physiology and behavior of ovulatory cycles in other mammals, such as elephants and horses. Currently, this approach is also known as double stimulation and sequential stimulation.

Using this novel approach, our first live birth was reported in 2006 at NHFC New York, and 2012 in NHFC Mexico, becoming the first group to achieve a live birth through luteal phase stimulation in the American continent.

34.2 Case Descriptions

Case 1:

During stimulation in the follicular phase of day 15, a 38-year-old patient with diminished ovarian reserve achieved development of three follicles larger than 16 mm. She was triggered with hCG and 36 h later, during her egg retrieval, three metaphase (MII) oocytes were retrieved. All three oocytes were arrested on day 3 after normal fertilization.

The day after egg retrieval, the patient underwent stimulation in the luteal phase with clomiphene citrate 50 mg daily dose and 75 IU FSH on days 18–23 of the cycle. On day 24, 36 h after the HCG trigger injection, one metaphase II oocyte was

J. Zhang (✉)
New Hope Fertility Center, New York, USA

© The Author(s), under exclusive license to Springer Nature Switzerland AG 2022
M. von Wolff (ed.), *Natural Cycle and Minimal Stimulation IVF*,
https://doi.org/10.1007/978-3-030-97571-5_34

retrieved, which achieved blastocyst development. PGT-A was performed with an euploid result. A live birth was achieved following a frozen embryo transfer.

Case 2:

On cycle day 10 of follicular stimulation, a 40-year-old patient with primary infertility was taking clomiphene. She developed three follicles of 20, 15, and 14 mm, and ovulation was triggered. On the day of oocyte retrieval, two metaphase II oocytes are retrieved and three smaller follicles at 13, 12, and 10 mm were left to continue stimulation. Three eggs were retrieved and fertilized and one reached blastocyst stage, however PGT-A showed aneuploidy.

Luteal phase stimulation began on the same day of oocyte retrieval where daily dose of clomiphene 50 mg was given for two consecutive days (day 12 and 13 of the cycle) and 150 IU HMG on day 13 of cycle.

On cycle day 14, follicles size reached 18, 15, and 11 mm and the patient was triggered with HCG and two metaphase II oocytes were retrieved, resulting in a blastocyst embryo with euploid PGT-A result.